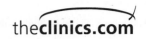

SURGICAL CLINICS
OF NORTH AMERICA

Advances in Abdominal Wall Hernia Repair

GUEST EDITORS
Kamal M.F. Itani, MD
Mary T. Hawn, MD, FACS

CONSULTING EDITOR
Ronald F. Martin, MD

February 2008 • Volume 88 • Number 1

SAUNDERS

An Imprint of Elsevier, Inc.
PHILADELPHIA   LONDON   TORONTO   MONTREAL   SYDNEY   TOKYO

W.B. SAUNDERS COMPANY
A Division of Elsevier Inc.

1600 John F. Kennedy Blvd., Suite 1800, Philadelphia, PA 19103-2899

http://www.theclinics.com

SURGICAL CLINICS OF NORTH AMERICA
February 2008
Editor: Catherine Bewick

Volume 88, Number 1
ISSN 0039–6109
ISBN-10: 1-4160-5803-6
ISBN-13: 978-1-4160-5803-8

The ideas and opinions expressed in *The Surgical Clinics of North America* do not necessarily reflect those of the Publisher. The Publisher does not assume any responsibility for any injury and/or damage to persons or property arising out of or related to any use of the material contained in this periodical. The reader is advised to check the appropriate medical literature and the product information currently provided by the manufacturer of each drug to be administered to verify the dosage, the method and duration of administration, or contraindications. It is the responsibility of the treating physician or other health care professional, relying on independent experience and knowledge of the patient, to determine drug dosages and the best treatment for the patient. Mention of any product in this issue should not be construed as endorsement by the contributors, editors, or the Publisher of the product or manufacturers' claims.

Surgical Clinics of North America (ISSN 0039–6109) is published bimonthly by Elsevier Inc., 360 Park Avenue South, New York, NY 10010-1710. Months of publication are February, April, June, August, October, and December. Business and Editorial Offices: 1600 John F. Kennedy Blvd., Suite 1800, Philadelphia, PA 19103-2899. Customer Service Office: 6277 Sea Harbor Drive, Orlando, FL 32887-4800. Periodicals postage paid at New York, NY and additional mailing offices. Subscription prices are $238.00 per year for US individuals, $382.00 per year for US institutions, $119.00 per year for US students and residents, $292.00 per year for Canadian individuals, $466.00 per year for Canadian institutions, $309.00 for international individuals, $466.00 per year for international institutions and $154.00 per year for Canadian and foreign students/residents. To receive student/resident rate, orders must be accompanied by name of affiliated institution, date of term, and the *signature* of program/residency coordinator on institution letterhead. Orders will be billed at individual rate until proof of status is received. Foreign air speed delivery is included in all *Clinics* subscription prices. All prices are subject to change without notice. POSTMASTER: Send address changes to *Surgical Clinics*, Elsevier Journals Customer Service, 6277 Sea Harbor Drive, Orlando, FL 32887-4800. **Customer Service: 1-800-654-2452 (US). From outside of the US, call 1-407-563-6020. Fax: 1-407-363-9661**. E-mail: JournalsCustomerService-usa@elsevier.com.

The Surgical Clinics of North America is also published in Spanish by McGraw-Hill Interamericana Editores S.A., P.O. Box 5-237 06500 Mexico D.F. Mexico; and in Portuguese by Interlivros Edicoes Ltda., Rua Comandante Coelho 1085, CEP 21250, Rio de Janeiro, Brazil; and in Greek by Paschalidis Medical Publications, Athens Greece.

The Surgical Clinics of North America is covered in *Index Medicus, EMBASE/Excerpta Medica, Current Contents/Clinical Medicine, Current Contents/Life Sciences, Science Citation Index*, and *ISI/BIOMED*.

Printed in the United States of America.

CONSULTING EDITOR

RONALD F. MARTIN, MD, Staff Surgeon, Marshfield Clinic, Marshfield; and Clinical Associate Professor, University of Wisconsin School of Medicine and Public Health, Madison, Wisconsin; Lieutenant Colonel, Medical Corps, United States Army Reserve

GUEST EDITORS

KAMAL M.F. ITANI, MD, Professor of Surgery, Boston University; Chief of Surgery, Boston Veterans Affairs Health Care System, West Roxbury; and Associate Chief of Surgery, Boston Medical Center and Brigham and Women's Hospital, Boston, Massachusetts

MARY T. HAWN, MD, FACS, Associate Professor of Surgery; Chief of the Section of Gastrointestinal Surgery, University of Alabama at Birmingham, Birmingham, Alabama

CONTRIBUTORS

GEORGES AL-KHOURY, MD, Pittsburgh, Pennsylvania

PATRICIO ANDRADES, MD, Research and Clinical Fellow, Division of Plastic Surgery; and Division of Transplant Immunology, University of Alabama at Birmingham, Birmingham, Alabama

SHARON BACHMAN, MD, Assistant Professor of Clinical Surgery, Department of General Surgery, University of Missouri-Columbia, Columbia, Missouri

MARY L. BRANDT, MD, Professor and Vice Chair, Michael E. DeBakey Department of Surgery, Texas Children's Hospital, Baylor College of Medicine, Houston, Texas

JORGE DE LA TORRE, MD, Professor of Plastic Surgery, Program Director, Division of Plastic Surgery, University of Alabama at Birmingham, Birmingham, Alabama

QUAN-YANG DUH, MD, Professor, Surgical Services, Veterans Affairs Medical Center, Department of Surgery, University of California San Francisco, San Francisco, California

DAVID B. EARLE, MD, FACS, Assistant Professor of Surgery, Tufts University School of Medicine; and Director of Minimally Invasive Surgery, Baystate Medical Center, Springfield, Massachusetts

ERIC EDWARDS, MD, St. Mary Medical Center, Langhorne, Pennsylvania

GEORGE S. FERZLI, MD, FACS, Chairman, Department of Surgery, Lutheran Medical Center; Professor of Surgery, Department of Surgery, SUNY Health Sciences Center at BKLYN, Brooklyn, New York

ROBERT J. FITZGIBBONS, Jr, MD, FACS, Harry E. Stuckenhoff Professor of Surgery, Department of Surgery, Creighton University School of Medicine, Omaha, Nebraska

MICHAEL G. FRANZ, MD, Associate Professor of Surgery, Chief, Division of Minimally Invasive Surgery, Department of Surgery, University of Michigan School of Medicine, Ann Arbor, Michigan

STEPHEN H. GRAY, MD, MSPH, General surgical resident, University of Alabama at Birmingham, Birmingham, Alabama

ROSEMARIE HARDIN, MD, Department of Surgery, SUNY Health Sciences Center at Brooklyn, Brooklyn, New York

MARY T. HAWN, MD, FACS, Associate Professor of Surgery; Chief of the Section of Gastrointestinal Surgery, University of Alabama at Birmingham, Birmingham, Alabama

LEIF A. ISRAELSSON, MD, PhD, Associate professor, Department of Surgery and Perioperative Science, Umeå University, Umeå, Sweden; and Kirurgkliniken, Sundsvalls sjukhus, Sundsvall, Sweden

KAMAL M.F. ITANI, MD, Professor of Surgery, Boston University; Chief of Surgery, Boston Veterans Affairs Health Care System, West Roxbury; and Associate Chief of Surgery, Boston Medical Center and Brigham and Women's Hospital, Boston, Massachusetts

LISA A. MARK, MD, Minimally Invasive Surgery Fellow, Department of Surgery, Baystate Medical Center, Springfield, Massachusetts

LEIGH NEUMAYER, MD, MS, Professor of Surgery, University of Utah, Salt Lake; and Professor of Surgery VA Healthcare System, Salt Lake City, Utah

ADRIAN E. PARK, MD, FRCCS, FACS, Campbell and Jeanette Plugge Professor of Surgery, Head, Division of General Surgery, and Vice Chair, Department of Surgery, University of Maryland School of Medicine, Baltimore, Maryland

VARUN PURI, MBBS, MS, Surgical Resident, Department of Surgery, Creighton University School of Medicine, Omaha, Nebraska

BRUCE RAMSHAW, MD, Chief of General Surgery & Associate Professor, Department of General Surgery, University of Missouri-Columbia, Columbia, Missouri

J.R. SALAMEH, MD, FACS, Clinical Associate Professor of Surgery, Georgetown University, Washington, DC; and Surgical Associates at Virginia Hospital Center, Arlington, Virginia

DAN H. SHELL IV, MD, Plastic Surgery Resident, Division of Plastic Surgery, University of Alabama at Birmingham, Birmingham, Alabama

MARK C. TAKATA, MD, Division of General Surgery, Scripps Clinic, La Jolla, California

KIRAN TURAGA, MBBS, MPH, Surgical Resident, Department of Surgery, Creighton University School of Medicine, Omaha, Nebraska

PATRICIA L. TURNER, MD, Assistant Professor of Surgery, Department of Surgery, University of Maryland School of Medicine, Baltimore, Maryland

LUIS O. VASCONEZ, MD, Professor of Plastic Surgery, Chief, Division of Plastic Surgery, University of Alabama at Birmingham, Birmingham, Alabama

BENJAMIN WOODS, BS, MS, Research Assistant in Surgery, University of Utah, Salt Lake City, Utah

CONTENTS

> Abdominal wall hernias occur when tissue structure and function are lost at the load-bearing muscle, tendon, and fascial layer. The fundamental biologic mechanisms are primary fascial pathology or surgical wound failure. In both cases, cellular and extracellular molecular matrix defects occur. Primary abdominal wall hernias have been associated with extracellular matrix diseases. Incisional hernias and recurrent inguinal hernias more often involve a combination of technical and biologic limitations. Defects in wound healing and extracellular matrix synthesis contribute to the high incidence of incisional hernia formation following laparotomy.

> The goals of this article are to describe the history of hernia repair and how innovations in surgical technique, prosthetics, and technology have shaped current practice.

> Almost all groin hernias in children are indirect inguinal hernias and occur as a result of incomplete closure of the processus

vaginalis. The treatment is repair by high ligation of the hernia sac, which can be done by an open or laparoscopic technique. The contralateral side can be explored by laparoscopy or left alone; open exploration is no longer indicated due to the potential risk of infertility. Umbilical hernias are common in infants but usually close with time. Surgery is indicated if the umbilical hernia is symptomatic or if the fascial defect fails to decrease in size over time.

Primary ventral hernias can be congenital or acquired, but are not associated with a fascial scar or related to a trauma. Some ventral hernias such as Spigelian, lumbar, or obturator hernias represent a diagnostic challenge, given their relative rarity and their unusual anatomic locations. The article presents the etiology, clinical presentation, and diagnosis of these hernias, and briefly describes the various surgical approaches, including open and laparoscopic.

Despite advances in many fields of surgery, incisional hernias still remain a significant problem. There is a lack of general consensus among surgeons regarding optimal treatment. A surgeon's approach is often based on tradition rather than clinical evidence. The surgeon's treatment plan should be comprehensive, with attention focused not merely on restoration of structural continuity. An understanding of the structural and functional anatomy of the abdominal wall and an appreciation of the importance of restoring dynamic function are necessary for the successful reconstruction of the abdominal wall.

Abdominal wall hernias are a familiar surgical problem. Millions of patients are affected each year, presenting most commonly with primary ventral, incisional, and inguinal hernias. Whether symptomatic or asymptomatic, hernias commonly cause pain or are aesthetically distressing to patients. These concerns, coupled with the risk of incarceration, are the most common reasons patients seek surgical repair of hernias. This article focuses on incisional hernias, reported to develop in 3% to 29% of laparotomy incisions.

Prosthetic Material in Ventral Hernia Repair: How Do I Choose?

Sharon Bachman and Bruce Ramshaw

Several factors must be considered in deciding which mesh to use for a ventral hernia repair. Open hernia repairs with no exposure of mesh to viscera can be performed with unprotected synthetic mesh, preferably a "lightweight" option. For open repair with high risk for fascial dehiscence and visceral exposure to mesh, and for open underlay repair and laparoscopic underlay repair, recommendations call for a tissue-separating mesh that prevents ingrowth of intra-abdominal contents into the mesh. Although no long-term data are available about biologic (acellular collagen scaffold) meshes, these may have good results when used in contaminated or well-drained infected fields, and do best when used according to the principles of a high-quality synthetic mesh repair (wide mesh overlap, frequent fixation points). Evidence is still insufficient to support the use of biologic materials for primary hernia repair.

Parastomal Hernias

Leif A. Israelsson

The incidence of parastomal hernias is probably 30% to 50%. Suture repair of a parastomal hernia or relocation of the stoma results in a high recurrence rate, whereas with mesh repair recurrence rates are lower. Several mesh repair techniques are used in open and laparoscopic surgery, but randomized trials comparing various techniques and with long-term follow-up are needed for better evidence.

Inguinal Hernias: Should We Repair?

Kiran Turaga, Robert J. Fitzgibbons, Jr, and Varun Puri

This review examines available data concerning the natural history of treated and untreated inguinal hernias. The incidence of complications with either treatment strategy is discussed using historical information from a time before herniorrhaphy became routine and contemporary data from two recently completed randomized controlled trials comparing routine repair using a tension-free technique with watchful waiting.

Open Repair of Inguinal Hernia: An Evidence-Based Review

Benjamin Woods and Leigh Neumayer

This article provides an evidence-based review of open hernia repair. Technical considerations in general, including perioperative management of the patient, and the most currently used open repairs are addressed. Outcomes after repair are reviewed using the latest available literature. Current recommendations from this review include the routine use of mesh in primary repair of inguinal hernia and the need to counsel patients preoperatively about the risk of chronic postoperative groin pain.

The safest and most effective inguinal hernia repair (laparoscopic versus open mesh) is being debated. As the authors point out, the former accounts for the minority of hernia repairs performed in the United States and around the world. The reasons for this are a demonstration in the literature of increased operative times, increased costs, and a longer learning curve. But the laparoscopic approach has clear advantages, including less acute and chronic postoperative pain, shorter convalescence, and earlier return to work. This article describes the transabdominal preperitoneal and totally extraperitoneal techniques, provides indications and contra-indications for laparoscopic repair, discusses the advantages and disadvantages of each technique, and provides an overview of the literature comparing tension-free open and laparoscopic inguinal hernia repair.

With numerous prosthetic options and a changing landscape of prosthetic development, a systematic approach to choosing a prosthetic is more sensible than trying to memorize all the details of each prosthetic. The surgeon should hone a single technique for the vast majority of inguinal hernia repairs to maximize profi-ciency. This limits the number of prosthetics to those suitable for that technique. Narrowing the choice further should be based on the likelihood that a given prosthetic will achieve the preoperative goals of the hernia repair. For alternative clinical scenarios, the surgeon should know one to two additional techniques, which may require a different prosthetic. The surgeon should use existing experimental and clinical data to estimate long-term benefits of any new prosthetic.

Groin pain following inguinal hernia repair remains a challenge to most general surgeons. Prevention of groin pain may be the most effective solution to this management problem and necessitates careful anatomic dissection and precise knowledge of surgical anatomy of the groin as well as potential pitfalls of surgical intervention. When complications arise, a period of watchful waiting is warranted, but surgical intervention with triple neurectomy offers the most definitive resolution of symptoms. This article aims to provide a thorough review of pertinent anatomic landmarks for the proper identification of the nerves that, if injured, result in chronic groin pain and to provide a treatment algorithm for patients suffering with this morbidity.

FORTHCOMING ISSUES

RECENT ISSUES

The Clinics are now available online!

www.theclinics.com

ELSEVIER
SAUNDERS

Surg Clin N Am 88 (2008) xiii–xv

SURGICAL
CLINICS OF
NORTH AMERICA

Foreword

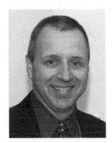

Ronald F. Martin, MD
Consulting Editor

A number of years ago, when I was just a few years into practice, I was asked to be a participant for a symposium on minimally invasive surgery. I thought that would be great. After all, I was building a practice and had been doing a number of operations laparoscopically that were fairly new to our area. This might not only be a good opportunity to learn and educate, but might even drum up some referrals—what could be better? So I agreed and asked what the moderator would like me to speak about, thinking maybe it would be laparoscopic splenectomy, or adrenalectomy, or common bile duct exploration. The topic I was assigned was "The defense of the open inguinal hernia repair." I was puzzled, but said that I would do it. As I thought about the topic after I hung up the phone, I started to wonder what that kind of request was all about. Then I learned that I was the only person on the panel who was assigned a "nonvideoscopic" topic. Now, a more paranoid individual than I might have sensed some sabotage in a challenging and competitive market place. And I will confess, the more I thought about it, the more the doubts crept into my mind. After all, my senior partner and I had performed the first laparoscopic inguinal hernia repair in our hospital and maybe our region. One would think that would have warranted some consideration. But no—defend open hernia repair it was.

After much thought and poring over the literature, it became clear to me that the assignment was more of a "legal argument" type problem that a "medical science" type problem. The studies were all over the map in

0039-6109/08/$ - see front matter © 2008 Elsevier Inc. All rights reserved.
doi:10.1016/j.suc.2008.01.001   *surgical.theclinics.com*

terms of results. The data were of wildly varying degrees of quality, and biases were evident to even the most casual of observers in any direction. My solution at the time was to do my own (probably poorly designed) study and throw myself on the mercy of the attendees at the conference. I collected all the data on every single patient that had undergone an inguinal hernia repair done in our area that was not performed as part of another procedure at either of the major hospitals in our city for an entire year. Data was collected on length of operation, cost (not charges) of materials, length of stay in recovery or admission, presence of trainees, type of repair, and short term complication rates. I did not have a mechanism to follow-up for long-term results or complications, nor could I tell if the patients had been readmitted or seen in another facility for problems.

What I learned was that the operations seemed to go as well in either group in terms of overall safety and complication rates. The laparoscopic hernias were considerably more expensive to the hospital (we later learned that differential reimbursement failed to cover this in most cases) and took considerably longer to perform. When complications did occur, they tended to be more devastating in the laparoscopic group, but the worst complications, though more rare, occurred in the open group.

I presented this data to our symposium. I felt assured that everybody would think, "Wow. That is quite startling. Maybe I'll rethink my practice patterns." I was so convinced that this was data worthy of concern that I even polled the audience to see if anybody thought this information would alter their practice choice. The resounding answer was, "No." Those who came in thinking that laparoscopic inguinal hernia repair was a good choice were not swayed. Those who felt open hernia repair was a good choice were similarly steadfast.

During the discussion part of the meeting, this topic was revived. I was still a little perplexed at my lack of persuasion but what happened next explained it all. Each person who commented made it clear that in his or her community, the decision of what type of hernia repair to offer was completely based upon the market forces in their locality. If the surgeon had a good grip on local market penetration, then he or she would do whichever operation was most comfortable to the operator. If, on the other hand, there were a number of competitors in the locality, then the surgeons in those towns tended to offer the "newer" procedure in higher percentages to maintain or improve market share. So much for data.

Now, if you are still reading this you might be wondering what this story has to do with a foreword: even though we are an imperfect group as surgeons, eventually the data will guide our practice. The truth shall out, as they say. But truth is an elusive concept. And what truth is largely depends upon how one wishes to apply it to reality. The issue before us is not necessarily to know which operation does what and for how much, but rather to define exactly what problem—if any—we are trying to resolve in the first place.

Are short postoperative stays in the order of a few hours after open inguinal hernia repairs onerous and, if so, are these improved upon by the laparoscopic approach? Are we serving an underserved group with new technology? Have we increased the safety of the procedure with a new approach? If we are spending more on new technology for equivalent results, are we getting a return on the investment that will help us save money for our patients in some other way? Is this the biggest problem we have to solve at this time?

Certainly these questions are not limited to inguinal hernia repair or other hernia repair. These questions apply to every change we make. Change is inevitable and change is generally good. But change for the sake of change is not. And it is there that we are obliged to look and see if the changes we make bring us the results that we thought they would. And if they do not, then we must decide whether we are on a good path and are traveling in a proper way.

The articles in this issue are well considered by authors who have mastered their subjects. They should provide an excellent base for understanding how the questions should be framed, and even give some opinion as to how the answers might appear. Whether you, the reader, use this information to guide your practice is, of course, up to you. We are all subject to forces in our lives that control our decision-making: some evidence based and others not.

I doubt very much that I changed anybody's mind that day at the symposium. Most likely, if I didn't it was because the data I had presented really did not address the concerns of the audience. As for the topic assignment and its political ramifications, the speaker presenting in favor of laparoscopic hernia repair (my opponent, as it were) was to become a practice partner of mine, and the presentation on laparoscopic bile duct exploration contained most of its graphics from an review article that had been published that month in the *World Journal of Surgery*, by Drs. Rosen, Rossi, and myself. It is hard to believe in coincidences in this business, but I am not paranoid enough to read too much into this.

I would like to thank Drs. Itani and Hawn, as well as their colleagues, for an excellent contribution this series.

Ronald F. Martin, MD
Department of Surgery
Marshfield Clinic
1000 North Oak Avenue
Marshfield, WI 54449, USA

E-mail address: Martin.ronald@marschfieldclinic.org

ELSEVIER
SAUNDERS

Surg Clin N Am 88 (2008) xvii–xix

SURGICAL
CLINICS OF
NORTH AMERICA

Preface

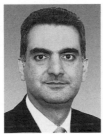 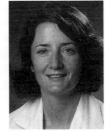

Kamal M.F. Itani, MD   Mary T. Hawn, MD, FACS
Guest Editors

In the field of general surgery, hernia surgery remains the most common surgical procedure performed, with inguinal hernias leading the pack. While surgeons spent the early part of the twentieth century improving the technique of primary repair, the latter half was focused on developing techniques of mesh repair, minimizing incisions, and maximizing comfort. As in the majority of studies in general surgery, most hernia reports were observational, retrospective, single center or single surgeon studies. It has not been until the last 10 years that well planned, prospective randomized trials have started to emerge, providing higher level evidence for the practice of hernia surgery. Despite these clinical trials, there is still no final consensus on timing of treatment, technique to be used, material, and mesh position.

We know from various observational studies that certain extrinsic conditions predispose a patient to hernia formation. Dr. Michael Franz, in the first article of this issue, delves into patient intrinsic factors that might lead to hernia formation and the body's reaction to prosthetics. In the second article, the editors present an overview of the surgical innovations in adult hernia repair over the last 120 years, since Bassini described his original repair. Away from the University hospital and the large medical centers, routine

0039-6109/08/$ - see front matter © 2008 Elsevier Inc. All rights reserved.
doi:10.1016/j.suc.2008.01.002   *surgical.theclinics.com*

pediatric surgery is performed by general surgeons. The pediatric hernia is treated differently from the adult hernia, and the editors devote a separate article to this topic, which is addressed by Dr. Brandt. The field of primary and unusual abdominal wall hernias is presented by Dr. Salameh.

Ventral incisional hernias are presented in the next four articles. While awaiting the results of prospective randomized trials comparing open repair to laparoscopic repair, Dr. Schell and colleagues present the various techniques of open ventral incisional hernia repair and the advantages and disadvantages of each, while Drs. Turner and Parks present the pros and cons of laparoscopic ventral incisional hernia repair. The ever-expanding field of prosthetic material to be used in ventral incisional hernia is presented by Drs. Bachman and Ramshaw. Although ventral incisional hernias are the most common of the ventral hernias, general surgeons encounter other types of ventral hernias that are sometimes very challenging to repair. The editors thought that parastomal hernias present a unique set of challenges, are common enough, and thus deserve to be presented separately; this is done by Dr. Israelson.

In the subsequent five articles, an in-depth review of inguinal hernias is presented by various leaders in the field. Although the presence of an inguinal hernia was always considered to be an indication for surgery, Dr. Fitzgibbons, in his prospective randomized trial, questions that dogma and presents in his article the evidence for his argument. Dr. Neumayer, who performed the largest trial in inguinal hernia surgery comparing open to laparoscopic repair, together with Dr. Woods, reviews the evidence behind various techniques in open hernia surgery. Dr. Duh, a noted laparoscopic surgeon who participated in Dr. Neumayer's trial, presents with Dr. Takata the evidence behind laparascopic repair and its various techniques. The various prostheses available for repair of an inguinal hernia are presented by Drs. Mark and Earle. One of the most debilitating and feared complications of inguinal hernia repair is after-herniorrhaphy groin pain; in their monograph, Dr. Ferzli and his colleagues give us clear guidelines on how to avoid this complication and how best to treat it when it happens.

Although recurrence remains the most important end point in hernia surgery, investigators in the twenty-first century started focusing on patient-centered outcome as recurrence rates decreased to an all time low. In addition to complications, postoperative pain, health related quality of life, caregiver burden, and patient satisfaction are now essential domains in the field of hernia surgery outcomes. With the continued evolution of minimally invasive surgery, the learning experience of surgeons and residents and the creation of more expensive prosthesis, health economics becomes another domain to address. The Neumayer trial addressed several of those domains, and there is no doubt that the next 10 years will continue to see a focus on patient centered outcomes, health economics, and improved prosthetic material.

Kamal M.F. Itani, MD
Department of Surgery
VA Boston Health Care System and Boston University
1400 VFW Parkway
Boston, MA 02132, USA

E-mail address: kitani@med.va.gov

Mary T. Hawn, MD, FACS
Department of Surgery
University of Alabama at Birmingham
KB 429, 1530 3rd Avenue South
Birmingham, AL 35294, USA

E-mail address: mhawn@uab.edu

Surg Clin N Am 88 (2008) 1–15

The Biology of Hernia Formation

Michael G. Franz, MD

*Division of Minimally Invasive Surgery, Department of Surgery, University of Michigan
School of Medicine, 2922H Taubman Center, 1500 East Medical Center Drive,
Ann Arbor, MI 48109-0331, USA*

Abdominal wall hernias occur when tissue structure and function are lost at the load-bearing muscle, tendon, and fascial layer. The fundamental biologic mechanisms are primary fascial pathology or surgical wound failure. In both cases, cellular and extracellular molecular matrix defects occur.

Abnormal collagen metabolism was an early biologic mechanism proposed for the development of primary and incisional hernias [1,2]. Immature collagen isoforms were measured in patients with inguinal and incisional hernias [3,4]. Importantly, the collagen abnormality was detected in skin biopsies remote from the hernia site, supporting a genetic basis for hernia formation, although a large, population-based study of collagen expression in surgical patients needs to be done. Acquired collagen defects were ascribed to cigarette smoking or nutritional deficiencies.

Secondary fascial pathology occurs following acute laparotomy wound failure. This is in large part due to the replacement of fascial planes with scar tissue. It is well known that the incidence of recurrent incisional hernia increases with each attempt at repair [5,6]. Fibroblast and wound collagen disorders were observed in scar from incisional hernia patients. There is also evidence that mechanical strain, like coughing and weight lifting, can induce secondary changes in tissue fibroblast function within load-bearing tissues [7,8]. It is possible that chronic loading induces pathologic changes in structural tissue cellular and molecular function, without an a priori biologic defect.

Laparotomy wound failure and the loss of normal wound-healing architecture may induce the selection of an abnormal population of wound repair fibroblasts, as occurs in chronic wounds [9,10]. This could result in the expression of abnormal structural collagen and also explain the high incidence

This work was supported by grant no. R01 GM078288 from the National Institutes of Health.

E-mail address: mfranz@umich.edu

of recurrent incisional hernias. One mechanism for phenotypic selection of abnormal laparotomy wound repair fibroblasts is the loss of abdominal wall load-force signaling as the incision mechanically fails. It is recognized that mechanical load forces stimulate the repair of tendons [11]. Wound ischemia also ensues during early acute wound failure, propagating deficient soft-tissue repair. The best studies of incisional hernia formation confirm that *early* laparotomy wound failure is an important mechanism of incisional hernia formation (Table 1) [12]. It is likely that early mechanical failure of the laparotomy wound induces pathologic function of wound repair fibroblasts. By this mechanism, otherwise normal wound repair fibroblasts fail, without the primary expression of an extracellular matrix or wound repair disease. This hypothesis is now tested in at least one animal model where intentional mechanical laparotomy wound failure led to pathologic wound fibroblast function in vivo and in vitro [10]. It is possible that a subset of incisional hernia patients expresses a defect in extracellular matrix and/or wound repair function. It is hard to resolve that mechanism with the fact that the majority of surgical patients have no history of a wound-healing defect (making them surgical candidates) and also do not express a defect at the primary surgical site (gastrointestinal tract, vascular system, solid organs, and so forth). It is possible that mechanical failure is the major mechanism for incisional hernia formation and that the loss of mechanical load signaling or some other acute wound-healing pathway induces defects in repair fibroblast biology. As the tissue fibroblast is the major source for collagen synthesis and turnover, defects in fibroblast function are an important mechanism for subsequent tissue collagen disease.

With the limited information available, it is likely that primary hernias are the result of a connective tissue disorder, whereas secondary hernias (eg, incisional hernias) are most frequently due to technical failure, inducing a chronic wound. Recurrent hernias likely are a combination of both mechanisms.

Extra-cellular matrix and collagen disease

Medicine provides many clues for the role of the extracellular matrix during hernia formation. Lathyrism is an acquired disorder of the connective tissue that predisposes to hernia formation. A diet high in chickpeas inhibits collagen cross-linking leading to a laxity in fascial planes [13]. Ehlers-Danlos syndrome is a collection of collagen isoform disorders, also predisposing to

Table 1
Occult laparotomy wound dehiscence by postoperative day 30

Outcome at 43 m	Less than 12-mm gap	More than 12-mm gap
% Healed	95% (140/147)	6% (1/18)
% Incisional hernia	5% (7/140)	94% (17/18)

hernia formation. There is growing evidence that patients with large-vessel aneurysmal disease express pathologic extracellular matrix metabolism, predisposing to dilated aortas and hernias. Early studies found that the rectus sheath of direct inguinal hernia patients was thinned, displayed disordered collagen fibers, and impaired hydroxylation of the collagen [1].

Increased proteolytic activity may cause weakness in structural tissue. Matrix metallo-protease (MMP)-2 overexpression was measured in fibroblasts of patients with direct inguinal hernias, and MMP-13 overexpression was detected in patients with recurrent inguinal hernias [14,15]. Studies like these are observational, and it is not clear whether increased MMP expression leads to direct inguinal hernia formation. Alternatively, failing groin tissue may secondarily express increased MMP levels.

Many studies associate incisional hernias with impaired collagen and protease metabolism. Tissue from incisional hernias expressed more soluble (immature) collagen, increased ratios of early wound matrix collagen isoforms (collagen III), and increased tissue matrix metalloprotease levels [4,16]. A decreased ratio of type I: type III collagen mRNA and protein was measured in the hernia ring and skin specimens obtained from patients with incisional hernias. Morphologic changes were present not only in the fascial tissue, but also in the hernia sac, skin specimens, and scar tissue surrounding explanted meshes of hernia patients. These studies were the most compelling for the presence of a genetic collagen defect in patients that develop incisional hernias.

Surgical wound healing

The mechanism of primary hernia formation is important to understand to improve diagnosis, to provide prognosis, and when modifying risks for hernia formation. Tissue matrix disorders that lead to primary hernia formation probably also impair surgical wound healing. Surgeons fundamentally seek a better understanding of the mechanism of successful and failed hernia repairs.

Acute wounds are defined by the loss of normal tissue structure and function in otherwise normal tissue where normal wound healing is expected to occur. An inter-regulated series of cellular and molecular events must be activated and modulated during the organization of a surgical wound matrix (Fig. 1) [17]. It is the integrated summation of each pathway along the continuum of this host response to injury that results in acute wound healing. The phases of acute wound healing are described as hemostasis, inflammation, fibro-proliferation (scar formation), and wound remodeling. A defect or delay in the activation of any of the repair pathways expressed during normal laparotomy and hernia repair may lead to hernia formation. Wound infection, wound ischemia, and steroids all delay parts of the surgical wound-healing pathway [18].

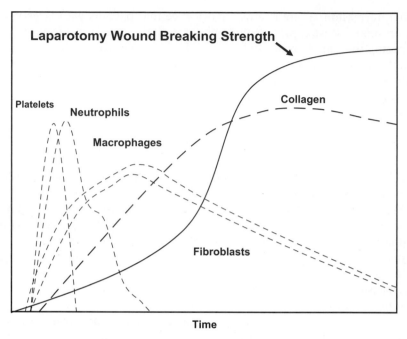

Fig. 1. A normal wound-healing cascade. In otherwise normal tissue, without impediments to wound healing, sequential cellular and molecular elements of tissue repair are activated.

Abnormal wound matrix structure also contributes to the mechanism of recurrent hernias. Ideally, normal-appearing aponeurotic and fascial structures would regenerate following hernia repairs. Smoking and malnutrition can impair collagen structure [1]. Biologic approaches for "normal" laparotomy wounds might be guided by information gained from identified genetic or epigenetic pathways associated with hernia formation such as abnormal collagen matrix structure in Ehlers-Danlos syndrome or MMP/TIMP (tissue inhibitors of the MMP) expression in abdominal aortic aneurysm disease or in other chronic wounds.

Early mechanical wound failure (fascial dehiscence)

Growing evidence supports that incisional hernias and recurrent hernias are most often the result of early surgical wound-healing failure. The majority of incisional hernias appear to develop following the mechanical disruption of laparotomy wounds occurring during the initial "lag phase" of the wound-healing trajectory (Fig. 2). Clinically evident laparotomy wound failure is a rare event, with reported dehiscence rates of 0.1% [19]. Prior literature examining wound healing concluded that incisional hernias were the result of late laparotomy wound failure and scar breakdown [2]. This concept was challenged by clinical studies of incisional hernias that recorded

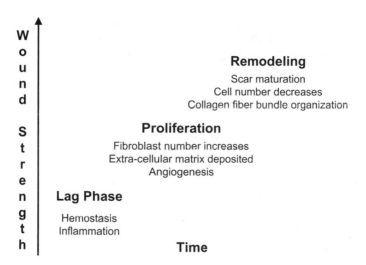

Fig. 2. During the initial "lag phase" of healing, the laparotomy wound is mechanically weakest. As surgical patients recover, increasing abdominal wall loads can cause acute wound failure.

high primary and secondary recurrence rates after short-term follow-up—typically only 2 to 4 years [6]. Prospective studies find that the true rate of laparotomy wound failure is closer to 11%, and that the majority of these (94%) go on to form incisional hernias during the first 3 years after abdominal operations [12]. The real laparotomy wound failure rate is therefore 100 times what most surgeons think it is. By this mechanism, most incisional hernias and recurrent inguinal hernias originate from clinically occult dehiscences. The overlying skin wound heals, concealing the underlying myofascial defect. This mechanism of early mechanical laparotomy wound failure is more consistent with modern acute wound-healing science. There are no other models of acute wound healing, suggesting that a successfully healed acute wound goes on to break down and mechanically fail at a later date.

Incisional hernias occur when the laparotomy wound fails to heal. The fundamental mechanism may be an underlying wound-healing defect or inadequate surgical technique. When a laparotomy wound fails due to inadequate surgical technique, selective changes occur involving the wound fibroblasts and extracellular matrix molecules, leading to a pathologic chronic wound.

The mechanism of incisional hernia formation

Biologic components

Laparotomy wounds are totally dependent on suture until breaking strengths are achieved that are capable of offsetting the increased loads placed across an acute wound by a recovering patient. Tensile strength normalizes breaking strength to the surface area of the wound edge, thereby measuring a physical property of the particular wound and scar (tensile strength = breaking strength/wound-edge surface area). Wound-breaking strength is more relevant for tissues placed under high loads. Burst abdomens, or acute fascial dehiscence with evisceration, are an important extreme of acute wound failure. They are associated with mortalities of 50% or greater [20].

Acute wound healing fails when there is a deficient quantity or quality of tissue repair. Ultimately, it is the time required for the recovery of wound-breaking strength that determines the risk of acute wound failure. Inadequate hemostasis owing to platelet dysfunction or poor technique can result in hematoma formation with ensuing mechanical disruption of a provisional wound matrix. A delayed or deficient inflammatory response can result in wound contamination or infection with abnormal signaling for progression into the fibro-proliferative phase of acute tissue repair [21]. A prolonged inflammatory response owing to the presence of a foreign material, like a mesh implant, or wound infection will delay the progression of acute wound healing into the fibro-proliferative phase, where rapid gains in breaking strength should occur [22]. Delayed fibroblast responses in turn impede the synthesis of a provisional wound matrix, prolonging the period of time a surgical wound is subjected to increasing mechanical loads and dependent entirely on suture material and technique for strength.

Inflammation

Inflammatory cells marginate into injured tissue and an efflux of leukocytes and plasma proteins enter the wound site. Neutrophils arrive initially and function to phagocytose and debride the wound, but are not required for wound healing in clean wounds. Monocytes and tissue macrophages populate the inflammatory infiltrate within 2 to 3 days. Macrophages phagocytose injured tissue and debris as well as secrete multiple growth factors. The macrophage orchestrates tissue repair and appears to be the only inflammatory cell type absolutely required [23].

Overall tissue strength of a wound is essentially zero during this inflammatory phase, thus an excessive or prolonged inflammatory response as is seen with incisional foreign bodies, like suture or mesh material, or infections predispose to wound failure. Steroids can reduce wound inflammation, but also inhibit collagen synthesis and wound contraction, synergistically impeding tissue repair [24]. Interestingly, there is minimal inflammatory cell infiltration seen in fetal wound repair during which the epidermis and dermis are restored to normal architecture without scar formation [25].

Fibroblasts

Fibroblasts are responsible for collagen synthesis and the recovery of wound-breaking strength. Fibroblasts migrate into acute wounds within

2 days and are the major cell type in granulation tissue by the fourth day following injury. At first, fibroblasts populate the wound site through migration and increase in number by proliferation. Wound fibroblast migration and proliferation are both influenced by soluble growth factors and inflammatory mediators [26]. The chemical and structural composition of the provisional matrix on which fibroblasts move is equally important. Receptor-mediated interactions are increasingly described between the wound extracellular matrix and activated repair fibroblasts. Very little, however, is known about defective fibroblast function during acute wound failure. Even less is known about the function of repair fibroblasts in tissue other than skin. It is not known whether abdominal wall wound failure reflects a defect in tendon fibroblast recruitment and function during incisional hernia formation, or whether abnormal mechanical signals following laparotomy wound failure subsequently results in impaired fibroblast function.

In chronic ulcer studies, it was suggested that low wound-growth factor levels might result in dermal fibroblast quiescence and even senescence [27]. This may also be true in failing acute laparotomy and hernia wounds as an initially rapid rising growth factor signaling cascade became depleted. Relative fascial or tendon wound ischemia might also induce fibroblast cell-cycle arrest. This would occur, for example, when a suture line is closed too tight, or in a patient who is in shock and soft-tissue perfusion is reduced. An ischemic laparotomy repair might also be deficient in the components and cofactors required for DNA and protein synthesis, again resulting in repair fibroblast cell-cycle arrest. Finally, too little or too much tension across the laparotomy tendon repair may disturb the optimal set point of a normal mechano-transduction mechanism, again resulting in premature laparotomy wound fibroblast cell-cycle arrest.

The precise histologic origin of abdominal wall fibroblast repair cells in healed versus herniated wounds is also unknown. Differences may exist in the chemotactic response of ventral (anterior) myofascial versus mesothelial surface fibroblasts following midline incisions. It is known, for example, that peritoneal surface defects heal by simultaneously re-epithelializing the entire wound surface as opposed to establishing an advancing epithelial edge as occurs in the skin [28,29]. Because epidermal-to-dermal communication is known to occur during the healing of skin, it is possible that a similar mechanism may be active on the peritoneal surfaces of abdominal wall (fascial) wounds. Peritoneal fluid itself may modulate acute repair in the abdominal wall. During fetal wound healing, amniotic fluid can act to accelerate the recovery of wound-breaking strength in addition to minimizing the amount of scar formation.

Defects have been identified in the kinetic properties of fibroblasts cultured from laparotomy wound and hernia biopsies obtained from a rat model of incisional hernias [9]. It was observed that fibroblasts cultured from incisional hernias expressed a defect in causing the contraction of fibroblast-populated collagen lattices. Normally healing laparotomy wound fibroblasts caused 80% lattice contraction over 5 days, whereas hernia fibroblasts caused only 50% lattice contraction. The same studies found no difference in the level of collagen gene expression between herniated and healed laparotomy wounds after 28 days. The results suggested that any difference in collagen gene expression occurs earlier than postoperative day 28 in this laparotomy repair model, or that the defect in herniated wounds is not one of collagen gene expression. Other possibilities included down-stream abnormalities in collagen protein synthesis and assembly, early scar crystallization, and/or fibroblast remodeling activity.

Collagen

Collagen is the predominant structural protein, especially of abdominal wall fascial layers, comprising 80% or more of structural tissue dry weight. Defects result in either delayed or abnormal collagen synthesis or increased wound protease activity leading to collagen degradation. The result is an imbalance in repair collagen homeostasis leading to a reduction in wound collagen levels, wound tensile strength, and an increased risk of mechanical wound failure [30]. Lathyrism, a disorder of collagen cross-linking, and lathyrogens were shown to be associated with herniation. Reduced hydroxyproline and collagen levels were measured in structural tissues of patients with direct inguinal hernias [31]. Isolated fibroblasts from these patients expressed a proliferative defect and a reduced ability to translocate hydroxyproline. Subsequent to that work, apparent abnormalities in the ratios of collagen isoform expression, decreased collagen cross-linking, and increased collagen solubility were observed. A twofold increase in the amount of immature type III collagen was reported in the skin fibroblasts of patients with inguinal hernias when compared with nonhernia patients [15]. A genetic predisposition to the formation of abdominal wall hernias was also suggested in large, controlled series of abdominal aortic aneurysm patients, supporting the long-held impression of a common extracellular matrix defect in both vascular wall and abdominal wall collagen metabolism [32–35].

The mechanism by which the collagen-rich early laparotomy wound matrix attaches to uninjured tissue at the wound border is also poorly understood. This mechanism is important, as acute laparotomy wounds most often fail at the interface of scar to normal tissue [36]. Animal modeling shows that a provisional wound matrix mechanically fails within the scar itself only during the first 3 to 5 days after injury. After that, mechanical failure is more likely to occur at the interface of early scar to wound edge (Fig. 3). Different tissue also heals at different rates. Native tissues with collagen bundles organized in a parallel orientation, such as fascia, ligament, or tendon, regain breaking strength faster than tissue with a more complex, three-dimensional fiber network, such as in the dermis [37]. Another way to describe this is by measuring the recovery in relative breaking strength, where wound progress is normalized to the uninjured tissue collagen

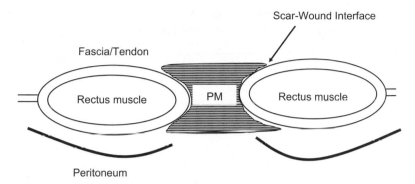

Fig. 3. Incisional hernias occur when suture fails, suture lines are too loose, or suture pulls through the tissue adjacent to the wound. This develops before the laparotomy wound scar is mechanically capable of withstanding the distractive forces. The provisional matrix (PM) is composed of immature and weak matrix glycoproteins and collagen isoforms. In addition, the scar-to-wound interface is not developed.

content. The time required to achieve 50% wound-breaking strength is greater in tissue with high collagen content—again, as in the case of dermis. Conversely, more "simply" arranged soft tissues (eg, abdominal wall fascia) with lower tissue collagen content but organized in a purely parallel manner along lines of tension should achieve uninjured breaking strength faster.

Growth factors

Growth factors are tissue repair signaling peptides upregulated initially during the inflammatory phase of laparotomy wound healing. Five to 7 days are required, however, before peak levels of fibro-proliferative growth factors such as transforming growth factor-beta are reached within acute wounds [38–40]. It is not known whether delays in the appearance of fibro-proliferative growth factors contribute to the development of incisional hernias. Surgical wound therapy with proliferative growth factors is known to stimulate the appearance of fibroblasts and collagen into the wound, thereby accelerating the gain in wound-breaking strength [41].

Nutrition

Tissue repair is an anabolic process that requires both energy and adequate nutritional building blocks. Patients who are malnourished or actively catabolic, such as in the systemic inflammatory response syndrome, demonstrate impaired healing. The National Surgery Quality Improvement Program, sponsored by the Veterans Administration, consistently measures low serum albumen as a risk factor for perioperative complications, including incisional hernia formation [42]. Inadequate nutrition also impairs the immune response-limiting opsonization of bacterial and sterilization of wounds. Several vitamin and mineral deficiencies also have been described that predispose to altered wound repair. Vitamins C, A, and B6 each are required for collagen synthesis and cross-linking. Deficiencies in vitamins B1 and B2 as well as zinc and copper cause syndromes associated with poor wound repair. Finally, essential fatty acids are required for cell synthesis, particularly in areas of high cell turnover such as healing wounds [43].

Tissue perfusion

Perioperative shock is a well-recognized risk factor for incisional hernia formation [44]. Tissue oxygen levels of 30-mm Hg are required for healing to occur. Besides systemic hypotension, a too-tight continuous suture line closure may exacerbate laparotomy wound ischemia. Emergency operations may also be associated with wound contamination and altered surgical technique. Laparotomies following gunshot wounds to the abdomen or for perforated viscous may leave devitalized tissue and high levels of bacteria in the surgical wound. High wound bacterial counts are known to lead to wound failure, and in this case, incisional hernia formation [45]. During emergency operations, midline incisions are most common and they are usually longer than during elective procedures. There is evidence that midline incisions herniate more frequently than transverse incisions [20]. The collagen bundles of the abdominal wall are predominantly oriented transversely [46]. A transverse suture line is therefore mechanically more stable, as it encircles tissue collagen bundles, rather than splitting them.

The effect of surgical technique on the biology of laparotomy and hernia repair

Most studies designed to improve laparotomy and hernia wound outcomes have focused on surgical technique and the mechanical properties of suture material and mesh [2,47,48]. During the evolution of inguinal hernia repairs, it was assumed that a strong, stout tissue such as the conjoined tendon rigidly sutured to a similar structure like Cooper's ligament would produce a reliable hernia repair. Purely surgical approaches like this proved unreliable for many surgeons, and recurrence rates remained unacceptably high.

Surgical wound failure is most often due to suture pulling through adjacent tissue and not suture fracture or knot slippage [20]. Tissue failure occurs in a metabolically active zone adjacent to the acute wound edge where proteases activated during normal tissue repair result in a loss of native tissue integrity at the point where sutures are placed. The breakdown of the tissue matrix adjacent to the wound appears to be part of the mechanism for mobilizing the cellular elements of tissue repair.

Abdominal wall tendons and fascia are connective tissues placed under intrinsic and extrinsic loads that are likely dependant on mechanical signals to regulate fibroblast homeostasis. Mechano-transduction pathways are being described in greater detail in ligament, tendon, and bone repair [7,36,49]. Mechanical signals are transmitted to the structural cell via integrin receptors, for example, and subsequently effect repair cell metabolism through the modulation of cytoskeleton anchoring proteins. In brief, a load imparted on a soft tissue or bone is transmitted to structural cells through the extracellular matrix via transmembrane integrin receptors located on the cell surface. In one proliferative pathway, subsequent activation of the focal adhesion kinase complex leads to cytoskeletal changes and the further activation of downstream signaling tyrosine kinases like c-src and the mitogen-activated protein kinase proliferation pathway [49].

The varying mechanical forces exerted across anatomically different celiotomy incisions such as midline versus transverse therefore may affect repair fibroblast activation, provisional matrix assembly and collagen deposition, and, ultimately, the temporal recovery of laparotomy wound tensile strength. Surgical experience has long held that transverse abdominal wall incisions oriented parallel to the predominant myofascial fibers regain unwounded tissue strength faster, but a clear benefit on wound outcomes has never been proven [20].

Biology or surgery?

Optimized laparotomy wound healing therefore depends on the normal assimilation of both biologic and mechanical signals. Factors that interfere with either or both of these pathways will result in delays or defects in the early phases of acute wound healing. From the "biologic" perspective, this most commonly includes infection, ischemia, malnutrition, and pharmacologic inhibitors. From the "mechanical" perspective, this involves the reinforcing cycle of wound failure with a loss in optimal strain loads and a down-regulation of the mechano-transduction pathways normally activated to signal tissue repair. In one extreme, this is due to acute wound overload and overt mechanical failure, and in the other extreme may be due to acute wound underload due to a poor suturing technique or even the placement of a bridging mesh implant.

Preliminary observations found for the first time that an interactive biomechanical mechanism may be activated during acute laparotomy wound failure. In other words, mechanical failure alone might result in the abnormal function of repair cells. Fibroblasts isolated from otherwise normal rat hernias were observed to cause 50% to 75% less contraction of a fibroblast-populated collagen lattice than those fibroblasts isolated from a normally healing wound. One possible mechanism for this loss in repair fibroblast kinetic and proliferative activity may be the reduction in mechanical signals that occurs as a structural soft tissue fails. As already discussed, it is known in tendon and ligament repair that mechano-transduction is an important pathway for setting fibroblast repair function [49]. From this perspective, an abdominal wall laparotomy wound behaves more like a ligament or tendon than skin during repair.

Abdominal wall physiology

As described above, well-controlled, prospective studies conclude that most laparotomy wound disruptions progressing to incisional hernias begin to form within 30 days of laparotomy wound closure [12]. In the animal models of hernia formation, laparotomy wounds are temporarily repaired with rapidly absorbed suture. Laparotomy wound-edge separation occurs early, resulting in incisional hernias due to incompletely supported mechanical loads. The incisional hernias that develop have well-defined hernia rings, hernia sacs, and visceral adhesions, all characteristic of the incisional hernias that develop in humans (Fig. 4).

The function of intact abdominal wall structures during laparotomy repair and following hernia formation can be measured. This includes effects

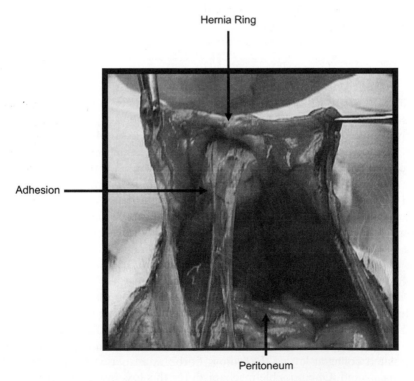

Fig. 4. The peritoneal view of a rodent model of incisional hernias. The hernias develop well-defined hernia rings, hernia sacs, and visceral adhesions, all characteristic of the incisional hernias that develop in humans. Modeling like this confirms biologic limits of laparotomy wound repair and suggests that pathologic changes occur in the wound and musculature of the abdominal wall following wound failure in otherwise normal tissue.

of the distractive load forces generated by the lateral oblique and midline rectus muscle and fascial components. When the midline laparotomy mechanically fails, pathologic disuse atrophy, fibrosis, and muscle fiber type changes occur in the abdominal wall muscles [50]. This pathologic change in the lateral abdominal wall musculature supports the important role that load signaling may play in abdominal wall wound repair. The observation is not surprising given the important function of the abdominal wall to support and animate the torso and to protect intra-abdominal organs. Surgically, it is equally likely that these pathologic changes cause reduced abdominal wall compliance and contribute to the difficulty in achieving durable incisional hernia repairs.

Most evidence supports that primary hernia formation derives from a biologic deficiency of the extracellular matrix of most patients. It is a soft-tissue disease. Risk factors like cigarette smoking and the metabolic syndrome likely contribute to the pathology. Once surgically repaired, the fundamental mechanism for recurrent hernia disease includes inadequate surgical technique and how that interacts with the biologic limits of wound healing. Incisional hernias may be considered chronic wounds expressing abnormal tissue repair pathways.

Summary

The fundamental mechanism of abdominal wall hernia formation is the loss of structural integrity at the musculo-tendinous layer. This results in the inability to contain abdominal organs, support upright posture, and maintain increased intraperitoneal pressure during Valsalva. Primary abdominal wall hernias have been associated with extracellular matrix diseases. Incisional hernias and recurrent inguinal hernias more often involve a combination of technical and biologic limitations. Defects in wound healing and extracellular matrix synthesis contribute to the high incidence of incisional hernia formation following laparotomy.

References

[1] Read RC. Introduction. Hernia 2006;10(6):454–5.
[2] Peacock J. Fascia and muscle. In: Peacock J, editor. Wound repair. 3rd edition. Philadelphia: W.B. Saunders; 1984. p. 332–62.
[3] Junge K, Klinge U, Rosch R, et al. Decreased collagen type I/III ratio in patients with recurring hernia after implantation of alloplastic prostheses. Langenbecks Arch Surg 2004;389(1): 17–22.
[4] Klinge U, Zheng H, Si ZY, et al. Synthesis of type I and III collagen, expression of fibronectin and matrix metalloproteinases–1 and–13 in hernial sac of patients with inguinal hernia. Int J Surg Investig 1999;1(3):219–27.
[5] Flum DR, Horvath K, Koepsell T. Have outcomes of incisional hernia repair improved with time? A population based analysis. Ann Surg 2003;237(1):129–35.

[6] Luijendijk RW, Hop WCJ, van den Tol P, et al. A comparison of suture repair with mesh repair for incisional hernia. N Engl J Med 2000;343(6):392–8.

[7] Skutek M, van Griensven M, Zeichen J, et al. Cyclic mechanical stretching modulates secretion pattern of growth factors in human tendon fibroblasts. Eur J Appl Physiol 2001;86(1): 48–52.

[8] Katsumi A, Naoe T, Matsushita T, et al. Integrin activation and matrix binding mediate cellular responses to mechanical stretch. J Biol Chem 2005;280(17):16546–9.

[9] Franz MG, Smith PD, Wachtel TL, et al. Fascial incisions heal faster than skin: a new model of abdominal wall repair. Surgery 2001;129(2):203–8.

[10] Dubay DA, Wang X, Adamson BS, et al. Progressive fascial wound failure impairs subsequent abdominal wall repairs: a new animal model of incisional hernia formation. Surgery 2005;137(4):463–71.

[11] Benjamin M, Hillen B. Mechanical influences on cells, tissues and organs—'mechanical morphogenesis'. Eur J Morphol 2003;41(1):3–7.

[12] Pollock AV, Evans M. Early prediction of late incisional hernias. Br J Surg 1989;76:953–4.

[13] Conner WT, Peacock EE Jr. Some studies on the etiology of inguinal hernia. Am J Surg 1973; 126(6):732–5.

[14] Bellon JM, Bajo A, Ga-Honduvilla N, et al. Fibroblasts from the transversalis fascia of young patients with direct inguinal hernias show constitutive MMP-2 overexpression. Ann Surg 2001;233(2):287–91.

[15] Zheng H, Si Z, Kasperk R, et al. Recurrent inguinal hernia: disease of the collagen matrix? World J Surg 2002;26(4):401–8.

[16] Rosch R, Junge K, Knops M, et al. Analysis of collagen-interacting proteins in patients with incisional hernias. Langenbecks Arch Surg 2003;387(11–12):427–32.

[17] Dubay DA, Franz MG. Acute wound healing: the biology of acute wound failure. Surg Clin North Am 2003;83(3):463–81.

[18] Robson MC, Hill DP, Woodske ME, et al. Wound healing trajectories as predictors of effectiveness of therapeutic agents. Arch Surg 2000;135:773–7.

[19] Santora TA, Roslyn JJ. Incisional hernia. Surg Clin North Am 1993;73(3):557–70.

[20] Carlson MA. Acute wound failure. Surg Clin North Am 1997;77(3):607–36.

[21] Robson MC, Steed DL, Franz MG. Wound healing: biologic features and approaches to maximize healing trajectories. Curr Probl Surg 2001;38(2):72–140.

[22] Robson MC, Shaw RC, Heggers JP. The reclosure of postoperative incisional abscesses based on bacterial quantification of the wound. Ann Surg 1970;171:279–82.

[23] Riches DWH. Macrophage involvement in wound repair, remodeling and fibrosis. In: Clark RAF, editor. The cellular and molecular biology of wound healing. 2nd edition. New York: Plenum Press; 1995. p. 95–141.

[24] Levenson SM, Demetriou AA. Metabolic factors. In: Cohen IH, Diegelmann RF, Lindblad WJ, editors. Wound healing: biochemical and clinical aspects. Philadelphia: Saunders; 2001. p. 248–73.

[25] Ferguson MW, Whitby DJ, Shah M. Scar formation: the spectral nature of fetal and adult wound repair. Plast Reconstr Surg 1996;97:854–60.

[26] Morgan CJ, Pledger WJ. Fibroblast proliferation. In: Cohen IH, Diegelmann RF, Lindblad WJ, editors. Wound healing: biochemical and clinical aspects. 1st edition. Philadelphia: Saunders; 1992. p. 63–76.

[27] Vande BJ, Rudolph R, Hollan C, et al. Fibroblast senescence in pressure ulcers. Wound Repair Regen 1998;6(1):38–49.

[28] Ellis H, Harrison W, Hugh TB. The healing of peritoneum under normal and pathological conditions. Br J Surg 1965;52:471–6.

[29] Hubbard TB Jr, Khan MZ, Carag VR. The pathology of peritoneal repair: its relation to the formation of adhesions. Ann Surg 1967;165:908–16.

[30] Prockop DJ, Kivirikko KI, Tuderman L, et al. The biosynthesis of collagen and its disorders. NEJM 1979;301:13–23.

[31] Jorgensen LN, Kellehave F, Karlsmark T, et al. Reduced collagen accumulation after major surgery. Br J Surg 1996;83:1591–4.

[32] Hall KA, Peters B, Smyth SH. Abdominal wall hernias in patients with abdominal aortic aneurysm versus aortoiliac occlusive disease. Am J Surg 1995;170:572–5.

[33] Ayde B, Luna G. Incidence of abdominal wall hernia in aortic surgery. Am J Surg 1998;175: 400–2.

[34] Lehnert B, Wadouh F. High coincidence of inguinal hernias and abdominal aortic aneurysms. Ann Vasc Surg 1992;6:134–7.

[35] Friedman DW, Boyd CD, Norton P. Increases in type III collagen gene expression and protein synthesis in patients with inguinal hernias. Ann Surg 1993;218:754–60.

[36] Viidik A, Gottrup F. Mechanics of healing soft tissue wounds. In: Schmidt-Schonbein GW, Woo SLY, Zweifach BW, editors. Frontiers in biomechanics. New York: Springer; 1986. p. 263–79.

[37] Viidik A. The dynamic connective tissue. Kaupa J, editor. Malmo (Sweden): Foerlags AB Eesti Post; Annals of Estonia Medical Association. 1975. p. 155–69.

[38] Cromack DT, Sporn MB, Roberts AB, et al. Transforming growth factor beta levels in rat wound chambers. J Surg Res 1987;42:622–8.

[39] Franz MG, Kuhn MA, Nguyen K, et al. Transforming growth factor β_2 lowers the incidence of incisional hernias. J Surg Res 2001;97(2):109–16.

[40] Roberts AB. Transforming growth factor beta; activity and efficacy in animal models of wound healing. Wound Repair Regen 1995;3(4):408–18.

[41] Mustoe TA, Pierce GF, Thomason A, et al. Accelerated healing of incisional wounds in rats induced by transforming growth factor-α. Science 1987;237:1333–6.

[42] Best WR, Khuri SF, Phelan M, et al. Identifying patient preoperative risk factors and postoperative adverse events in administrative databases: results from the department of veterans affairs national surgical quality improvement program. J Am Coll Surg 2002;194(3):257–66.

[43] Williams JG, Barbul A. Nutrition and wound healing. Surg Clin North Am 2003;83:571–96.

[44] Mudge M, Hughes LE. Incisional hernia: a 10 year prospective study of incidence and attitudes. Br J Surg 1985;72(1):70–1.

[45] Robson MC. Infection in the surgical patient: an imbalance in the normal equilibrium. Clin Plast Surg 1979;6:493–503.

[46] Korenkov M, Beckers A, Koebke J, et al. Biomechanical and morphological types of the linea alba and its possible role in the pathogenesis of midline incisional hernia. Eur J Surg 2001;167(12):909–14.

[47] Jenkins TPN. Incisional hernia repair: a mechanical approach. Br J Surg 1980;67(5):335–6.

[48] Nilsson E. The relative rate of wound healing in longitudinal and transverse incisions. Acta Chir Scand 1982;148:251–6.

[49] Schmidt C, Pommerenke H, Durr F. Mechanical stressing of integrin receptors induces enhanced tyrosine phosphorylation of cytoskeletally anchored proteins. J Biol Chem 1998;273: 5081–5.

[50] Dubay DA, Choi W, Urbanchek MG, et al. Incisional herniation induces decreased abdominal wall compliance via oblique muscle atrophy and fibrosis. Ann Surg 2007;245(1):140–6.

ELSEVIER
SAUNDERS

Surg Clin N Am 88 (2008) 17–26

SURGICAL
CLINICS OF
NORTH AMERICA

Surgical Progress in Inguinal and Ventral Incisional Hernia Repair

Stephen H. Gray, MD, MSPH[a],
Mary T. Hawn, MD, FACS[a],*,
Kamal M.F. Itani, MD[b,c]

[a]Section of Gastrointestinal Surgery, University of Alabama at Birmingham,
KB 429, 1530 3rd Avenue South, Birmingham, AL 35294, USA
[b]Boston Veterans Affairs Health Care System, 1400 VFW Parkway,
West Roxbury, MA 02132, USA
[c]Boston University, One Boston Medical Center Place/C500, Boston, MA 02118, USA

Repair of abdominal wall hernias represents the most common group of operations performed by general surgeons. In 2003 it was estimated that over 700,000 inguinal hernia repairs and over 100,000 ventral incisional hernia repairs were performed [1]. The field of hernia repair has evolved as a result of surgical innovation and has benefited significantly from technologic improvements. The tension-free repair is one of the key concepts that have revolutionized hernia surgery. The use of a mesh prosthesis to approximate the fascial defect has resulted in a decrease in recurrence rates for inguinal and incisional hernias. More recently, laparoscopic approaches to the inguinal and incisional hernia have extended the options and approaches for repairing the fascial defect. As opposed to tension-free repair, the results of laparoscopic approaches for inguinal and incisional hernia repair have been mixed, and these approaches have not been rapidly embraced by surgeons. The goals of this article are to describe the history of hernia repair and how innovations in surgical technique, prosthetics, and technology have shaped current practice.

Open techniques

In 1887, the Bassini inguinal hernia repair heralded the beginning of contemporary inguinal hernia surgery. Numerous modifications to the Bassini repair emerged in an attempt to decrease the recurrence rate. High

* Corresponding author.
E-mail address: mhawn@uab.edu (M.T. Hawn).

0039-6109/08/$ - see front matter. Published by Elsevier Inc.
doi:10.1016/j.suc.2007.11.007
surgical.theclinics.com

recurrence rates due to tension at the repair site were addressed with a variety of innovations. First, a relaxing incision to reduce tension was included in the repair and is still performed commonly today in a McVay [2] (Cooper's ligament) repair. Another modification of the Bassini repair, the Shouldice repair, achieved excellent results in the hand of its originators; however, the Shouldice repair failed to gain widespread use due to its technical difficulties and inconsistent results outside the Shouldice clinic [3,4]. Stoppa described a preperitoneal approach in 1975 for complicated and recurrent hernias. The Stoppa repair used a large mesh in the preperitoneal space to support the fascial defect, which is the concept upon which the laparoscopic inguinal hernia repair is based. In 1986, the tension-free inguinal hernia repair with mesh was described by Lichtenstein [5,6]. The Lichtenstein repair has become the most popular open technique for inguinal hernia repair and has been shown to have superior recurrence rates when compared with tissue-based hernia repair [7–9]. The Lichtenstein repair is attractive to many surgeons because of the simplicity of the repair, the reproducible low recurrence rates, and the decreased postoperative pain experienced by patients.

The concept of plugging the inguinal canal with foreign material and tissue to repair defects began in the mid-nineteenth century (Fig. 1). In 1987, Gilbert refined the mesh plug technique into the cone or umbrella shape, which Rutkow and Robbins developed into the preformed cone that is now commercially available [10–12]. A recent randomized controlled trial found the mesh plug and Lichtenstein repair to have comparable recurrence rates [13].

Further developments of the mesh repair have sought to combine the anterior approach as used by Lichtenstein with a posterior reinforcement as used in the laparoscopic and Stoppa repair. One such product popularized by Gilbert is the Prolene Hernia System (Ethicon, Cincinanitti, Ohio) that combines two sheets of mesh linked by a connector. The posterior sheet of mesh is placed into the preperitoneal space, and the anterior mesh reinforces the repair. Results from a retrospective study suggest that the Prolene Hernia System may represent a superior alternative for open repair of inguinal hernias [14]. Further prospective randomized trials are necessary to confirm or refute these findings.

Although advances in inguinal hernia repair have resulted in significant improvements in surgical and patient reported outcomes, the repair of ventral incisional hernia has been more challenging. Recent data from a prospective randomized controlled trial of suture versus mesh repair in ventral incisional hernia revealed superior results with the mesh repair [15]. Analysis of a population-based registry revealed that the rate of mesh placement for ventral incisional hernia repair has increased from 35% in 1987 to 66% in 1999 [16]. Current practice for the repair of incisional hernias is the selective placement of mesh in patients based on the surgeon's preference and experience [17]. Fear of mesh infection and fistula

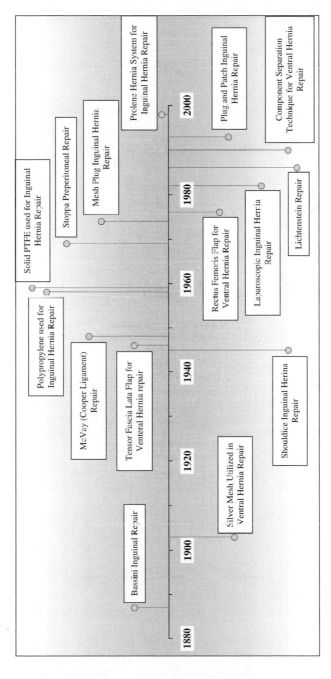

Fig. 1. Timeline of hernia repair.

formation continue to limit the systematic use of mesh in ventral incisional hernia repair. Innovative techniques in the repair of ventral incisional hernias that reduce tension without the use of prosthetic material include the component separation technique and the use of preoperative tissue expansion. The component separation technique was initially reported in 1990 and is based on enlargement of the abdominal wall surface by separation of the anterior abdominal muscular layers [18]. Because no prosthetic material is required, this technique can be used in contaminated wounds [18,19]. Recently published interim data demonstrate favorable outcomes when comparing component separation with prosthetic mesh repair [19].

Preoperative tissue expansion can be used to facilitate reapproximation of tissue without tension. Two reported methods of tissue expansion consist of progressive pneumoperitoneum and implantation of tissue expanders. Progressive pneumoperitoneum has been described in case reports and case series. Advantages include the detection of multiple fascial defects, approximation of natural tissues without tension, and preoperative lysis of adhesions [20,21]. Progressive pneumoperitoneum is achieved by insufflation of air at regular intervals via percutaneous puncture or indwelling intra-abdominal catheters [22]. The use of implanted tissue expanders was first described to repair congenital and posttraumatic defects [23]. Gradual expansion is thought to provide natural innervated healthy tissue that can be used for reapproximation of the fascial defect. Expanders can be placed in the subcutaneous, intermuscular, intramuscular, and intra-abdominal positions.

More complex abdominal wall reconstructions have been described. Use of the tensor fascia lata flap was described to close lower abdominal wall defects in 1946 and use of the rectus femoris in 1977 [24,25]. Recently, use of a free vascularized composite anterolateral thigh flap with tensor fascia lata has been described [26]. Complications associated with flaps include donor site morbidity, flap necrosis, flap shrinkage, and hernia recurrence [25,27].

Prosthetic material

Synthesis of plastic began in the twentieth century, and nylon was the first material widely available as suture. Publications document the use of nylon mesh during World War II in France [28]. Unfortunately, nylon loses tensile strength due to hydrolysis and denaturation and is associated with hernia recurrence. During the 1950s and 1960s, polypropylene and Dacron were introduced [28]. Usher used polypropylene prosthesis in 1958 for inguinal and incisional hernia repair. In the repair of incisional hernias, he placed oversized mesh deep to the abdominal wall musculature to allow for adequate overlap. By 1962, a survey documented that 20% of general surgeons were using techniques advocated by Usher [29]. Polypropylene is inexpensive, easy to handle, and incorporates well into the abdominal wall. Clinical experience with polypropylene has demonstrated some complications when it is placed intraperitoneally, including adhesion formation, erosion into abdominal viscera, and fistula formation [30–33].

Direct contact between abdominal viscera and prosthetic material can cause an inflammatory reaction leading to adhesion formation [34,35]. The development of postoperative adhesions has significant clinical consequences. Intestinal adhesions not only result in future bowel obstructions, female infertility, and abdominal pain but also increase the risk of bowel injury during subsequent abdominal surgery [36,37]. Postoperative adhesions have been shown to increase subsequent operative time, the conversion rates from laparoscopic to open procedures, and the incidence of postoperative complications [37–40].

To reduce these complications, solid polytetrafluoroethylene (PTFE) was used for the first time in hernia surgery in 1959. Solid PTFE was plagued by high recurrence rates due to low tensile strength and lack of incorporation within tissue [41]. Expanded PTFE (ePTFE) was later developed in Japan and was used mainly in the intraperitoneal position [28]. Unlike polypropylene, ePTFE has a low incidence of visceral erosion, bowel obstruction, fistulization, abscess formation, and, due to rapid coverage with mesothelium, less adhesion formation [42–44].

Another strategy to reduce adhesion formation and visceral erosion is the use of composite meshes which have been shown to form fewer adhesions of weaker strength [45]. Composite meshes generally consist of two sides— a "non-tissue ingrowth" side that faces viscera and a "tissue incorporating" side against the abdominal wall. Animal studies have demonstrated decreased rates of adhesion formation 1 year after implantation of composite mesh when compared with polypropylene mesh [30].

The implantation of mesh and the resultant inflammatory reaction may also lead to the formation of a rigid scar plate with loss of abdominal wall pliability and changes in abdominal wall compliance. Patients may complain of a sensation of stiffness, physical discomfort, and limitations in activities of daily living. Light weight meshes with reduced polypropylene content and larger pore size have demonstrated reduced inflammation and improved integration into surrounding tissues in animal studies [46]. In addition, light weight meshes have been associated with decreased complaints of pain, paresthesias, and improved abdominal wall compliance [47]. Animal studies demonstrate that light weight polypropylene mesh results in less restriction of abdominal wall compliance while providing adequate repair strength [48].

Recently, several absorbable and biologic prostheses have become commercially available. Hernia repair in the setting of a contaminated surgical field requires either a staged repair or primary tissue repair. Absorbable polyglactin (Vicryl) prosthetics have been used for hernia repair associated with contaminated operative fields [49]. The hypothesis behind using absorbable prosthetic material is that the mesh can support the ingrowth of host repair tissues and then degrade when the repair is functionally stable. Biologic prostheses are useful when the wound is contaminated or the risk of infection is high. Acellular dermal matrix, porcine intestinal mucosa, and porcine dermal collagen have been used safely and effectively as an alternative to traditional mesh to successfully repair hernias in contaminated operative fields and in conditions that would not have been safe for traditional permanent mesh prosthesis [50–53]. Long-term data on hernia outcomes using these expensive biologic mesh products are lacking.

Laparoscopic hernia repair

The first laparoscopic inguinal hernia repair was performed in 1982 and consisted of intra-abdominal closure of the neck of the hernia sac [54]. In 2003, 14% of 800,000 groin hernias were repaired laparoscopically [1]. There are two accepted approaches to laparoscopic inguinal hernia repair: (1) the totally extraperitoneal (TEP) approach using the principles of preperitoneal repair originally described by Stoppa, and (2) the transabdominal preperitoneal repair (TAPP). The major difference between the TEP and TAPP technique is the access to the preperitoneal space. The TEP repair does not violate the peritoneal cavity and is thought to decrease the risk of bowel and bladder injury. A recent meta-analysis could not find evidence to support either technique as superior [55].

There is considerable debate about which patients should undergo laparoscopic inguinal hernia repair. The results of the multicenter, randomized Department of Veterans Affairs Cooperative study found a higher recurrence and complication rate among patients who had laparoscopic inguinal hernia repair [56]. In addition, the study found that patients who underwent laparoscopic inguinal hernia repair had less initial pain and returned to normal activities faster than patients who underwent an open repair. Although some studies suggest that laparoscopic inguinal hernia repair is not cost effective [57,58], the Veterans Affairs study revealed that laparoscopic repair while not cost effective overall is a cost-effective option for unilateral hernia repair [59]. A Swedish multicenter trial of inguinal hernia repair reported similar recurrence rates among patients who underwent laparoscopic or Shouldice repair [60]. The Veterans Affairs study also illustrates the learning curve associated with laparoscopic inguinal hernia repair as evidenced by the significantly lower recurrence rate among surgeons who have completed greater than 250 laparoscopic repairs [56].

There is significant debate among experts regarding the optimal approach for ventral incisional hernia. Advocates of laparoscopic repair argue that it is a better approach because it does not require extensive subcutaneous tissue dissection and postoperative drainage. In addition, sublay mesh placement appears to be the most physiologic method of ventral incisional hernia repair [61]. Studies have associated laparoscopic repair with a shorter length of hospitalization, lower wound infection rates, shorter operative time, and earlier return to work [62–64]. Recently published studies have found that laparoscopic repair of ventral hernias in obese patients and patients with large fascial defects is safe and associated with a low recurrence and complication rate [62–64]. The most common complication of laparoscopic ventral incisional hernia repair is seroma formation, which occurs in 10% to 15% of cases. The occurrence of an unrecognized enterotomy or bowel injury resulting in sepsis or death is the most feared complication of ventral incisional hernia repair [65]. Rates of bowel injury during laparoscopic and open ventral hernia repair range from 7.2% to 9% [40,66].

Summary and future directions

Contemporary repair of abdominal wall hernias is supported by strong evidence and calls for a tension-free repair with placement of mesh in the majority of cases. Laparoscopic repair demands significant expertise to achieve outcomes comparable with those of open repair. In ventral incisional hernias, placement of the mesh in a sublay position has been found to be effective and to have a low recurrence rate, although randomized trials have not been performed [67].

In a paradigm shift, the necessity of inguinal hernia repair upon diagnosis in relatively asymptomatic men is now questioned [68]. With improvements in recurrence and complications, emphasis is now placed on patient-centered outcomes and increasing the benefits of surgery over the risks and complications while obtaining the best physiologic outcome [69].

Several milestones were achieved with the use of prosthetic material, and the new bioprostheses hold promise in decreasing inflammatory reaction and improving physiologic results. Future research will continue to focus on the indications for surgery as well as on surgical techniques and materials to achieve the best patient-centered outcomes and functionality.

References

[1] Rutkow IM. Demographic and socioeconomic aspects of hernia repair in the United States in 2003. Surg Clin North Am 2003;83(5):1045–51, v–vi.

[2] McVay CB. Inguinal hernioplasty: common mistakes and pitfalls. Surg Clin North Am 1966; 46(5):1089–100.

[3] Hay JM, Boudet MJ, Fingerhut A, et al. Shouldice inguinal hernia repair in the male adult: the gold standard? A multicenter controlled trial in 1578 patients. Ann Surg 1995;222(6): 719–27.

[4] Kingsnorth AN, Gray MR, Nott DM. Prospective randomized trial comparing the Shouldice technique and plication darn for inguinal hernia. Br J Surg 1992;79(10):1068–70.

[5] Lichtenstein IL, Shulman AG, Amid PK, et al. The tension-free hernioplasty. Am J Surg 1989;157(2):188–93.

[6] Lichtenstein IL, Shulman AG. Ambulatory outpatient hernia surgery: including a new concept, introducing tension-free repair. Int Surg 1986;71(1):1–4.

[7] Nordin P, Bartelmess P, Jansson C, et al. Randomized trial of Lichtenstein versus Shouldice hernia repair in general surgical practice. Br J Surg 2002;89(1):45–9.

[8] Danielsson P, Isacson S, Hansen MV. Randomised study of Lichtenstein compared with Shouldice inguinal hernia repair by surgeons in training. Eur J Surg 1999;165(1):49–53.

[9] McGillicuddy JE. Prospective randomized comparison of the Shouldice and Lichtenstein hernia repair procedures. Arch Surg 1998;133(9):974–8.

[10] Gilbert AI. Overnight hernia repair: updated considerations. South Med J 1987;80(2): 191–5.

[11] Gilbert AI. Sutureless repair of inguinal hernia. Am J Surg 1992;163(3):331–5.

[12] Robbins AW, Rutkow IM. Mesh plug repair and groin hernia surgery. Surg Clin North Am 1998;78(6):1007–23, vi–vii.

[13] Frey DM, Wildisen A, Hamel CT, et al. Randomized clinical trial of Lichtenstein's operation versus mesh plug for inguinal hernia repair. Br J Surg 2007;94(1):36–41.

[14] Awad SS, Yallalampalli S, Srour AM, et al. Improved outcomes with the Prolene Hernia System mesh compared with the time-honored Lichtenstein onlay mesh repair for inguinal hernia repair. Am J Surg 2007;193(6):697–701.

[15] Luijendijk RW, Hop WC, van den Tol MP, et al. A comparison of suture repair with mesh repair for incisional hernia. N Engl J Med 2000;343(6):392–8.

[16] Flum DR, Horvath K, Koepsell T. Have outcomes of incisional hernia repair improved with time? A population-based analysis. Ann Surg 2003;237(1):129–35.

[17] Courtney CA, Lee AC, Wilson C, et al. Ventral hernia repair: a study of current practice. Hernia 2003;7(1):44–6.

[18] Ramirez OM, Ruas E, Dellon AL. "Components separation" method for closure of abdominal-wall defects: an anatomic and clinical study. Plast Reconstr Surg 1990;86(3): 519–26.

[19] de Vries Reilingh TS, van Goor H, Rosman C, et al. "Components separation technique" for the repair of large abdominal wall hernias. J Am Coll Surg 2003;196(1):32–7.

[20] Mansuy MM, Hager HG Jr. Pneumoperitoneum in preparation for correction of giant hernias. N Engl J Med 1958;258(1):33–4.

[21] Raynor RW, Del Guercio LR. Update on the use of preoperative pneumoperitoneum prior to the repair of large hernias of the abdominal wall. Surg Gynecol Obstet 1985;161(4): 367–71.

[22] Mayagoitia JC, Suarez D, Arenas JC, et al. Preoperative progressive pneumoperitoneum in patients with abdominal-wall hernias. Hernia 2006;10(3):213–7.

[23] Hobar PC, Rohrich RJ, Byrd HS. Abdominal-wall reconstruction with expanded musculofascial tissue in a posttraumatic defect. Plast Reconstr Surg 1994;94(2):379–83.

[24] Wangensteen O. Repair of abdominal defects by pedicled fascial flaps. Surg Gynecol Obstet 1946;82:144–50.

[25] McCraw JB, Dibbell DG, Carraway JH. Clinical definition of independent myocutaneous vascular territories. Plast Reconstr Surg 1977;60(3):341–52.

[26] Kuo YR, Kuo MH, Lutz BS, et al. One-stage reconstruction of large midline abdominal wall defects using a composite free anterolateral thigh flap with vascularized fascia lata. Ann Surg 2004;239(3):352–8.

[27] O'Hare PM, Leonard AG. Reconstruction of major abdominal wall defects using the tensor fasciae latae myocutaneous flap. Br J Plast Surg 1982;35(3):361–6.

[28] Read RC. Milestones in the history of hernia surgery: prosthetic repair. Hernia 2004;8(1): 8–14.

[29] Adler RH. An evaluation of surgical mesh in the repair of hernias and tissue defects. Arch Surg 1962;85:836–44.

[30] Novitsky YW, Harrell AG, Cristiano JA, et al. Comparative evaluation of adhesion formation, strength of ingrowth, and textile properties of prosthetic meshes after long-term intraabdominal implantation in a rabbit. J Surg Res 2007;140(1):6–11.

[31] Robinson TN, Clarke JH, Schoen J, et al. Major mesh-related complications following hernia repair: events reported to the Food and Drug Administration. Surg Endosc 2005; 19(12):1556–60.

[32] Losanoff JE, Richman BW, Jones JW. Entero-colocutaneous fistula: a late consequence of polypropylene mesh abdominal wall repair. Case report and review of the literature. Hernia 2002;6(3):144–7.

[33] Miller K, Junger W. Ileocutaneous fistula formation following laparoscopic polypropylene mesh hernia repair. Surg Endosc 1997;11(7):772–3.

[34] Law NW, Ellis H. Adhesion formation and peritoneal healing on prosthetic materials. Clin Mater 1988;3(2):95–101.

[35] Luijendijk RW, de Lange DC, Wauters CC, et al. Foreign material in postoperative adhesions. Ann Surg 1996;223(3):242–8.

[36] DeCherney AH, diZerega GS. Clinical problem of intraperitoneal postsurgical adhesion formation following general surgery and the use of adhesion prevention barriers. Surg Clin North Am 1997;77(3):671–88.

[37] Coleman MG, McLain AD, Moran BJ. Impact of previous surgery on time taken for incision and division of adhesions during laparotomy. Dis Colon Rectum 2000;43(9):1297–9.

[38] Oliveira L, Reissman P, Nogueras J, et al. Laparoscopic creation of stomas. Surg Endosc 1997;11(1):19–23.

[39] van der Voort M, Heijnsdijk EA, Gouma DJ. Bowel injury as a complication of laparoscopy. Br J Surg 2004;91(10):1253–8.

[40] Gray S, Vick C, Graham L, et al. Enterotomy or unplanned bowel resection during elective hernia repair increases complications. Arch Surg, in press.

[41] Ambrosiani N, Harb J, Gavelli A, et al. [Failure of the treatment of eventrations and hernias with the PTFE plate (111 cases)]. Ann Chir 1994;48(10):917–20 [French].

[42] Sikkink CJ, Vries de Reilingh TS, Malyar AW, et al. Adhesion formation and reherniation differ between meshes used for abdominal wall reconstruction. Hernia 2006;10(3):218–22.

[43] Koehler RH, Begos D, Berger D, et al. Minimal adhesions to ePTFE mesh after laparoscopic ventral incisional hernia repair: reoperative findings in 65 cases. JSLS 2003;7(4):335–40.

[44] Bauer JJ, Salky BA, Gelernt IM, et al. Repair of large abdominal wall defects with expanded polytetrafluoroethylene (PTFE). Ann Surg 1987;206(6):765–9.

[45] Franklin ME Jr, Gonzalez JJ Jr, Glass JL, et al. Laparoscopic ventral and incisional hernia repair: an 11-year experience. Hernia 2004;8(1):23–7.

[46] Conze J, Rosch R, Klinge U, et al. Polypropylene in the intra-abdominal position: influence of pore size and surface area. Hernia 2004;8(4):365–72.

[47] Welty G, Klinge U, Klosterhalfen B, et al. Functional impairment and complaints following incisional hernia repair with different polypropylene meshes. Hernia 2001;5(3):142–7.

[48] Cobb WS, Burns JM, Peindl RD, et al. Textile analysis of heavy weight, mid-weight, and light weight polypropylene mesh in a porcine ventral hernia model. J Surg Res 2006;136(1):1–7.

[49] Tobias AM, Low DW. The use of a subfascial Vicryl mesh buttress to aid in the closure of massive ventral hernias following damage-control laparotomy. Plast Reconstr Surg 2003;112(3):766–76.

[50] Kim H, Bruen K, Vargo D. Acellular dermal matrix in the management of high-risk abdominal wall defects. Am J Surg 2006;192(6):705–9.

[51] Patton JH Jr, Berry S, Kralovich KA. Use of human acellular dermal matrix in complex and contaminated abdominal wall reconstructions. Am J Surg 2007;193(3):360–3 [discussion: 3].

[52] Ansaloni L, Catena F, Gagliardi S, et al. Hernia repair with porcine small-intestinal submucosa. Hernia 2007;11(4):321–6.

[53] Gagliardi S, Ansaloni L, Catena F, et al. Hernioplasty with Surgisis Inguinal Hernia Matrix (IHM) trade mark. Surg Technol Int 2007;16:128–33.

[54] Swanstrom LL. Laparoscopic herniorrhaphy. Surg Clin North Am 1996;76(3):483–91.

[55] Wake BL, McCormack K, Fraser C, et al. Transabdominal pre-peritoneal (TAPP) vs totally extraperitoneal (TEP) laparoscopic techniques for inguinal hernia repair. Cochrane Database Syst Rev 2005;1:CD004703.

[56] Neumayer L, Giobbie-Hurder A, Jonasson O, et al. Open mesh versus laparoscopic mesh repair of inguinal hernia. N Engl J Med 2004;350(18):1819–27.

[57] Vale L, Grant A, McCormack K, et al. Cost-effectiveness of alternative methods of surgical repair of inguinal hernia. Int J Technol Assess Health Care 2004;20(2):192–200.

[58] Vale L, Ludbrook A, Grant A. Assessing the costs and consequences of laparoscopic vs. open methods of groin hernia repair: a systematic review. Surg Endosc 2003;17(6):844–9.

[59] Hynes DM, Stroupe KT, Luo P, et al. Cost effectiveness of laparoscopic versus open mesh hernia operation: results of a Department of Veterans Affairs randomized clinical trial. J Am Coll Surg 2006;203(4):447–57.

[60] Arvidsson D, Berndsen FH, Larsson LG, et al. Randomized clinical trial comparing 5-year recurrence rate after laparoscopic versus Shouldice repair of primary inguinal hernia. Br J Surg 2005;92(9):1085–91.

[61] Novitsky YW, Porter JR, Rucho ZC, et al. Open preperitoneal retrofascial mesh repair for multiply recurrent ventral incisional hernias. J Am Coll Surg 2006;203(3):283–9.

[62] Lomanto D, Iyer SG, Shabbir A, et al. Laparoscopic versus open ventral hernia mesh repair: a prospective study. Surg Endosc 2006;20(7):1030–5.

[63] Heniford BT, Park A, Ramshaw BJ, et al. Laparoscopic ventral and incisional hernia repair in 407 patients. J Am Coll Surg 2000;190(6):645–50.

[64] McGreevy JM, Goodney PP, Birkmeyer CM, et al. A prospective study comparing the complication rates between laparoscopic and open ventral hernia repairs. Surg Endosc 2003;17(11):1778–80.

[65] Perrone JM, Soper NJ, Eagon JC, et al. Perioperative outcomes and complications of laparoscopic ventral hernia repair. Surgery 2005;138(4):708–16.

[66] Itani KM, Neumayer L, Reda D, et al. Repair of ventral incisional hernia: the design of a randomized trial to compare open and laparoscopic surgical techniques. Am J Surg 2004; 188(6A Suppl):22S–9S.

[67] Kurzer M, Kark A, Selouk S, et al. Open mesh repair of incisional hernia using a sublay technique: long-term follow-up. World J Surg 2008;32(1):31–6.

[68] Fitzgibbons RJ Jr, Giobbie-Hurder A, Gibbs JO, et al. Watchful waiting vs repair of inguinal hernia in minimally symptomatic men: a randomized clinical trial. JAMA 2006;295(3): 285–92.

[69] Witt WP, Gibbs J, Wang J, et al. Impact of inguinal hernia repair on family and other informal caregivers. Arch Surg 2006;141(9):925–30.

ELSEVIER
SAUNDERS

SURGICAL
CLINICS OF
NORTH AMERICA

Surg Clin N Am 88 (2008) 27–43

Pediatric Hernias

Mary L. Brandt, MD

Michael E. DeBakey Department of Surgery, Texas Children's Hospital,
Baylor College of Medicine, One Baylor Plaza, Houston, TX 77030, USA

Indirect inguinal herniorrhaphy is one of the most frequently performed surgical procedures in children. The overall incidence of inguinal hernias in childhood ranges from 0.8% to 4.4% [1,2]. The incidence is up to 10 times higher in boys than in girls [3]. The incidence is much higher in premature infants; inguinal hernias develop in 13% of infants born before 32 weeks gestation and in 30% of infants weighing less than 1000 g [4].

Embryology of indirect inguinal hernias

Indirect inguinal hernias in children are basically an arrest of embryologic development rather than an acquired weakness, which explains the increased incidence in premature infants. The formation of inguinal hernias in children is directly linked to descent of the developing gonads. The descent of the testes from the embryologic retroperitoneum begins early in gestation. In this early stage, testicular position is not so much a descent as a parting of the ways with the developing kidney. As the mesonephros (developing kidney) ascends into its usual position in the retroperitoneum, the testes remain at the level of the internal rings. The final descent of the testes into the scrotum occurs late in gestation between weeks 28 and 36. The testes are preceded in this descent by the gubernaculum and a "finger" of peritoneum, which ultimately forms the processus vaginalis. This finger or "diverticulum" of peritoneum is first visible around the 12th week of gestation [4]. In normal development, the processus vaginalis closes, obliterating the peritoneal opening of the internal ring between the 36th and 40th week of gestation [5]. The distal portion of the processus vaginalis obliterates, except for the part that becomes the tunica vaginalis. This process is often incomplete, leaving a small patent processus in many newborns. However, closure continues postnatally, and the rate of patency is inversely

E-mail address: brandt@bcm.edu

proportional to the age of the child [1,6,7]. Although the data are somewhat variable, approximately 40% of patent processus vaginalis close during the first months of life and an additional 20% close by 2 years of age [7]. This closure is asymmetric; the left testis descends before the testis on the right. The closure of the patent processus vaginalis on the left also precedes closure on the right; therefore, it is not surprising that 60% of indirect inguinal hernias occur on the right side [4].

Much of the confusion about indirect inguinal hernias in children stems from the assumption that a patent processus vaginalis is the same as an inguinal hernia. The presence of a patent processus vaginalis is a necessary but not sufficient variable in developing a congenital indirect inguinal hernia. In other words, all congenital indirect inguinal hernias are preceded by a patent processus vaginalis, but not all patent processus vaginalis go on to become inguinal hernias. The classic teaching has been that approximately 20% of boys have a patent processus vaginalis at 2 years of age [7]. It is assumed that closure will continue during childhood for some but not all patients. Van Veen and colleagues [8] studied over 300 adults undergoing unilateral hernia repair. These patients had laparoscopic exploration of the contralateral side; 12% of these patients had a patent processus vaginalis. With a 5.5-year average follow-up, inguinal hernias developed in 12% of adult patients with a patent processus vaginalis, a rate four times greater than in the adults in the study who had a closed ring. An incidence of 12% to 14% has been confirmed in other studies of adults as well [9]. Because the overall incidence of indirect inguinal hernias in the population is approximately 1% to 2% and the incidence of a patent processus vaginalis is approximately 12% to 14%, clinically appreciable inguinal hernias should develop in approximately 8% to 12% of patients with a patent processus vaginalis.

Although the embryology is well described, the molecular basis for closure of the patent processus vaginalis is not known. Work by Tanyel has suggested that failure of regression of smooth muscle (present to provide the force for testicular descent) may have a role in the development of indirect inguinal hernias [10,11]. Smooth muscle is present in inguinal hernia sacs in children but absent in the wall of hydroceles and hernia sacs associated with undescended testes [10,12]. The mechanism for disappearance of the smooth muscle is not yet elucidated, although mediators of autonomic tone have been suggested to have a role [11,13,14]. Several studies have investigated genes involved in the control of testicular descent for their role in closure of the patent processus vaginalis, for example, hepatocyte growth factor [14,15] and calcitonin gene-related peptide [14,16,17]. Unlike in adult hernias, there does not appear to be any change in collagen synthesis associated with inguinal hernias in children [12].

The genetics of inguinal hernias, like the molecular biology, are also poorly understood. There is some genetic risk incurred for siblings of patients with inguinal hernias; the sisters of affected girls are at the highest risk with a relative risk of 17.8 [18]. In general, the risk for brothers of a sibling is around 4 to 5, as is the risk for a sister of an affected brother [18]. Both a multifactorial threshold model and autosomal dominance with incomplete penetrance and sex influence have been suggested as an explanation for this pattern of inheritance [19,20].

Diagnosis

The diagnosis of inguinal hernias in children is traditionally suggested by the history of a bulge in the groin with crying and is confirmed on physical examination (Fig. 1). For children too small to cough on command, other methods can be used to increase intra-abdominal pressure. For babies, holding their legs and arms gently against the examination table so they cannot move invariably results in crying. For slightly older children, blowing bubbles, tickling them to make them laugh, or having them blow up balloons (eg, examination gloves) will increase intra-abdominal pressure [3]. Despite these maneuvers, it is not uncommon for the surgeon not to see the bulge. Although some surgeons will operate based on a classic description by parents or a referring physician, most, having been tricked by a retractile testes, will insist on seeing the hernia themselves.

The use of the "silk purse" or "silk glove" sign has been suggested as an alternative to seeing the bulge. This sign can be elicited by gently rolling the cord structures across the pubic tubercle. The feeling of the sac moving on itself during this maneuver is considered a positive finding. Published reports from the 1950s to 1970s showed a wide variation in diagnostic accuracy using the silk purse sign [6]; however, a recent prospective study from China of 1040 patients showed this physical finding to have a sensitivity of 91% and specificity of 97.3% in diagnosing inguinal hernias [21]. Currently, the most reasonable approach is to consider the silk purse sign as supporting but not conclusive evidence that there is an inguinal hernia.

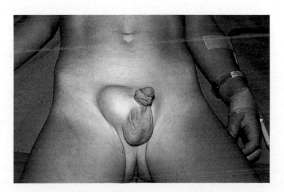

Fig. 1. Inguinal bulge seen with inguinal hernias.

An interesting new approach to diagnosis that has been used primarily in Asia is the performance of office ultrasound to differentiate between a patent processus vaginalis and an inguinal hernia [22]. Chen and colleagues were able to use office ultrasound to increase diagnostic accuracy from 84% (on physical examination alone) to 97.9% [23,24]. Erez performed preoperative ultrasound on 642 children scheduled for inguinal hernia repair and showed, by comparing preoperative and operative findings, that a hypoechoic structure in the midinguinal canal measuring 4 to 6 mm was a patent processus vaginalis, and that structures greater than 6 mm were hernias [23].

Isolated congenital hydroceles, that is, hydroceles present at birth, usually resolve in the first 2 years of life and do not necessarily increase the likelihood that a patent processus vaginalis or hernia is present [25]; however, hydroceles that develop after birth are more likely to be associated with a patent processus vaginalis that is less likely to close [25]. Communicating hydroceles can be distinguished from noncommunicating hydroceles by a history of enlargement in the evening (with standing) and a smaller size in the morning (after being supine). On physical examination, the sensation of fluid passing into the abdomen with scrotal pressure may be appreciated as well. If a hydrocele is communicating, it should be considered a hernia, and repair is indicated regardless of the age. For noncommunicating hydroceles, most pediatric surgeons recommend waiting until the child is between 1 and 2 years of age because spontaneous resolution is the rule rather than the exception.

Treatment

Open repair of inguinal hernias

Once an inguinal hernia is diagnosed, the treatment is surgical repair. Unlike in adults, all hernias in children are repaired at the time they are diagnosed, even if they are asymptomatic. Although inguinal hernia repair is not by any definition an emergency, repair should take place in a timely manner to eliminate any risk of incarceration, particularly in infants less than 12 months of age [26]. The initial description of repair of a pediatric inguinal hernia was by Celsus in 25 A.D. who removed the sac and the testes through a scrotal incision [3]. The classic contemporary description of the repair of indirect inguinal hernias in children is attributed to Potts, although the original description of high ligation of the sac was by Czerny in 1887 [3,27]. High ligation of the sac is practiced by all pediatric surgeons. Even though minor changes in technique have evolved, the current technique is directly descended from the procedure taught by Ladd and Gross, the founders of North American pediatric surgery [28].

A skin incision is made in the inguinal crease overlying the internal ring. Scarpa's fascia and the external oblique are opened. The cremasteric fibers are bluntly dissected until the sac can be seen. The sac is then gently separated from the cord structures, divided, dissected to the level of the internal ring, and ligated at this level. In patients with a dilated internal ring, a Marcy repair (closure of a widely dilated internal ring) can be added to the high ligation [29]. Hydroceles, which are present 19% of the time, are either split anteriorly or excised [30]. In one prospective randomized trial of excision versus splitting of a distal sac/hydrocele, there was no difference in recurrence of the hydrocele or complications, suggesting that simply opening the anterior wall is effective [31]. Skin closure in children can be done with subcuticular sutures or Dermabond; however, two different prospective studies have shown that Dermabond has no improved outcome, takes longer than subcuticular sutures, and has slightly more complications [32,33]. The use of an "L-stitch" may decrease the risk of stitch abscess after subcuticular closure [30,34]. Anesthesia and pain control during and after inguinal hernia repair have evolved with contemporary techniques of pediatric anesthesia. Caudal blocks are used routinely in most children's hospitals because they result in decreased emergence time and better pain control [35]. Intraoperative injection of the ilioinguinal nerve (lateral to the internal ring) and the ileohypogastric nerve (beneath the external oblique) can be performed in patients who do not undergo a caudal block [30]. Postoperatively, most children do well with acetominophen alone, although the addition of codeine may be necessary for some.

The classic open repair with high ligation of the sac has excellent results. In the largest series reported by a single surgeon (6361 patients), there was a 1.2% recurrence rate, a 1.2% wound infection rate, and a 0.3% rate of testicular atrophy. Other series report a recurrence rate of approximately 1% as well [30,36,37]. Factors that may contribute to recurrence in open inguinal hernia repair in children include failure to ligate the sac high enough, an excessively dilated internal ring injury to the floor of the canal (with subsequent development of a direct inguinal hernia), and the presence of comorbid conditions (eg, collagen disorders, malnutrition, or pulmonary disease) [38]. Other complications that occur after inguinal hernia repair in children include testicular atrophy, injury to the vas deferens, and iatrogenic cryptorchidism. Testicular atrophy occurs in 1% to 2% and decreased testicular size in 2.7% to 13% of patients [39]. Iatrogenic cryptorchidism occurs in 0.6% to 2.9% of patients [39]. Injury to the vas deferens has been reported to occur in as many as 1.6% of patients based on findings on pathology [39]. A more realistic risk of injury to the vas deferens is 0.13% to 0.53% [40–42]. Higher numbers may represent inexperienced surgeons or pathologists, because embryologic remnants may be misinterpreted as vas deferens [41,42]. Although extremely rare, infertility as a result of injury to the fallopian tubes has been reported in girls as well [43,44]. Mesh repair in children is ill advised and may even be contraindicated. Although there are conflicting data [45], many animal studies have demonstrated that polypropylene mesh results in an inflammatory reaction which causes changes in the vas deferens and testes [46,47]. In addition, infertility in men as a direct result of herniorrhaphy with mesh has been reported [48].

Contralateral exploration in children with unilateral hernias

In 1952 Duckett reported that contralateral hernias were present in as many as 30% of children presenting with unilateral hernias. We now know that these "hernias" were often the processus vaginalis and that, had they been left alone, many would not have become clinically significant hernias. Duckett's report was followed by an article in 1955 by Rothenberg who recommended "prophylactic" contralateral exploration in all children [49]. These reports became the basis for the recommendation that all children undergo a contralateral exploration when a unilateral hernia was diagnosed. This standard of care persisted until the 1990s when this classic teaching began to be questioned. The debate about contralateral exploration involves a choice between treating only obvious hernias (and dealing with a metachronous hernia later) versus preventing metachronous hernias by closing any patent processus vaginalis that is found. After weighing the risks and benefits, most pediatric surgeons now believe that routine open contralateral exploration is not indicated. Testicular atrophy occurs in 2% to 30% of children undergoing open groin exploration or hernia repair [50]. Open exploration is associated with an increased risk of infertility; as many as 40% of infertile males who had bilateral hernia repairs as children have bilateral obstruction of the vas deferens [51] Vas deferens injury can also result in sperm-agglutinating antibodies which influence fertility [52]. Even minor inadvertent pinching of the vas or stretching of the cord can result in injury, which also increases the risk of infertility [53–56] This inadvertent injury may be more likely when there is no true hernia sac present because the vas is more exposed. When boys were studied 8 to 20 years after inguinal hernia repair, 5.8% of them had decreased testicular size on the side of the repair and 1% had testicular atrophy [37].

For surgeons who opt to treat only the symptomatic side and to follow the patient for a possible metachronous hernia, the benefit is avoiding any risk of injury to cord structures, which might affect future fertility. The risk of this approach is that the patient will develop a metachronous hernia with an accompanying, albeit small, risk of incarceration. Incarceration may also lead to infertility through vascular compromise to the testes [57]. In 1997 Miltenberg and colleagues [58] published a meta-analysis of over 13,000 patients who had undergone repair of a unilateral hernia. The rate of metachronous hernia in children undergoing unilateral repair in this large meta-analysis was 7%. The risk was slightly higher if the initial presenting hernia was on the left (11%). Other large studies have shown that metachronous hernias occur in 3.6% to 11.6% of children after unilateral inguinal hernia repair [1,22,30,39,59–62]. In a study from New Zealand following the publication of Miltenberg's study, 264 patients were followed prospectively after unilateral hernia repair rather than routinely exploring the contralateral side. Metachronous hernias developed in 5% of these patients. This approach also resulted in decreased operating room time and decreased overall cost [1].

The advent of laparoscopic exploration has added a middle ground to the debate, because the laparoscope allows evaluation of the contralateral side without significant risk of injury to the vas and vessels. The percentage of pediatric surgeons using laparoscopic exploration is increasing [37]. The downside of this approach is that laparoscopic exploration cannot differentiate between a patent processus vaginalis and a true hernia. Some surgeons use a "significant" peritoneal opening [59], lack of termination of the visualized opening [59], or the visualization of bubbles internally with external pressure [59] as demonstration of a true hernia (Figs. 2 and 3). Most surgeons proceed with repair if there is any finding of patency, regardless of whether it is thought to be a patent processus vaginalis or true hernia. Approximately 50% of these procedures will be "unnecessary" because the findings would have remained an asymptomatic patent processus vaginalis. Alternatively, this approach avoids the small risk of incarceration of a metachronous hernia as well as the cost and anxiety of a second operation [3,50]. Different techniques have been described for exploring the contralateral internal ring, including placing an umbilical port for a 5-mm laparoscope, placing an umbilical port for the laparoscope and using a "probe" placed through a 14-gauge Angiocath to assess patency [63], insufflation through the ipsilateral sac and then placement of a lateral upper port (16-gauge Angiocath) for in-line inspection with a 1.2-mm camera [64], and insertion of a 30-, 70-, or 120-degree laparoscope through the ipsilateral hernia sac [59,65]. Other approaches to evaluate the contralateral side, which should be mentioned for historical interest only, include herniography, the use of Bakes dilators, and the Goldstein test (diagnostic pneumoperitoneum) [66,67].

Currently, both unilateral repair with waiting or laparoscopic exploration with repair of a patent processus vaginalis or hernia are considered the standard of care. The most ethical approach in the setting of inadequate data is to present the pros and cons of each approach to the families and allow them to participate in the decision. In some situations, the risk-benefit ratio may warrant the more aggressive approach of laparoscopic exploration

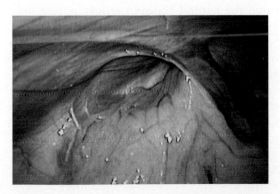

Fig. 2. Laparoscopic view of a left inguinal hernia.

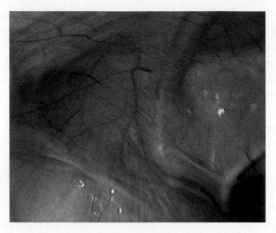

Fig. 3. Laparoscopic view of a normal left internal ring.

rather than opting to observe the contralateral side. For example, preterm infants have an additional risk of postoperative apnea and higher risk of incarceration; therefore, they should probably undergo laparoscopic exploration. Exploration may also be justified in patients known to be at higher risk for bilateral hernias or at increased operative risk, such as patients with cystic fibrosis, ventriculoperitoneal shunts, peritoneal dialysis catheters, or connective tissue disorders [59,65].

The preterm infant

The preterm infant represents a unique combination of operative and perioperative risks, which changes the basic algorithm for management. Hernias are more common in premature infants, and there is an increased risk of incarceration, as high as 31% in some series [5,68]; however, other studies have suggested that the risk may not be as great as previously thought. In one prospective study of 51 premature infants who were observed to watch the natural history of their patent processus vaginalis and hernias, only 1 (2%) experienced an incarceration [5]. The hernia sac in premature infants is more fragile than in older infants and children, and, not surprisingly, the recurrence rate and complication rate after repair are slightly higher [69]. In addition, premature infants have an added risk of postoperative apnea and bradycardia. This risk decreases as the infant matures. There are limited data based on prospective studies, but current recommendations include using regional anesthesia to limit or eliminate the need for general anesthesia, and admission for observation for infants less than 46 weeks postconceptional age [70]. Children under 60 weeks postconceptional age who have a history of lung disease, apnea at home, or other comorbidities also should be monitored after surgery. Balancing the increased risk of incarceration against the risk of perioperative

the potential risk of infertility. Umbilical hernias are common in infants but usually close with time. Surgery is indicated if the umbilical hernia is symptomatic or if the fascial defect fails to decrease in size over time.

References

[1] Manoharan S, Samarakkody U, Kulkarni M, et al. Evidence-based change of practice in the management of unilateral inguinal hernia. J Pediatr Surg 2005;40(7):1163–6.

[2] Glick PL, Boulanger S. Inguinal hernias and hydroceles. In: Grosfeld JL, O'Neill J, Coran A, et al, editors. Pediatric surgery. Philadelphia: Elsevier; 2006. p. 1172–92.

[3] Lloyd D. Inguinal and femoral hernia. In: Ziegler M, Azizkhan R, Weber T, editors. Operative pediatric surgery. New York: McGraw-Hill; 2003. p. 543–54.

[4] Kurkchubasche A, Tracy T. Unique features of groin hernia repair in infants and children. In: Fitzgibbons R, Greenburg A, editors. Nyhus and Condon's hernia. Philadelphia: Lippincott Williams & Wilkins; 2002. p. 435–51.

[5] Toki A, Watanabe Y, Sasaki K, et al. Adopt a wait-and-see attitude for patent processus vaginalis in neonates. J Pediatr Surg 2003;38(9):1371–3.

[6] Miltenburg DM, Nuchtern JG, Jaksic T, et al. Laparoscopic evaluation of the pediatric inguinal hernia: a meta-analysis. J Pediatr Surg 1998;33(6):874–9.

[7] Rowe MI, Copelson LW, Clatworthy HW. The patent processus vaginalis and the inguinal hernia. J Pediatr Surg 1969;4(1):102–7.

[8] van Veen RN, van Wessem KJ, Halm JA, et al. Patent processus vaginalis in the adult as a risk factor for the occurrence of indirect inguinal hernia. Surg Endosc 2007;21(2):202–5.

[9] van Wessem KJ, Simons MP, Plaisier PW, et al. The etiology of indirect inguinal hernias: congenital and/or acquired? Hernia 2003;7(2):76–9.

[10] Tanyel FC, Dagdeviren A, Muftuoglu S, et al. Inguinal hernia revisited through comparative evaluation of peritoneum, processus vaginalis, and sacs obtained from children with hernia, hydrocele, and undescended testis. J Pediatr Surg 1999;34(4):552–5.

[11] Tanyel FC, Okur HD. Autonomic nervous system appears to play a role in obliteration of processus vaginalis. Hernia 2004;8(2):149–54.

[12] Hosgor M, Karaca I, Ozer E, et al. Do alterations in collagen synthesis play an etiologic role in childhood inguinoscrotal pathologies: an immunohistochemical study. J Pediatr Surg 2004;39(7):1024–9.

[13] Hosgor M, Karaca I, Ozer E, et al. The role of smooth muscle cell differentiation in the mechanism of obliteration of processus vaginalis. J Pediatr Surg 2004;39(7):1018–23.

[14] Cook BJ, Hasthorpe S, Hutson JM. Fusion of childhood inguinal hernia induced by HGF and CGRP via an epithelial transition. J Pediatr Surg 2000;35(1):77–81.

[15] Ting AY, Huynh J, Farmer P, et al. The role of hepatocyte growth factor in the humoral regulation of inguinal hernia closure. J Pediatr Surg 2005;40(12):1865–8.

[16] Hutson JM, Albano FR, Paxton G, et al. In vitro fusion of human inguinal hernia with associated epithelial transformation. Cells Tissues Organs 2000;166(3):249–58.

[17] Clarnette TD, Hutson JM. The genitofemoral nerve may link testicular inguinoscrotal descent with congenital inguinal hernia. Aust N Z J Surg 1996;66(9):612–7.

[18] Jones ME, Swerdlow AJ, Griffith M, et al. Risk of congenital inguinal hernia in siblings: a record linkage study. Paediatr Perinat Epidemiol 1998;12(3):288–96.

[19] Gong Y, Shao C, Sun Q, et al. Genetic study of indirect inguinal hernia. J Med Genet 1994; 31(3):187–92.

[20] Czeizel A, Gardonyi J. A family study of congenital inguinal hernia. Am J Med Genet 1979; 4(3):247–54.

[21] Luo CC, Chao HC. Prevention of unnecessary contralateral exploration using the silk glove sign (SGS) in pediatric patients with unilateral inguinal hernia. Eur J Pediatr 2007;166(7): 667–9.

[22] Toki A, Watanabe Y, Sasaki K, et al. Ultrasonographic diagnosis for potential contralateral inguinal hernia in children. J Pediatr Surg 2003;38(2):224–6.

[23] Erez I, Rathause V, Vacian I, et al. Preoperative ultrasound and intraoperative findings of inguinal hernias in children: a prospective study of 642 children. J Pediatr Surg 2002;37(6): 865–8.

[24] Chen KC, Chu CC, Chou TY, et al. Ultrasonography for inguinal hernias in boys. J Pediatr Surg 1998;33(12):1784–7.

[25] Katz DA. Evaluation and management of inguinal and umbilical hernias. Pediatr Ann 2001;30(12):729–35.

[26] Stylianos S, Jacir NN, Harris BH. Incarceration of inguinal hernia in infants prior to elective repair. J Pediatr Surg 1993;28(4):582–3.

[27] Potts WJ, Riker WL, Lewis JE. The treatment of inguinal hernia in infants and children. Ann Surg 1950;132(3):566–76.

[28] Levitt MA, Ferraraccio D, Arbesman MC, et al. Variability of inguinal hernia surgical technique: a survey of North American pediatric surgeons. J Pediatr Surg 2002;37(5):745–51.

[29] Yokomori K, Ohkura M, Kitano Y, et al. Modified Marcy repair of large indirect inguinal hernia in infants and children. J Pediatr Surg 1995;30(1):97–100.

[30] Ein SH, Njere I, Ein A. Six thousand three hundred sixty-one pediatric inguinal hernias: a 35-year review. J Pediatr Surg 2006;41(5):980–6.

[31] Gahukamble DB, Khamage AS. Prospective randomized controlled study of excision versus distal splitting of hernial sac and processus vaginalis in the repair of inguinal hernias and communicating hydroceles. J Pediatr Surg 1995;30(4):624–5.

[32] Ong CC, Jacobsen AS, Joseph VT. Comparing wound closure using tissue glue versus subcuticular suture for pediatric surgical incisions: a prospective, randomised trial. Pediatr Surg Int 2002;18(5–6):553–5.

[33] van den Ende ED, Vriens PW, Allema JH, et al. Adhesive bonds or percutaneous absorbable suture for closure of surgical wounds in children: results of a prospective randomized trial. J Pediatr Surg 2004;39(8):1249–51.

[34] Mahabir RC, Christensen B, Blair GK, et al. Avoiding stitch abscesses in subcuticular skin closures: the L-stitch. Can J Surg 2003;46(3):223–4.

[35] Conroy JM, Othersen HB Jr, Dorman BH, et al. A comparison of wound instillation and caudal block for analgesia following pediatric inguinal herniorrhaphy. J Pediatr Surg 1993; 28(4):565–7.

[36] Ozgediz D, Roayaie K, Lee H, et al. Subcutaneous endoscopically assisted ligation (SEAL) of the internal ring for repair of inguinal hernias in children: report of a new technique and early results. Surg Endosc 2007;21(8):1327–31.

[37] Antonoff MB, Kreykes NS, Saltzman DA, et al. American Academy of Pediatrics section on surgery hernia survey revisited. J Pediatr Surg 2005;40(6):1009–14.

[38] Grosfeld JL, Minnick K, Shedd F, et al. Inguinal hernia in children: factors affecting recurrence in 62 cases. J Pediatr Surg 1991;26(3):283–7.

[39] Tackett LD, Breuer CK, Luks FI, et al. Incidence of contralateral inguinal hernia: a prospective analysis. J Pediatr Surg 1999;34(5):684–7 [discussion: 687–8].

[40] Partrick DA, Bensard DD, Karrer FM, et al. Is routine pathological evaluation of pediatric hernia sacs justified? J Pediatr Surg 1998;33(7):1090–2 [discussion: 1093–4].

[41] Popek EJ. Embryonal remnants in inguinal hernia sacs. Hum Pathol 1990;21(3):339–49.

[42] Steigman CK, Sotelo-Avila C, Weber TR. The incidence of spermatic cord structures in inguinal hernia sacs from male children. Am J Surg Pathol 1999;23(8):880–5.

[43] Hansen KA, Eyster KM. Infertility: an unusual complication of inguinal herniorrhaphy. Fertil Steril 2006;86(1):217–8.

[44] Urman BC, McComb PF. Tubal occlusion after inguinal hernia repair: a case report. J Reprod Med 1991;36(3):175–6.

[45] Kolbe T, Lechner W. Influence of hernioplastic implants on male fertility in rats. J Biomed Mater Res B Appl Biomater 2007;81(2):435–40.

[46] Maciel LC, Glina S, Palma PC, et al. Histopathological alterations of the vas deferens in rats exposed to polypropylene mesh. BJU Int 2007;100(1):187–90.

[47] Peiper C, Junge K, Klinge U, et al. Is there a risk of infertility after inguinal mesh repair? Experimental studies in the pig and the rabbit. Hernia 2006;10(1):7–12.

[48] Shin D, Lipshultz LI, Goldstein M, et al. Herniorrhaphy with polypropylene mesh causing inguinal vasal obstruction: a preventable cause of obstructive azoospermia. Ann Surg 2005; 241(4):553–8.

[49] Rothenberg RE, Barnett T. Bilateral herniotomy in infants and children. Surgery 1955; 37(6):947–50.

[50] Marulaiah M, Atkinson J, Kukkady A, et al. Is contralateral exploration necessary in preterm infants with unilateral inguinal hernia? J Pediatr Surg 2006;41(12):2004–7.

[51] Matsuda T, Muguruma K, Hiura Y, et al. Seminal tract obstruction caused by childhood inguinal herniorrhaphy: results of microsurgical reanastomosis. J Urol 1998;159(3):837–40.

[52] Friberg J, Fritjofsson A. Inguinal herniorrhaphy and sperm-agglutinating antibodies in infertile men. Arch Androl 1979;2(4):317–22.

[53] Ceylan H, Karakok M, Guldur E, et al. Temporary stretch of the testicular pedicle may damage the vas deferens and the testis. J Pediatr Surg 2003;38(10):1530–3.

[54] Abasiyanik A, Guvenc H, Yavuzer D, et al. The effect of iatrogenic vas deferens injury on fertility in an experimental rat model. J Pediatr Surg 1997;32(8):1144–6.

[55] Janik JS, Shandling B. The vulnerability of the vas deferens (II): the case against routine bilateral inguinal exploration. J Pediatr Surg 1982;17(5):585–8.

[56] Shandling B, Janik JS. The vulnerability of the vas deferens. J Pediatr Surg 1981;16(4): 461–4.

[57] Le Coultre C, Cuendet A, Richon J. Frequency of testicular atrophy following incarcerated hernia. Z Kinderchir 1983;38(Suppl):39–41.

[58] Miltenburg DM, Nuchtern JG, Jaksic T, et al. Meta-analysis of the risk of metachronous hernia in infants and children. Am J Surg 1997;174(6):741–4.

[59] Sözubır S, Ekingen G, Senel U, et al. A continuous debate on contralateral processus vaginalis: evaluation technique and approach to patency. Hernia 2006;10(1):74–8.

[60] Nassiri SJ. Contralateral exploration is not mandatory in unilateral inguinal hernia in children: a prospective 6-year study. Pediatr Surg Int 2002;18(5–6):470–1.

[61] Kemmotsu H, Oshima Y, Joe K, et al. The features of contralateral manifestations after the repair of unilateral inguinal hernia. J Pediatr Surg 1998;33(7):1099–102 [discussion: 1102–3].

[62] Given JP, Rubin SZ. Occurrence of contralateral inguinal hernia following unilateral repair in a pediatric hospital. J Pediatr Surg 1989;24(10):963–5.

[63] Geiger JD. Selective laparoscopic probing for a contralateral patent processus vaginalis reduces the need for contralateral exploration in inconclusive cases. J Pediatr Surg 2000; 35(8):1151–4.

[64] Bhatia AM, Gow KW, Heiss KF, et al. Is the use of laparoscopy to determine presence of contralateral patent processus vaginalis justified in children greater than 2 years of age? J Pediatr Surg 2004;39(5):778–81.

[65] Tamaddon H, Phillips JD, Nakayama DK. Laparoscopic evaluation of the contralateral groin in pediatric inguinal hernia patients: a comparison of 70- and 120-degree endoscopes. J Laparoendosc Adv Surg Tech A 2005;15(6):653–60.

[66] Timberlake GA, Ochsner MG, Powell RW. Diagnostic pneumoperitoneum in the pediatric patient with a unilateral inguinal hernia. Arch Surg 1989;124(6):721–3.

[67] Christenberry DP, Powell RW. Intraoperative diagnostic pneumoperitoneum (Goldstein test) in the infant and child with unilateral inguinal hernia. Am J Surg 1987;154(6):628–30.

[68] Rajput A, Gauderer MW, Hack M. Inguinal hernias in very low birth weight infants: incidence and timing of repair. J Pediatr Surg 1992;27(10):1322–4.

[69] Rathauser F. Historical overview of the bilateral approach to pediatric inguinal hernias. Am J Surg 1985;150(5):527–32.

[70] Walther-Larsen S, Rasmussen LS. The former preterm infant and risk of postoperative apnoea: recommendations for management. Acta Anaesthesiol Scand 2006;50(7):888–93.

[71] Gonzalez Santacruz M, Mira Navarro J, Encinas Goenechea A, et al. Low prevalence of complications of delayed herniotomy in the extremely premature infant. Acta Paediatr 2004;93(1):94–8.

[72] Misra D. Inguinal hernias in premature babies: wait or operate? Acta Paediatr 2001;90(4): 370–1.

[73] Uemura S, Woodward AA, Amerena R, et al. Early repair of inguinal hernia in premature babies. Pediatr Surg Int 1999;15(1):36–9.

[74] Marinkovic S, Kantardzic M, Bukarica S, et al. When to operate nonreducible ovary? Med Pregl 1998;51(11–12):537–40.

[75] Boley SJ, Cahn D, Lauer T, et al. The irreducible ovary: a true emergency. J Pediatr Surg 1991;26(9):1035–8.

[76] Kaya M, Huckstedt T, Schier F. Laparoscopic approach to incarcerated inguinal hernia in children. J Pediatr Surg 2006;41(3):567–9.

[77] Spurbeck WW, Prasad R, Lobe TE. Two-year experience with minimally invasive herniorrhaphy in children. Surg Endosc 2005;19(4):551–3.

[78] Montupet P, Esposito C. Laparoscopic treatment of congenital inguinal hernia in children. J Pediatr Surg 1999;34(3):420–3.

[79] Schier F. Laparoscopic inguinal hernia repair: a prospective personal series of 542 children. J Pediatr Surg 2006;41(6):1081–4.

[80] Chan KL, Hui WC, Tam PK. Prospective randomized single-center, single-blind comparison of laparoscopic vs open repair of pediatric inguinal hernia. Surg Endosc 2005;19(7):927–32.

[81] Schier F. Laparoscopic surgery of inguinal hernias in children: initial experience. J Pediatr Surg 2000;35(9):1331–5.

[82] Gorsler CM, Schier F. Laparoscopic herniorrhaphy in children. Surg Endosc 2003;17(4): 571–3.

[83] Zallen G, Glick PL. Laparoscopic inversion and ligation inguinal hernia repair in girls. J Laparoendosc Adv Surg Tech A 2007;17(1):143–5.

[84] Becmeur F, Philippe P, Lemandat-Schultz A, et al. A continuous series of 96 laparoscopic inguinal hernia repairs in children by a new technique. Surg Endosc 2004;18(12):1738–41.

[85] Yip KF, Tam PK, Li MK. Laparoscopic flip-flap hernioplasty: an innovative technique for pediatric hernia surgery. Surg Endosc 2004;18(7):1126–9.

[86] Oak SN, Parelkar SV, K R, et al. Large inguinal hernia in infants: is laparoscopic repair the answer? J Laparoendosc Adv Surg Tech A 2007;17(1):114–8.

[87] Takehara H, Yakabe S, Kameoka K. Laparoscopic percutaneous extraperitoneal closure for inguinal hernia in children: clinical outcome of 972 repairs done in 3 pediatric surgical institutions. J Pediatr Surg 2006;41(12):1999–2003.

[88] Schier F, Klizaite J. Rare inguinal hernia forms in children. Pediatr Surg Int 2004;20(10): 748–52.

[89] Schier F. Direct inguinal hernias in children: laparoscopic aspects. Pediatr Surg Int 2000; 16(8):562–4.

[90] Ollero Fresno JC, Alvarez M, Sanchez M, et al. Femoral hernia in childhood: review of 38 cases. Pediatr Surg Int 1997;12(7):520–1.

[91] Al-Shanafey S, Giacomantonio M. Femoral hernia in children. J Pediatr Surg 1999;34(7): 1104–6.

[92] Haberlik A, Sauer H. [Treatment of femoral hernia in children]. Chirurg 1990;61(4):289–91.

[93] Ceran C, Koyluoglu G, Sonmez K. Femoral hernia repair with mesh-plug in children. J Pediatr Surg 2002;37(10):1456–8.

[94] Lee SL, DuBois JJ. Laparoscopic diagnosis and repair of pediatric femoral hernia: initial experience of four cases. Surg Endosc 2000;14(12):1110–3.

[95] Ikossi DG, Shaheen R, Mallory B. Laparoscopic femoral hernia repair using umbilical ligament as plug. J Laparoendosc Adv Surg Tech A 2005;15(2):197–200.

[96] Cilley R. Disorders of the umbilicus. In: Grosfeld JL, O'Neill J, Coran A, et al, editors. Pediatric surgery. Philadelphia: Elsevier; 2006. p. 1143–56.

[97] Kokoska E, Weber T. Umbilical and supraumbilical disease. In: Ziegler M, Azizkhan R, Weber T, editors. Operative pediatric surgery. New York: McGraw-Hill; 2003. p. 543–54.

[98] Brown RA, Numanoglu A, Rode H. Complicated umbilical hernia in childhood. S Afr J Surg 2006;44(4):136–7.

[99] Fall I, Sanou A, Ngom G, et al. Strangulated umbilical hernias in children. Pediatr Surg Int 2006;22(3):233–5.

[100] Meier DE, OlaOlorun DA, Omodele RA, et al. Incidence of umbilical hernia in African children: redefinition of "normal" and reevaluation of indications for repair. World J Surg 2001;25(5):645–8.

[101] Ikeda H, Yamamoto H, Fujino J, et al. Umbilicoplasty for large protruding umbilicus accompanying umbilical hernia: a simple and effective technique. Pediatr Surg Int 2004; 20(2):105–7.

[102] el-Dessouki NI, Shehata SM, Torki AM, et al. Double half-cone flap umbilicoplasty: a new technique for the proboscoid umbilical hernia in children. Hernia 2004;8(3):182–5.

[103] Merei JM. Umbilical hernia repair in children: is pressure dressing necessary. Pediatr Surg Int 2006;22(5):446–8.

[104] Coats RD, Helikson MA, Burd RS. Presentation and management of epigastric hernias in children. J Pediatr Surg 2000;35(12):1754–6.

[105] Albanese CT, Rengal S, Bermudez D. A novel laparoscopic technique for the repair of pediatric umbilical and epigastric hernias. J Pediatr Surg 2006;41(4):859–62.

[106] Graivier L, Bronsther B, Feins NR, et al. Pediatric lateral ventral (spigelian) hernias. South Med J 1988;81(3):325–6.

[107] Losanoff JE, Richman BW, Jones JW. Spigelian hernia in a child: case report and review of the literature. Hernia 2002;6(4):191–3.

[108] Wakhlu A, Wakhlu AK. Congenital lumbar hernia. Pediatr Surg Int 2000;16(1–2):146–8.

[109] Pul M, Pul N, Gürses N. Congenital lumbar (Grynfelt-Lesshaft) hernia. Eur J Pediatr Surg 1991;1(2):115–7.

ELSEVIER
SAUNDERS

SURGICAL
CLINICS OF
NORTH AMERICA

Surg Clin N Am 88 (2008) 45–60

Primary and Unusual Abdominal Wall Hernias

J.R. Salameh, MD, FACS[a,b,*]

[a]*Georgetown University, Washington, DC, USA*
[b]*Surgical Associates at Virginia Hospital Center, 1625 North George Mason Drive,
Suite 334, Arlington, VA 22205, USA*

Primary ventral hernias are abdominal wall hernias that occur spontaneously and are not associated with a fascial scar or related to a trauma. Groin hernias are among the most common primary abdominal wall hernias but are not discussed here. This article covers the various aspects of other common primary hernias and those in unusual anatomic locations, including umbilical, epigastric, Spigelian, lumbar, obturator, supravesical, perineal, and sciatic hernias. Many of these hernias remain a diagnostic challenge for primary health care physicians because of their relative rarity, leading to a delay in presentation and management. In addition, most of them carry a relatively high risk of incarceration because of the frequently associated tight fascial defect.

Hernias are sometimes "unusual" because of the contents of their sacs, such as a Meckel's diverticulum (Littre's hernia), a segment of the antimesenteric border of the intestinal wall (Richter's hernia), or the vermiform appendix (Amyand's hernia). The clinical characteristics and the management of these hernias are beyond the scope of this article.

Umbilical hernia

Umbilical hernias are hernias that occur at the umbilicus. Umbilical hernias can be infantile or adult, based on their onset. The infantile umbilical hernia is a result of an abnormally large or weak umbilical ring in an otherwise normal abdominal wall; the defect is covered by skin. In most children, the umbilical ring progressively diminishes in size and eventually closes. Defects less than 1 cm in diameter close spontaneously by 5 years of age in 95% of cases [1]. However, a ring greater than 1.5 cm in diameter seldom closes spontaneously [2].

---

* Surgical Associates at Virginia Hospital Center, 1625 North George Mason Drive, Suite 334, Arlington, VA 22205.

E-mail address: salamehj@yahoo.com

0039-6109/08/$ - see front matter © 2008 Elsevier Inc. All rights reserved.
doi:10.1016/j.suc.2007.10.004   *surgical.theclinics.com*

The adult umbilical hernia occurs through the umbilical canal, which is bordered by the umbilical fascia posteriorly, the linea alba anteriorly, and the medial edges of the two rectus sheaths on each side [1]. It does not usually result from persistence of infantile hernias, but is acquired in almost 90% of cases and is due to a gradual yielding of the cicatricial tissue that closes the umbilical ring, secondary to increasing intra-abdominal pressure. Predisposing factors include obesity, multiple pregnancies, cirrhosis with ascites, and large abdominal tumors.

Clinical presentation and diagnosis

It is estimated that as many as 10% of all infants are born with an umbilical hernia; the incidence is as high as 20% in African-American infants versus 3% in white neonates, and is increased in association with certain disease states (Beckwith-Wiedemann syndrome, Down's syndrome) [2]. The incidence of umbilical hernia is also markedly increased in premature babies and may be seen in as many as 75% of infants under 1500 g [2]. There are no significant gender differences. Infantile umbilical hernias are most often asymptomatic and, in contrast to inguinal hernias, rarely incarcerate.

Adult umbilical hernias are more common in women than men and are most likely to occur in the fifth and sixth decades of life. They usually present as a bulge at the umbilicus that is usually asymptomatic but can cause discomfort or pain. Diagnosis is almost always clinical. Complications of umbilical hernias are few, with strangulation, incarceration, or evisceration being reported in 5% of patients in large series [3]. Hernias smaller than 1.5 cm in diameter become incarcerated twice as often as do larger hernias. In cirrhotic patients with ascites, skin ulceration and necrosis may lead to rupture with chronic ascitic fluid leak or peritonitis.

Treatment

Infantile umbilical hernias can be safely managed with observation and usually resolve spontaneously by the time the child reaches 5 years of age. Hernias that are symptomatic, extremely large, or persisting beyond age 5 should be repaired. Most defects can be managed with simple primary closure [2].

Adult umbilical hernias should be surgically repaired as early as possible. The presence of cirrhosis and ascites should not discourage repair, as strangulation, incarceration, and rupture are particularly dangerous in patients with these disorders. Significant ascites, however, should first be thoroughly treated, and nutrition optimized as morbidity and recurrence rate are much higher after hernia repair in these patients.

The modern adult umbilical hernia repair is attributed to William J. Mayo [4], who used the technique of overlapping abdominal wall fascia in a "vest-over-pants" manner. Currently, however, a mesh repair, using either a mesh plug or a mesh sheet based on the size of the hernia, is favored. In a randomized clinical trial comparing primary suture herniorrhaphy with mesh hernioplasty in 200 adult patients with a primary umbilical hernia followed for 64 months, the hernia recurrence rate was significantly higher after suture repair (11%) than after mesh repair (1%); there did not appear to be a significant relationship between recurrence rate and size of the hernia [5].

In the last decade, laparoscopic ventral hernia repairs have been shown to be safe and effective techniques and have been used for large adult umbilical hernias. In one retrospective comparative study of 32 laparoscopic repairs and 20 open-mesh repairs for umbilical hernias, laparoscopy resulted in shorter operating time, less use of postoperative drains, lower complication rates, and shorter return to normal activities [6]. Laparoscopic repair is an attractive option for umbilical hernias larger than 3 cm in diameter and in recurrent hernias of any size.

Epigastric hernia

Epigastric hernias are hernias of the linea alba occurring between the umbilicus and the xiphoid. Although congenital epigastric hernias have been described in infants [7], they are usually considered an acquired condition.

A number of theories have been suggested to explain the origin and development of epigastric hernias, but controversies still prevail. The first, and most likely, hypothesis links the cause of epigastric hernias to the vascular lacunae that form when the small neurovascular bundles that run between the transversalis fascia and the peritoneum, perforate the linea alba [8,9]. Over periods of increased abdominal tension, preperitoneal fat derived from the falciform ligament is forced along these blood vessels enlarging the fascial defect, and an epigastric hernia is eventually formed. Another hypothesis proposed by Askar [10] and widely quoted relates to an intrinsic weakness in the linea alba fibers. Askar [10,11] noted that the linea alba is formed by the decussation of the tendinous aponeurotic fibers of the muscular layers passing from one side to the other, and that epigastric hernias occur exclusively in patients who had single, instead of triple, anterior and posterior lines of decussation. This finding could not, however, be confirmed by other investigators [12]. Instead, Korenkov and colleagues [12] found that the biomechanical characteristics of the linea alba are not governed by the number of aponeurotic crossings but by the thickness and density of the fibers, and that the weak type of linea alba aponeurosis may be a predisposing factor for the development of a hernia.

About 20% of epigastric hernias are multiple and about 80% are located just off the midline [1]. Fascial defects vary in size from only millimeters to several centimeters. Most epigastric hernias, however, are small and are made up of preperitoneal fat only with no peritoneal sac; these are especially prone to incarceration and strangulation. Frequently, the preperitoneal fat herniating through this small defect grows over time and becomes chronically incarcerated. Larger hernias with a peritoneal sac most commonly contain omentum, but can contain any upper intraperitoneal organ such as small bowel, colon, or stomach; these hernias seldom incarcerate or strangulate.

Clinical presentation and diagnosis

Epigastric hernias account for 1.6% to 3.6% of all abdominal wall hernias [9] and are three times more common in men than in women. Most of them present themselves between the third to fifth decade of life, with a noticeable drop in incidence after the sixth decade [13]. These findings suggest that epigastric hernias are a condition closely related to physical activity of an individual and not a degenerative disease as in other types of hernia.

Symptoms are related to the defect size and the hernia content. Small hernias typically present with epigastric pain that is usually related to the compression of the neurovascular bundle by the herniated preperitoneal fat [14]. The pain may be associated with an epigastric mass, which can be difficult to palpate in obese individuals. Chronically incarcerated hernias are often confused with lipomas. Most large reducible hernias, on the other hand, are asymptomatic or may cause minimal discomfort. Incarceration produces an acutely painful mass along with symptoms related to the involved organs and their viability.

The diagnosis is usually easy to make on physical examination. Epigastric hernias should be distinguished from diasthesis recti, which is a weakening and broadening of the entire linea alba above the umbilicus. Occasionally, when the diagnosis is uncertain, especially in obese patients, ultrasonography or CT scan may be used to detect the hernia defects.

Treatment

Epigastric hernias, even if asymptomatic, should be repaired at time of diagnosis because of the risk of incarceration. The current literature on the outcome of epigastric hernia repair is scant, given that most are reported as part of series of ventral and incisional hernia repairs.

Most epigastric hernias, especially the small and single ones, and those that are acutely or chronically incarcerated are usually repaired through an open approach. A targeted midline incision is used. The presence of other occult fascial defects should be ruled out as recurrence may be occasionally due to failure to recognize and repair multiple small defects [1]. The preperitoneal fat or hernia sac is reduced or excised without enlarging the defect. If the defects are multiple and contiguous, the fascial bridges between the necks should be left in place if possible—but more often than not, the defects are connected together. The fascia around the defect is often thin and weak, and primary repair is not advised unless the defect is less than 3 mm [14]. A mesh repair is otherwise always performed; adequate options include an underlay mesh, a mesh plug, or a combination of onlay and underlay mesh [1,14,15]. In one series of 57 epigastric hernias ranging in size from 0.5 cm to 5 cm and repaired under local anesthesia with a mesh plug in all but 4 cases, no recurrences were noted, with follow-up ranging from 4 to 60 months [1].

Laparoscopic epigastric hernia repair is a good alternative to open repair in larger hernias and in those that are multiple. The falciform ligament and the peritoneum must be taken down to allow the visualization of the entire epigastric fascia and the identification of hernias only containing preperitoneal fat. There are no published series of laparoscopic epigastric hernia repair. If results are extrapolated from umbilical hernia repairs [6], laparoscopy may be expected to have lower complication rate and faster recovery than open repairs in large epigastric hernias, as well as a superior cosmetic result.

Spigelian hernia

A Spigelian hernia, also known as "spontaneous lateral ventral hernia," is a hernia through the spigelian fascia, which is the aponeurotic layer between the lateral edge of the rectus abdominis muscle medially and the semilunar line laterally (Fig. 1). It is named after the Belgian anatomist Adriaan van den Spieghel [16], who was the first to describe the semilunar line or linea Spigeli, in 1645. This line represents the transition between the muscular and aponeurotic portions of the transversus abdominis muscle. A Spigelian hernia is generally an interparietal hernia, meaning that the preperitoneal fat and/or the hernia sac penetrate the transversus abdominis and internal oblique muscles but remain behind the external oblique aponeurosis (Fig. 2).

Although Spigelian hernias can occur at any point along the spigelian fascia, they almost always develop at or below the arcuate line, probably because of the absence of posterior rectus sheath at that level. In addition, the fibers of the spigelian aponeurosis run in a parallel fashion below the umbilicus instead of crossing one another at right angles, becoming vulnerable to separation by preperitoneal fat. In fact, 90% of Spigelian hernias are found within the Spigelian hernia belt of Spangen [17], which is a 6-cm transverse strip above the line joining both anterior superior iliac spines, and where the spigelian fascia is wider and weaker (see Fig. 1). Lower hernias are rare and should be differentiated from direct inguinal or supravescical hernias. In most cases, the hernia defect is small—less than 2 cm—with well-defined and firm margins.

Spigelian hernias are normally acquired conditions, although congenital cases have been reported in children. Predisposing factors include morbid obesity, multiple pregnancies, rapid weight loss, chronic obstructive pulmonary disease, chronic constipation, prostatic enlargement, ascitis, trauma, and previous surgery weakening the semilunar line.

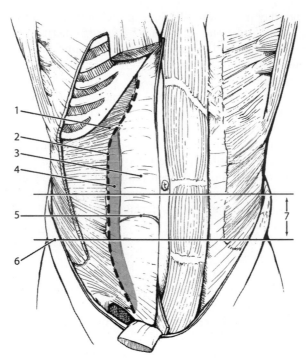

Fig. 1. View of the anterior abdominal wall with the external oblique, internal oblique, and rectus abdominus muscles peeled away on the left. (*1*) transverses muscle, (*2*) semilunar line, (*3*) posterior rectus sheath, (*4*) spigelian aponeurosis, (*5*) arcuate line, (*6*) anterior superior iliac spine, (*7*) spigelian hernia belt.

Clinical presentation and diagnosis

Spigelian hernias represent 0.12% to 2.4% of all abdominal wall hernias, although their incidence appears to be increasing, given the improved detection on cross-sectional imaging. They present most commonly in the fifth and sixth decades of life, but can be seen at any age. They have a slightly higher preponderance in women (female to male ratio, 1.4: 1) [17].

The diagnosis of a Spigelian hernia is elusive and requires a high index of suspicion, given its rarity, the vague associated abdominal complaints, and the frequent lack of consistent physical findings.

The clinical presentation varies, depending on the size, the type, and the contents of the hernia. In patients with a reducible hernia, the most common symptoms are pain, which is usually intermittent and nonspecific, and a lateral bulge or mass when standing. Many patients, however, present with a hernia-related complication, given the small size of the hernia orifice; incarceration at the time of operation is seen in 17% to 24% of reported hernias [17,18].

Physical examination alone fails to detect any findings in 36% of patients [18] and can be falsely positive in up to 50% of cases [19]. Given

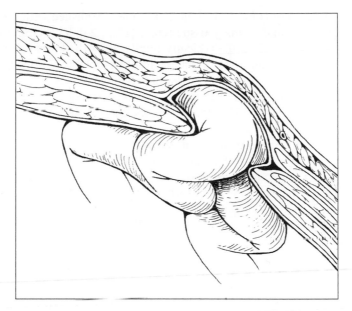

Fig. 2. Cross-sectional view of a Spiegelian hernia showing the relationship of the hernia sac to the anterior abdominal wall muscles and fascias.

that most hernias are small and covered by a usually intact external oblique aponeurosis, it is difficult to palpate a hernia or a hernia defect. Persistent point tenderness in the spigelian aponeurosis with a tensed abdominal wall is often the only sign upon physical examination that suggests the diagnosis [17].

Imaging is recommended before surgical exploration, especially when the diagnosis is in doubt. Ultrasonography is accurate in displaying defects in the spigelian fascia [20,21]; it is easy to perform and not expensive, but is operator dependent. CT scan also allows the diagnosis of Spigelian hernia and gives more detailed information on the contents of the sac than does ultrasonography [21,22]. The true sensitivity and specificity of these diagnostic techniques is, however, unknown; in one study, false-negative CT occurred in 32% (6/19) of patients with obvious findings of a Spigelian hernia at the time of operation [14]. Modern helical CT is probably more accurate, and it is currently uncommon not to be able to confirm the diagnosis before surgical exploration. Only occasionally is diagnostic laparoscopy required to establish the diagnosis in patients with unclear acute or chronic pain.

Treatment

Spigelian hernias should always be surgically repaired in view of the high frequency of incarceration. Various techniques have been described and are currently performed.

Repair of this hernia has traditionally been accomplished with a targeted transverse incision and primary tissue repair [17,18,23]. This is often possible with low tension, given the typically small size of the hernia defect, and the repair is relatively durable. In one institutional review of 70 primary repairs with a mean follow-up of 8 years, the recurrence rate was 4.3%, with recurrences occurring at an average of 3 years postoperatively [18]. However, in another report of 21 primary repairs, the recurrence rate was high at 14.3% [24].

The addition of mesh to the open repair of Spigelian hernias has led to improved outcomes [18,24–28]. The various reported techniques involving mesh include intra- and preperitoneal sublay mesh placement [24–26], obliteration of the ring by a preformed polypropelene mesh umbrella-type plug [27], or a combination of preperitoneal underlay mesh connected to an overlay mesh lying over the internal oblique muscle [26]. None of the published series using mesh report any recurrences with variable follow-up periods.

Laparoscopic repair was first reported in 1992 [29]. Intraperitoneal, transabdominal preperitoneal, and totally extraperitoneal laparoscopic techniques with underlay mesh placement have been described [26,29–31]. In a prospective randomized trial comparing 11 open and 11 laparoscopic (8 intraperitoneal, 3 totally extraperitoneal) Spigelian hernia repairs, laparoscopy was shown to have a significantly lower morbidity and shorter hospital length of stay; no recurrences were noted in either group, with mean follow-up of 3.4 years [28].

Lumbar hernia

Lumbar hernias are those that occur in the area of the posterior abdominal wall bounded by the 12th rib superiorly, the iliac crest inferiorly, the erector spinae muscles posteriorly, and the posterior border of the external oblique anteriorly. Primary lumbar hernias can be congenital (rare) or acquired. They occur within two distinct anatomic spaces: the inferior and the superior lumbar triangles.

- *Inferior lumbar triangle or Petit's triangle* is often simply called the lumbar triangle owing to its more superficial location and ease in demonstration. It lies in the posterolateral abdominal wall and is defined by the latissimus dorsi, the free margin of the external abdominal oblique muscle, and the iliac crest (Fig. 3). The floor of the inferior lumbar triangle is the internal abdominal oblique muscle. French surgeon Jean Louis Petit (1674–1750) is given credit for describing this triangle that bears his name. The triangle exists in 63% to 82.5% of the dissected cadavers [32,33] and its size varies a great deal, from merely a slit to a surface area greater than 12 cm^2, exposing a large component of the internal abdominal oblique muscle [32,33].

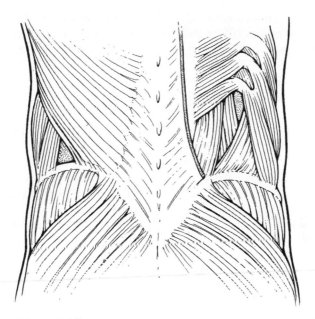

Fig. 3. On the left, inferior lumbar triangle of Petit (*dotted area*); on the right, latissimus dorsi peeled off showing the superior lumbar triangle of Grynfeltt (*dotted area*).

- *Superior lumbar triangle or Grynfeltt-Lesshaft triangle* lies deep to the latissimus dorsi. It usually has the shape of an inverted triangle and is defined by the 12th rib, the quadratus lumborum muscle, and the internal oblique muscle (see Fig. 3). The floor of the superior lumbar triangle is the transversalis fascia. Grynfeltt [34] first described a hernia through this lumbar triangle in 1866. The thickness of the aponeurosis varies in this space, but at its uppermost limit, the thinnest portion of the lumbar region is seen. In this thin area, the 12th intercostal vessels and nerves are usually found and it is in this region that hernias most often occur. Of the two lumbar triangles, the superior one is the more consistently found in cadavers (93.5%) and the more common site of herniation [32].

Predisposing factors in spontaneously acquired lumbar hernia are age, obesity, extreme thinness, chronic debilitating disease, muscular atrophy, intense slimming, chronic bronchitis, and strenuous physical activity [35]. It appears that the loss of fatty tissue facilitates the rupture of the neurovascular orifices that penetrate the lumbodorsal fascia; situations related to increased intra-abdominal pressure would act as factors that trigger the appearance of these hernias [35].

Clinical presentation and diagnosis

The clinical presentation of lumbar hernias depends on their size and contents. The most common clinical manifestation is a bulge that increases with coughing and strenuous activity and tends to disappear with the patient in the lateral decubitus position. Patients usually report nonspecific abdominal discomfort, fatigue, or back pain along the area of distribution of the sciatic nerve [35]. The diagnosis should be considered in young women and athletes with back pain [36].

In about 9% of cases, patients present acutely with an incarceration such as a small- or large-bowel obstruction or a painful irreducible mass [36]. Strangulation may occur but is uncommon. Other rare manifestations include urinary obstruction symptoms such as hematuria, oliguria, and colicky pain; pelvic mass; and retroperitoneal and gluteal abscess.

Although the diagnosis is typically clinical based on the patient's history, symptoms, and physical signs, the use of CT scan must be regarded as a routine exploratory technique in the preoperative evaluation of patients with lumbar hernias, to confirm the diagnosis, evaluate the abdominal wall muscles, reliably assess the anatomical relationships of the lumbar area, and identify the hernia contents [35,37].

Treatment

Lumbar hernias are difficult to repair because of their location and the surrounding bony structures [37]. Currently, there are two established possible surgical approaches, both performed with the patient in lateral decubitus: the anterior approach with lumbar incision and the laparoscopic approach.

The open anterior approach consists of an incision over the hernia site and extensive dissection, sometimes from the 12th rib to the iliac crest. In Grynfeltt hernias, the latissimus dorsi needs to be divided. Primary sutured repairs or the use of mesh plugs should not currently be recommended regardless of the size of the hernia defect, in view of the rigidity of the margins. Repairs are best performed using synthetic mesh placed in the extraperitoneal space, below the muscular layers, using a tension-free technique. The results of lumbar hernia treatment are difficult to analyze because of the limited experience of each surgeon. In one series of nine primary lumbar hernias (seven Grynfeltt hernias and two Petit hernias) repaired in this fashion, there were no cases of recurrence or postsurgical sequelae, such as pain or muscular weakness after a median follow-up period of 25 months [38].

The laparoscopic approach consists of either a transabdominal or a totally extraperitoneal technique [39,40]. The transabdominal approach is the more popular and usually requires mobilization of the colon and the kidney. The mesh can be secured to the costal margin superiorly, the iliac crest periosteum inferiorly, the erector spinae fascia medially, and external oblique fascia laterally [39]. In the posteromedial area, fixation of the mesh with intracorporeal suturing and avoiding tacks and transfascial sutures to prevent potential entrapment of the nerves that run in that area are advocated [37]. Advantages of the laparoscopic approach include excellent operative visualization and wide mesh coverage.

There are no published studies comparing these two techniques in primary lumbar hernias. However, in a prospective nonrandomized study of open versus laparoscopic repair of 16 secondary lumbar hernias, mean operating time, postoperative morbidity, mean hospital stay, consumption of analgesics, and time to return to normal activities were significantly lower in the laparoscopic group [41].

Obturator hernia

Obturator hernias are hernias through the obturator canal in the pelvis. This canal is the opening in the superior part of the obturator membrane covering the foramen formed by the union of the pubic bone and ischium, and through which the obturator nerve, artery, and vein pass from the pelvic cavity into the thigh (Fig. 4). Weakening of the obturator membrane may result in enlargement of the canal and formation of a hernia sac. The defect is usually located anterior and medial to the obturator neurovascular bundle [42]. The hernia is located deeply in the thigh between the pectineus and adductor longus muscles. The formation of these hernias is thought to begin with a "pilot tag" of properitoneal fat followed by the appearance of a peritoneal dimple that ultimately grows into a larger hernia sac that may

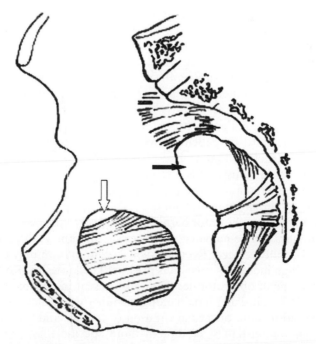

Fig. 4. View of the bony pelvis demonstrating the obturator canal (*arrow*) and the greater sciatic foramen (*solid arrow*).

contain small bowel, large bowel, omentum, fallopian tube, or appendix. The frequency of pilot tags in cadavers and the rarity of actual obturator hernias suggest that most obturator hernias do not progress beyond the early stages of development [43].

Obturator hernias are associated with profound asthenia and weight loss because of loss of the protective fat in the obturator canal. Women are affected more often than men because of their broader pelvis and larger obturator canal. Chronic lung disease, constipation, kyphoscoliosis, and pregnancy can predispose to obturator herniation by increasing intra-abdominal pressure [44].

Clinical presentation and diagnosis

Obturator hernias are rare, comprising approximately 0.073% of all hernias and occurring in approximately 0.4% of bowel obstructions [45]. They may occur bilaterally or in association with another hernia, most often a femoral hernia.

Obturator hernias typically affect elderly, frail, chronically ill, often institutionalized women; 85% of patients are female with mean age of 82 years and mean weight of 34.5 kg [46]. They characteristically affect the right side because the sigmoid colon tends to prevent it on the left side.

The diagnosis of an obturator hernia is difficult because it is rare, the symptoms are often vague, and the physical examination is rarely helpful, given that the hernia is concealed beneath the adductor muscles of the thigh; only 1 of 10 cases is correctly diagnosed preoperatively [45]. The classic symptom of groin pain radiating down the medial aspect of the thigh to the knee and caused by pressure on the obturator nerve, when present, is often overlooked or misinterpreted as arthritic pain in this often geriatric population.

More than 90% of patients with obturator hernia present with intestinal obstruction. One third of patients have a history of previous attacks of small-bowel obstruction that is likely secondary to transient herniation that resolved spontaneously. It is also common for nonspecific gastrointestinal symptoms, including anorexia, weight loss, and emaciation, to precede the diagnosis of hernia by many months.

Physical findings of obturator hernia are relatively nonspecific. Occasionally, a groin mass can be palpated with the patient supine, thigh flexed, adducted, and laterally rotated. Rectal or pelvic examination may confirm the diagnosis if a high index of suspicion is present. The Howship-Romberg sign is pathognomonic of obturator hernia and is present in approximately 50% of patients [42]. It is ipsilateral pain along the inner thigh that is exacerbated by extension, adduction, or medial rotation of the hip and relieved by flexion. The Hannington-Kiff sign, though more specific than the Howship-Romberg sign, is less widely known. It refers to an absent adductor reflex in the thigh [47]; a difference compared with the controlateral side and a normal ipsilateral patellar reflex are indicators of compression of the obturator nerve.

Definitive preoperative diagnosis is usually made possible by CT scan. It is likely that with increasing use of CT scan in patients with small-bowel obstruction and in those with nonspecific abdominal complaints, the diagnosis of obturator hernia will become more frequent.

Treatment

When the diagnosis of obturator hernia is known preoperatively and strangulation is not suspected, the posterior preperitoneal approach is preferred and provides direct access to the hernia. It can be performed either through an open approach using a lower midline or Pfannensteil incision, or laparoscopically [48]. If petechiae or dark bowel suggest necrotic bowel, the peritoneal cavity can be easily entered for bowel resection. Reduction of the hernia may occasionally require incision of the obturator membrane with care to avoid injury to the obturator nerve and vessels. Direct primary suture repair of the hernia defect is difficult because the foramen is bordered by bone and spanned by the tough, immobile obturator membrane. Repair using a plug in the obturator canal has the potential for aggravating the obturator neuralgia and should probably be avoided. The preferred repair technique consists of placing a large flat polypropylene mesh in the properitoneal space to cover the obturator orifice as well as the femoral and inguinal areas [45].

When the diagnosis is unclear or when strangulation is suspected, the abdominal approach is most often favored. The hernia may then be repaired as described above after opening the parietal peritoneum. In the cases of strangulated or perforated bowel, gross contamination, and/or bowel resection, there is reluctance in using a synthetic mesh. A biologic mesh may be placed or nearby tissue such as periosteal flaps, bladder wall, or uterine fundus or ligaments may be mobilized.

The morbidity and mortality of obturator hernia repair remain high owing to the frequently delayed recognition with resultant bowel strangulation, and to the high incidence of patients with concurrent medical illness.

Other unusual hernias

Supravesical hernia

Supravesical hernias are hernias that protrude through the supravesical fossa. They occur because of a weakness in the lower aspect of the transversus abdominis muscle and the transversalis fascia where both insert into Cooper's ligament [27]. According to their relationship with the vesical dome and the space of Retzius, they can be classified as prevesical, paravesical, intravesical, or retrovesical. They can be internal or external and may occasionally penetrate the inguinal, femoral, or obturator rings. These hernias are very rare—only 70 cases have been reported worldwide [27]. They occur most frequently in elderly, malnourished males.

Preoperative diagnosis is possible if a given groin hernia is associated with signs and symptoms of intestinal obstruction along with urinary disturbances. Symptoms can sometimes mimic those of prostatic obstruction. CT scan can provide the diagnosis. Repair is usually performed through an infraumbilical midline laparotomy, using mesh if the field is clean.

Perineal hernia

Perineal hernias are hernias that protrude through the pelvic diaphragm. An anterior and a posterior form can be distinguished based on their position relative to the transverse perineii muscle. Primary perineal hernias are rare, with about 100 cases reported in the literature [49]. They occur most commonly in older, multiparous women, and can be quite large. They manifest clinically as a unilateral bulge in the area of the labia or the gluteal or perineal region. The hernia is frequently detected on bimanual rectal-vaginal examination. The diagnosis can be supported by sonography or CT scan.

Perineal hernias can be repaired through a transabdominal, a perineal, or combined transabdominal and perineal approaches. After the sac contents are reduced, the pelvic floor defect should be repaired with either direct suture or implantation of a mesh, depending on its size, its margins, and its relationship with the rectum.

Sciatic hernia

Sciatic hernias occur through the greater sciatic foramen (see Fig. 4). They are extremely unusual, with only 53 documented cases [50]. They are frequently asymptomatic and undiagnosed until intestinal obstruction occurs. When present, the most common symptom is an uncomfortable or slowly enlarging mass in the gluteal area. Herniation of the ureter or the bladder may manifest as urinary tract symptoms [51]. On rare occasions, sciatic hernias may mimic sciatica, with back or leg pain, owing to compression of the sciatic nerve.

A transperitoneal approach is recommended in patients presenting with small-bowel obstruction, especially when bowel strangulation is suspected. On the other hand, a less invasive transgluteal approach, in the prone position, may be used if the diagnosis is certain and the hernia contents appear viable and reducible. Prosthetic mesh repair is usually preferred.

References

[1] Muschaweck U. Umbilical and epigastric hernia repair. Surg Clin North Am 2003;83(5): 1207–21.

[2] Snyder CL. Current management of umbilical abnormalities and related anomalies. Semin Pediatr Surg 2007;16(1):41–9.

[3] Nyhus LM, Pollack R. Epigastric, umbilical, and ventral hernias. In: Cameron J, editor. Current surgical therapy. St. Louis (MO): Mosby; 1992. p. 536–9.

[4] Mayo WJ. An operation for the radical cure of umbilical hernia. Ann Surg 1901;34:276–80.

[5] Arroyo A, García P, Pérez F, et al. Randomized clinical trial comparing suture and mesh repair of umbilical hernia in adults. Br J Surg 2001;88(10):1321–3.

[6] Gonzalez R, Mason F, Duncan T, et al. Laparoscopic versus open umbilical hernia repair. JSLS 2003;7(4):323–8.

[7] Coats RD, Helikson MA, Burd RS. Presentation and management of epigastric hernias in children. J Pediatr Surg 2000;35(12):1754–6.

[8] Moschowitz AV. The pathogenesis and treatment of herniae of the linea alba. Surg Gynecol Obstet 1914;18:504–7.

[9] Lang B, Lau H, Lee F. Epigastric hernia and its etiology. Hernia 2002;6(3):148–50.

[10] Askar OM. Aponeurotic hernias. Recent observations upon paraumbilical and epigastric hernias. Surg Clin North Am 1984;64(2):315–33.

[11] Askar OM. Surgical anatomy of the aponeurotic expansions of the anterior abdominal wall. Ann R Coll Surg Engl 1977;59(4):313–21.

[12] Korenkov M, Beckers A, Koebke J, et al. Biomechanical and morphological types of the linea alba and its possible role in the pathogenesis of midline incisional hernia. Eur J Surg 2001;167(12):909–14.

[13] Ponka JL, Mohr B. Epigastric hernia. In: Ponka JL, Mohr B, editors. Hernias of the abdominal wall. Philadelphia: Saunders; 1980.

[14] Deysine M. Epigastric hernias. In: Bendavid R, Abrahamson J, Arregui ME, et al, editors. Abdominal wall hernias: principles and management. 1st edition. New York: Springer-Verlag; 2001. p. 685–7.

[15] Khera G, Berstock DA. Incisional, epigastric and umbilical hernia repair using the Prolene Hernia System: describing a novel technique. Hernia 2006;10(4):367–9.

[16] Spieghel A. Opera quae extore omnia. Amsterdam: John Bloew; 1645.

[17] Spangen L. Spigelian hernia. World J Surg 1989;13:573–80.

[18] Larson DW, Farley DR. Spigelian hernias: repair and outcome for 81 patients. World J Surg 2002;26(10):1277–81.

[19] Stirnemann H. The Spigelian hernia: missed? rare? puzzling diagnosis? Chirurg 1982;53: 314–7.

[20] Nelson RL, Renigers SA, Nyhus LM, et al. Ultrasonography of the abdominal wall in the diagnosis of spigelian hernia. Am Surg 1980;46(7):373–6.

[21] Balthazar EJ, Subramanyam BR, Megibow A. Spigelian hernia: CT and ultrasonography diagnosis. Gastrointest Radiol 1984;9(1):81–4.

[22] Luedke M, Scholz FJ, Larsen CR. Computed tomographic evaluation of spigelian hernia. Comput Med Imaging Graph 1988;12(2):123–9.

[23] Artioukh DY, Walker SJ. Spigelian herniae: presentation, diagnosis and treatment. J R Coll Surg Edinb 1996;41(4):241–3.

[24] Mouton WG, Otten KT, Weiss D, et al. Preperitoneal mesh repair in Spigelian hernia. Int Surg 2006;91(5):262–4.

[25] Malazgirt Z, Topgul K, Sokmen S, et al. Spigelian hernias: a prospective analysis of baseline parameters and surgical outcome of 34 consecutive patients. Hernia 2006;10(4):326–30.

[26] Campanelli G, Pettinari D, Nicolosi FM, et al. Spigelian hernia. Hernia 2005;9:3–5.

[27] Montes IS, Deysine M. Spigelian and other uncommon hernia repairs. Surg Clin North Am 2003;83(5):1235–53.

[28] Moreno-Egea A, Carrasco L, Girela E, et al. Open vs laparoscopic repair of spigelian hernia: a prospective randomized trial. Arch Surg 2002;137(11):1266–8.

[29] Carter JE, Mizes C. Laparoscopic diagnosis and repair of Spigelian hernia: report of a case and technique. Am J Obstet Gynecol 1992;167:77–8.

[30] Felix EL, Michas C. Laparoscopic repair of spigelian hernias. Surg Laparosc Endosc 1994; 4(4):308–10.

[31] Palanivelu C, Vijaykumar M, Jani KV, et al. Laparoscopic transabdominal preperitoneal repair of spigelian hernia. JSLS 2006;10(2):193–8.

[32] Goodman EH, Speese J. Lumbar hernia. Ann Surg 1916;63(5):548–60.

[33] Loukas M, Tubbs RS, El-Sedfy A, et al. The clinical anatomy of the triangle of Petit. Hernia 2007;11(5):441–4.

[34] Grynfeltt J. La Hernie Lombaire. Montp Med 1866;16:329.

[35] Moreno-Egea A, Baena EG, Calle MC, et al. Controversies in the current management of lumbar hernias. Arch Surg 2007;142(1):82–8.

[36] Light HG. Hernia of the inferior lumbar space: a cause of back pain. Arch Surg 1983;118: 1077–80.

[37] Salameh JR, Salloum EJ. Lumbar incisional hernias: diagnostic and management dilemma. JSLS 2004;8(4):391–4.

[38] Cavallaro G, Sadighi A, Miceli M, et al. Primary lumbar hernia repair: the open approach. Eur Surg Res 2007;39(2):88–92.

[39] Heniford BT, Iannitti DA, Gagner M. Laparoscopic inferior and superior lumbar hernia repair. Arch Surg 1997;132(10):1141–4.

[40] Postema RR, Bonjer HJ. Endoscopic extraperitoneal repair of a Grynfeltt hernia. Surg Endosc 2002;16(4):716.

[41] Moreno-Egea A, Torralba-Martinez JA, Morales G, et al. Open vs laparoscopic repair of secondary lumbar hernias: a prospective nonrandomized study. Surg Endosc 2005;19(2): 184–7.

[42] Itani KMF. Uncommon abdominal wall hernias. In: Bland KI, editor. The practice of general surgery. 1st edition. Philadelphia: W.B. Saunders Company; 2002. p. 810–3.

[43] Skandalakis LJ, Androulakis J, Colborn GL, et al. Obturator hernia. Embryology, anatomy, and surgical applications. Surg Clin North Am 2000;80(1):71–84.

[44] Kozlowski JM, Beal JM. Obturator hernia: an elusive diagnosis. Arch Surg 1977;112: 1001–2.

[45] Bergstein JM, Condon RE. Obturator hernia: current diagnosis and treatment. Surgery 1996;119(2):133–6.

[46] Yip AW, AhChong AK, Lam KH. Obturator hernia: a continuing diagnostic challenge. Surgery 1993;113:266–9.

[47] Hannington-Kiff JG. Absent thigh adductor reflex in obturator hernia. Lancet 1980;1(8161): 180.

[48] Shapiro K, Patel S, Choy C, et al. Totally extraperitoneal repair of obturator hernia. Surg Endosc 2004;18(6):954–6.

[49] Preiss A, Herbig B, Dörner A. Primary perineal hernia: a case report and review of the literature. Hernia 2006;10(5):430–3.

[50] Skandalakis JE, Gray SW, Burns WB, et al. Internal and external supravesical hernia. Am Surg 1976;42:142–6.

[51] Yu PC, Ko SF, Lee TY, et al. Small bowel obstruction due to incarcerated sciatic hernia: ultrasound diagnosis. Br J Radiol 2002;75(892):381–3.

ELSEVIER
SAUNDERS

SURGICAL
CLINICS OF
NORTH AMERICA

Surg Clin N Am 88 (2008) 61–83

Open Repair of Ventral Incisional Hernias

Dan H. Shell IV, MD[a], Jorge de la Torre, MD[a],*,
Patricio Andrades, MD[a,b], Luis O. Vasconez, MD[a]

[a]Division of Plastic Surgery, University of Alabama at Birmingham,
510 20th Street S, Birmingham, AL 35294-3411, USA
[b]Division of Transplant Immunology, University of Alabama at Birmingham,
510 20th Street S, Birmingham, AL 35294-3411, USA

Incisional hernia is a common and often debilitating complication after laparotomy. Despite significant advances in many areas of surgery, correction of incisional hernias continues to be problematic, with recurrence rates ranging from 5% to 63% depending on the type of repair used [1–8]. Recurrence rates are likely underestimated because of a lack of long-term follow-up and objective criteria in the literature to determine true recurrence.

More than 2 million laparotomies are performed annually in the United States, with a reported 2% to 11% incidence of incisional hernia [1,5,9–11]. It is the most common complication after laparotomy by a 2:1 ratio over bowel obstruction and is the most common indication for reoperation by a 3:1 ratio over adhesive small bowel obstruction [12]. Approximately 100,000 hernia repairs are performed annually in the United States [13]. The associated morbidity secondary to incarceration, strangulation, and bowel obstruction is significant. In a retrospective review of 206 patients who underwent incisional hernia repair, Read and Yoder [9,10] found that strangulation or incarceration was the indication for repair in 17% of patients. The gradual enlargement of the hernia over time results in a relative loss of abdominal domain, with adverse effects on postural maintenance, respiration, micturition, defecation, and biomechanical properties, which have a profound impact on patients' overall physical capacity and quality of life. As patients are forced to alter their lifestyle, their ability to work becomes impaired, which has negative economic consequences. Progressive enlargement of the hernia also results in a cosmetic deformity, which is detrimental to patients' self-esteem.

---

* Corresponding author.
  E-mail address: jdlt@uab.edu (J. de la Torre).

Incisional hernias are the only abdominal hernias that are iatrogenic [10]. Controversy exists regarding the ideal treatment of incisional hernias. Nowhere in surgery does the phrase "if there are multiple ways of fixing a problem then there is not one good way" hold true more so than with incisional hernia repair. The approach to incisional hernia repair is often based on tradition rather than evidence. Several important contributions to the literature in recent years have helped our understanding of the causes of incisional hernia formation and the important physiologic and functional properties of the abdominal wall. An appreciation for the dynamic function of the abdominal wall has led to technical refinements and the recognition of important principles that are necessary for successful repair.

Etiology

Many patient-related risk factors have been implicated in the development of incisional hernias, including obesity, smoking, aneurismal disease, chronic obstructive pulmonary disease, male gender, malnourishment, corticosteroid dependency, renal failure, malignancy, and prostatism [1–8,10,11,14–23]. Many of these risk factors may contribute to the development of an incisional hernia, but no single factor is so regularly associated that it may be declared as serving a truly etiologic role [22].

In a study by Condon and colleagues [21] of complications associated with closure of 1000 midline laparotomies, no single factor was associated with incisional hernia on univariate analysis. On multivariate analysis, only the combination of reopening and reclosing previous incisions coupled with wound infection influenced the development of incisional hernia. Postoperative wound infection has been found in additional studies to be the single most significant prognostic factor in the development of incisional hernia [1,7,10,14,19,21]. Bucknall and colleagues [1] reported a 23% incidence of incisional hernia formation in patients who developed a wound infection.

Obesity often has been cited as a risk factor, with an incisional hernia rate of 15% to 20% [24–26]. In a prospective, randomized evaluation that compared fascial closure techniques, Brolin [24] found a reduction in incisional hernia occurrence from 18% to 10% with the use of double-stranded #1 PDS placed in continuous fashion compared with #1 Ethibond placed in interrupted figure-of-eight fashion. Aneurysmal disease also has been found in multiple studies to be an independent risk factor in the development of incisional hernias [22,27–29]. A recent multicenter, prospective study by Rafetto and colleagues [22] found a 28.2% incidence of incisional hernia formation in patients undergoing surgery for aortic aneurysm repair. After correcting for other risk factors, this figure represents a ninefold increase in the incidence of incisional hernia formation compared with surgery for aortic occlusive disease. It has been suggested that a defect in collagen metabolism with a decreased ratio of type I to type III procollagen may play a role; however, further studies are needed before a causal relationship can be established [22,30].

Incisional hernias differ from other abdominal wall hernias in their iatrogenic origin. Surgeon-related technical errors are responsible for most incisional hernias. Closure under tension results in fascial strangulation and hernia formation. Studies have shown that 50% of hernia recurrences are detected in the first postoperative year, 75% are detected at 2 years, and 90% are detected at 3 years, with continued failure rates of 2% per year thereafter [2,5,6,11]. These findings implicate technical factors in early wound failure and patient-related factors in late wound failure. Playforth and colleagues [31] applied radiopaque staples to the margins of incised fascia. Serial radiographs were taken at time intervals up to 1 year. In patients who developed incisional hernias at 1 year, there was separation of the staples at 1 week postoperatively. This finding supports faulty surgical technique as the primary cause of early wound failure. Poole [32] concluded in a comprehensive review that local technical factors were of greater significance than patient-related conditions in the development of incisional hernias. Given these findings, it is incumbent on surgeons to identify and use appropriate techniques and materials to minimize the incidence of incisional hernias.

Controversy exists regarding the optimal closure material and technique used to avoid incisional hernias. Carlson and colleagues [21] compared the incisional hernia rate of midline, transverse, and paramedian incisions. Midline incisions had the highest hernia rate—10.5% compared with 7.5% with transverse incisions and 2.5% with paramedian incisions. A meta-analysis of randomized, controlled trials that compared suture material and technique found that abdominal fascial closure with nonabsorbable monofilament suture in a continuous fashion had a significantly lower rate of incisional hernia [33]. In work that has been reinforced by others, Jenkins [34–36] found that a suture length-to-incision ratio of 4:1 was optimal for fascial closure. To use this length of suture, bites should encompass 1 cm of tissue at 1-cm intervals with attention to simply approximate the fascia. They also found nonabsorbable suture in continuous fashion to be the material and technique of choice.

Presentation and natural history

Patients typically present with a bulge in a portion of the healed surgical incision. Complaints of dull abdominal discomfort and associated nausea are common and are related to stretching of the bowel mesentery as it protrudes through the defect [10,11]. Bowel obstruction may result from incarceration in the hernia sac but is more often caused by twisting of the bowel around adhesions at the lateral margins of the hernia defect [10,11]. The natural history of incisional hernias is gradual enlargement. The linea alba serves as the midline anchor for the aponeurotic insertions of the rectus sheath and oblique musculature [37]. Disruption results in gradual enlargement of the hernia defect because of unopposed lateral contraction of the oblique musculature. As the hernia defect widens, task-dependent functions of the abdominal wall musculature are interfered with and significant physiologic derangements occur [11,38,39].

The abdominal wall has important functions in respiration. As the hernia defect widens, the diaphragm loses synergy with the abdominal wall, as evidenced by paradoxic abdominal respiratory motion [37]. Puckree and colleagues [39] demonstrated that the internal oblique and transversus abdominus muscles receive neural impulses from central expiratory neurons. Misuri and colleagues [40] demonstrated by ultrasound assessment that the transversus abdominus muscle is a major contributor to the generation of expiratory forces. Trunk motion abnormalities are common in patients with incisional hernias. Myrinkas and colleagues [41] measured stretch reflexes of the rectus abdominus muscles and found that a crossed monosynaptic communication exists between the right and left rectus muscles, which controls trunk flexion and extension. Trunk rotation results from joint contraction of one external oblique and the contralateral internal oblique. Blondeel and colleagues [42] demonstrated in isokinetic dynamometric studies that displacement of the oblique fibers insertions results in statistically significant reductions in trunk rotation.

The abdominal wall plays an important role in posture maintenance and support of the lumbar spine [43–45]. Patients with large incisional hernias often have significant lumbar lordosis and disabling back pain. Children with prune belly syndrome are functionally impaired by the associated scoliosis [45]. Ramirez and colleagues [46] demonstrated complete relief of back pain after repair of large incisional hernias by restoration of midline myofascial continuity. In a study by Toranto [43], resolution of back pain was observed in 24 of 25 patients after wide rectus plication. This resolution is postulated to result from a restoration of the counterbalancing effect of the abdominal wall muscles with the back musculature. The lateral pull of the internal oblique-transversus abdominus musculature on the lumbodorsal fascia is responsible for a reduction in intervertebral joint stress [46].

Expulsive functions are compromised and may become problematic as the hernia enlarges. Contraction of the abdominal wall musculature and generation of intra-abdominal pressure are important in functions such as coughing, micturition, and defecation.

Dermatologic changes may occur as the hernia enlarges. As the overlying skin is stretched, the subcutaneous tissue atrophies and the skin at the apex becomes ischemic, which renders it susceptible to ulceration and infection.

Repair principles

The presence of an incisional hernia is an indication for repair; the hernia will only enlarge in size and lead to progressive physiologic derangements.

The actual size of the hernia is defined by the size of the parietal defect to be repaired, which is often significantly larger than the palpable clinical defect. This includes all secondary hernias and zones of weakened fascia [47]. Multiple repair techniques have been used in the past; however, there is lack of a general consensus regarding the optimal technique. Several important principles have been defined to aid in the surgical approach to this difficult problem [48–51]. The goals of hernia repair should be as follows:

1. Prevention of visceral eventration
2. Incorporation of the remaining abdominal wall in the repair
3. Provision of dynamic muscular support
4. Restoration of abdominal wall continuity in a tension-free manner

The high recurrence rates with primary suture repair have led to an increased use of prosthetic mesh to provide for a "tension-free" repair. This approach has resulted in a decline in recurrence rates; however, mesh-related complications, such as infection, extrusion, and fistula formation, are significant problems. Recent emphasis on the importance of restoration of midline myofascial continuity and dynamic abdominal wall support has led to the application of numerous techniques of autologous reconstruction.

Primary suture repair

Until the 1990s, simple suture repair of incisional hernias was the gold standard. Multiple retrospective studies in the literature have demonstrated high recurrence rates (25%–63%) of primary suture repair of even small (< 5 cm) fascial defects [3,4,7,9,11]. Various techniques have been applied; however, the continued presence of tension at the site of repair has led to high recurrence rates (Table 1). Additional hernias and areas of fascial weakening may not be appreciated by the limited exposure of primary suture repair and may result in future recurrences. In a study of recurrent hernias by Girotto and colleagues [55], 50% of patients were noted to have more than one hernia at the time of exploration.

The high recurrence rates of primary suture repair were supported in a large, prospective, randomized trial by Luijendijk and colleagues [3]. In a study that compared mesh and primary suture repair for incisional hernias smaller than 6 cm in greatest dimension, they found a 46% recurrence rate in the primary suture repair group compared with 23% in the mesh repair group [3]. A long-term follow-up of the study by Burger and colleagues [4] revealed a 10-year cumulative rate of recurrence of 63% for the suture repair group compared with 32% for the mesh repair group, which led the authors to conclude that "primary suture repair of incisional hernias should be completely abandoned." An expert panel on incisional herniorrhaphy concluded that primary suture repair should be used only for small (< 5 cm) hernias and if the repair is oriented horizontally with nonresorbable, monofilament suture with a suture-to-wound length ratio of 4:1 [56].

Table 1
Results of primary suture repair techniques

Author/Year	N	Recurrence (%)	Follow-up (mo)
Langer, et al, 1985 [6]	154	31	48–120
George, et al, 1986 [2]	81	46	14
Van der Linden, et al, 1988 [52]	151	49	39
Read, et al, 1989 [9]	206	24.8	
Gecim, et al, 1996 [15]	109	45	7–92
Luijendijk, et al, 2000 [3]	97	46	36
Burger, et al, 2004 [4]	97	63	120
Sauerland, et al, 2005 [53]	305	18	60
Al-Salamah, et al, 2006 [54]	72	20.8	37.5

Adapted from Cassar K, Munro A. Surgical treatment of incisional hernia. Br J Surg 2002;89:534–45; with permission of Blackwell Science Ltd.

Mesh repair

High recurrence rates associated with primary suture repair have led to an increased application of prosthetic mesh for the repair of incisional hernias. The use of synthetic mesh in incisional hernia repairs increased from 34.2% in 1987 to 65.5% in 1999 [57]. The American Hernia Society has declared that the use of mesh currently represents the standard of care in incisional hernia repair [58]. Placement of mesh allows for a tension-free restoration of the structural integrity of the abdominal wall. Advantages to the use of mesh include availability, absence of donor site morbidity, and strength of the repair [59]. The ideal prosthetic material should be nontoxic, nonimmunogenic, and nonreactive [59,60]. The ultimate goal when using mesh is for it to become incorporated into the surrounding tissues.

Tensile strength is another important property of the synthetic material. Tensile strength of the abdominal wall may be calculated as the product of tension strength according to LaPlace's formula ($\Delta P = 2T/r$) and the area of cross-section of the abdomen [59]. In an average-sized human, the maximum required tensile strength to maintain abdominal closure is 16 N/cm [59]. In general, prosthetic materials have a tensile strength more than 32 N/cm [61]. Rarely is there a true failure of the mesh material. Recurrences seen after mesh repair typically occur laterally at the mesh-tissue interface. The physical properties of this interface are important in determining the ultimate strength and durability of the repair.

The two most commonly used permanent prosthetic materials are polypropylene and expanded polytetrafluoroethylene (ePTFE). Polypropylene was first introduced in the 1950s by Usher [62]. The large pore size of the polypropylene mesh allows for macrophage and neutrophil infiltration, which provides greater resistance to infection. Its porosity also allows for better fibrovascular ingrowth and a reduced incidence of seroma formation [59]. ePTFE (Goretex; W.L. Gore and Associates, Flagstaff, Arizona) has a microporous structure that minimizes cellular infiltration and tissue incorporation. Studies have shown ePTFE prosthesis to be stronger than marlex and equivalent to polypropylene in terms of suture retention strength [63]. As a result of its flexible, soft, and conforming qualities and minimal tissue ingrowth, it can be placed directly on bowel [59]. The disadvantages of ePTFE are related to its microporous structure. The material is virtually impenetrable, which prevents host tissue incorporation and leads to seroma formation. Once infected, ePTFE requires explantation. The micropores range from 3 to 41 μm in size, which are large enough for bacteria (1 μm) to infiltrate but too small for macrophages (> 50 μm) [59].

In an effort to reduce mesh-related complications and more closely duplicate abdominal wall physiology, research has focused on the development of composite materials that combine nonabsorbable and absorbable materials. Well-designed, comparative studies with long-term follow-up are still needed. Knowledge of the structural anatomy and an appreciation of the physiology of the abdominal wall are necessary for successful abdominal wall reconstruction. Recurrence after mesh repair is rarely caused by intrinsic failure of the prosthetic material. Failure to identify healthy fascia and technical error in securing the mesh to the fascia commonly lead to recurrence at the mesh-fascia interface (Table 2).

Several methods of securing the mesh to the fascia have been described, with the most common being mesh onlay, mesh inlay, retrorectus placement, and intraperitoneal underlay. The onlay technique (Fig. 1A) is popular among surgeons because it avoids direct contact with the bowel and imparts less tension on the repair. In a survey of more than 1000 surgeons, Milliken [11] reported that 50% of surgeons use this repair without closing the fascial defect. The disadvantages are that it requires wide tissue undermining, which may predispose to wound-related complications, and that the pressure required to disrupt the mesh from the anterior abdominal wall is less than other repairs. Chevrel and Rath [76,77] reported their results of 389 patients and found a recurrence rate of 18.4% ($n = 153$) without the use of mesh compared with 5.5% ($n = 133$) with the use of polypropylene onlay mesh and 0.97% ($n = 103$) with the use of fibrin glue in addition to the mesh. Their technique consisted of relaxing incisions in the anterior rectus sheath with primary approximation of the linea alba and medial turnover of the anterior rectus sheath followed by mesh placement.

The inlay technique involves excision of the hernia sac and identification of healthy fascial margins (Fig. 1B). This technique provides for a tensionless repair at the time of surgery and avoids the wide undermining of the onlay repair. Without the overlying support of the anterior abdominal wall, activities that increase intra-abdominal pressure impart significant tension to the mesh-fascial interface, which is the weakest point of the repair [76]. High recurrence rates of 10% to 20% have resulted in use of other techniques to optimize strength of the mesh-fascia interface [3,11]. Retrorectus placement of mesh, popularized by Rives and Stoppa, has been used with increasing frequency [11,78,79]. In this technique, the hernia sac is preserved and used as a buffer between the mesh and underlying viscera. The mesh is

Table 2
Results of open mesh repair of incisional hernias

Author	Year	N	Mesh	Technique	Recurrence (%)	Follow-up (mo)
McCarthy, et al [64]	1981	25	Polypropylene	Intraperitoneal 3-cm overlap	8	27
Matapurkar, et al [65]	1991	60	Polpropylene	Extraperitoneal 2-cm overlap	0	36–84
Temudom, et al [66]	1996	50	Polypropylene ePTFE	Extraperitoneal 4- to 6-cm overlap	4	24
Gillion, et al [67]	1997	158	PTFE		4	37
McLanahan, et al [68]	1997	106	Polypropylene	Extraperitoneal 4- to 6-cm overlap	4	24
Balen, et al [69]	1998	45	PTFE	Extraperitoneal 2-cm overlap	2	39
Turkcapar, et al [70]	1998	45	Polypropylene		2	36
Arnaud, et al [71]	1999	250	Dacron	Intraperitoneal 10-cm overlap	3	97
Bauer, et al [72]	1999	98	PTFE	Extraperitoneal	10	72
Utrera Gonzalez, et al [73]	1999	84	PTFE	Intraperitoneal 5- to 7-cm overlap	2	12–36
Chrysos, et al [74]	2000	52	PTFE		8	–
Luijendijk, et al [3]	2000	84	Polypropylene	Extraperitoneal 2- to 4-cm overlap	23	23
Burger, et al [4]	2004	84	Polypropylene	Extraperitoneal 2- to 4-cm overlap	32	120
Martin-Duce, et al [75]	2001	152	Polypropylene	Extraperitoneal	1	72

Adapted from Cassar K, Munro A. Surgical treatment of incisional hernia. Br J Surg 2002;89:534–45; with permission of Blackwell Science Ltd.

placed above the posterior rectus sheath and beneath the rectus muscle (Fig. 1C). Below the arcuate line, the mesh is placed in the preperitoneal space. It is generally recommended to place the mesh with at least 4 cm of contact between the mesh and fascia, which allows for distribution of pressure over a wider area (Pascal's principle), and the pressure-induced apposition promotes fibrous ingrowth at the mesh-fascial interface [59].

It has also been experimentally demonstrated that prolene may shrink up to 30% after implantation [80,81]. By placing the mesh beneath the abdominal wall, the repair is bolstered by the anterior abdominal wall, which provides for a more secure and physiologic repair. Recurrence rates of less than 10% have been reported with this technique [66,68]. Intraperitoneal underlay placement is a common technique used in open and laparoscopic approaches. Proponents of this technique cite that the ability to place the mesh with a large underlay allows for better tissue ingrowth and a more

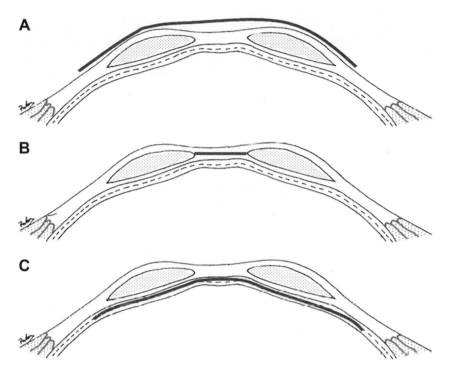

Fig. 1. Mesh placement techniques. (*A*) Onlay technique. (*B*) Inlay technique. (*C*) Retrorectus underlay technique.

secure mesh-fascial interface [11]. Fixation techniques vary from approximation at the fascial margins to full-thickness lateral fixation [82]. Recurrence rates of less than 5% have been reported with this technique [82].

Advances in laparoscopic surgery have led to an increased application of this technology to the treatment of incisional hernias. This technique involves intraperitoneal mesh placement, which is secured with either a tacking device or transabdominal sutures or both. Advocates of this technique cite lower recurrence rates of 2% to 4%, shorter hospital stay, decreased infection rate, and reduced wound complication rates as advantages. Several comparative studies have concluded that it is a superior technique [83–87]. Restoration of dynamic abdominal wall function by midline myofascial approximation and cosmetic improvement of the abdomen by excision of excess tissue and scar are important objectives of hernia repair that are not accomplished by the laparoscopic approach [58].

Although the application of mesh has resulted in a significant improvement in recurrence rates, the use of mesh is associated with specific complications that may range from being relatively minor to life threatening. Infection is one of the most feared complications after mesh placement. The average rate of early and late mesh infections is approximately 7% [8,59,72,88–90] and depends on the type of mesh used. The most common organisms are *Staphyloccocus aureus* and *Staphylococcus epidermidis* [59]. Reports exist in the literature of mesh salvage in the face of infection; however, in most cases mesh removal is required [91]. Law [92] examined the effects of infection on the mesh-fascial interface and found significant weakening, which predisposes to higher recurrence rates. Robertson and colleagues [93–106] demonstrated that isolation of the incision away from the hernia repair through an abdominoplasty approach is associated with lower complication and recurrence rates. It was particularly helpful in obese patients and patients with multiple or recurrent hernias.

Seroma is a common complication after hernia repair and comprises up to 16% of the overall complications [8,88,107]. Reduction of the hernia leaves a potential space for fluid accumulation. Combined with inflammation, disruption of lymphatics, and continued irritation caused by the foreign body reaction from the prosthetic material, this complication results in fluid accumulation [59]. Seromas often resolve with time; however, continued prosthetic irritation may result in persistent seroma requiring surgical drainage.

Inadequate soft tissue coverage may result in mesh extrusion. Less pliable materials, such as marlex, are associated with a higher extrusion rate. When extrusion is noted, most authors agree that mesh removal is indicated. Enteric fistula formation is a potentially devastating complication that occurs when the prosthetic material erodes into the underlying bowel. Leber and colleagues [8] demonstrated that excision of the hernia sac, lack of omental interposition, and the presence of a fascial gap were factors associated with a higher incidence of fistula formation.

Bioprosthetics

Justified concern regarding mesh-related complications has led to the search for more biocompatible prosthetic material. Advances in tissue engineering technology have led to the development of biomaterials derived from human and animal tissues. These materials differ in that they heal by a regenerative process rather than by scar tissue formation. The collagen-based extracellular matrix is preserved, which allows for maintenance of mechanical integrity while providing a scaffold for host tissue regeneration. These materials have demonstrated resistance to infection, tolerance of cutaneous exposure, and mechanical stability when used in incisional hernia repair. Disadvantages are the high cost and lack of long-term follow-up studies.

Components separation technique

A significant contribution to the repair of incisional hernias was the description by Ramirez and colleagues [46] of the components separation technique (Fig. 2). The evolution of the components separation technique is based on early descriptions by Vasconez and colleagues [108] of transverse

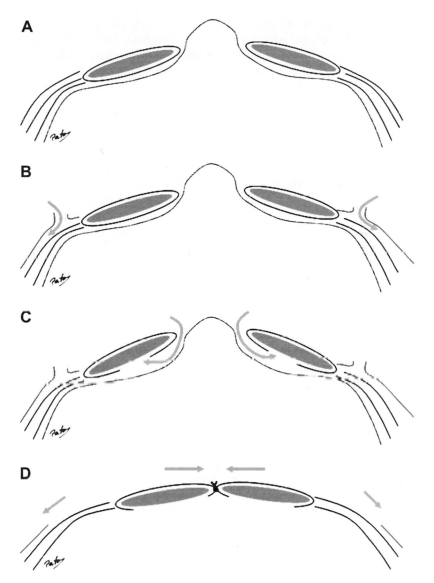

Fig. 2. Components separation technique. (A) The abdominal wall formed by overlapping muscle layers that may be separated. (B) Elevation of the external oblique off the internal oblique. (C) Rectus is released form the posterior sheath. (D) Medial advancement of rectus muscle and attached internal oblique–transversus abdominus complex.

rectus abdominus myocutaneous closure that involves separation of the external and internal oblique musculature and release of the posterior sheath. Ramirez and colleagues [46,51,109,110] noted that the abdominal wall is formed by overlapping muscle layers that may be separated while preserving their innervation and blood supply, specifically, elevation of the external oblique off the internal oblique while maintaining the neurovascular supply to the rectus abdominus, which travels in a segmental fashion between the internal oblique and transversus abdominus. The rectus then can be released from the posterior sheath. Once this procedure is accomplished, medial advancement of a compound flap of rectus muscle and attached internal oblique-transversus abdominus complex can be used to cover large midline abdominal defects. Unilateral advancement of 5 cm in the epigastric region, 10 cm at the umbilicus, and 3 cm in the suprapubic region has been described. Fabian and colleagues [111,112] described a modification that involved division of the internal oblique of the anterior rectus sheath, which allowed for unilateral advancement of 8 to 10 cm in the epigastric area, 10 to 15 cm in the mid abdomen, and 6 to 8 cm in the suprapubic region. A lower hernia recurrence rate, avoidance of prosthetic material, restoration of dynamic abdominal wall function, and improvement in back and postural abnormalities have been cited in the literature (Table 3). Wound-related complications have been problematic with this technique and are related to the wide undermining required. Recent work has demonstrated a reduction in wound-related complications with preservation of periumbilical perforators [121].

In a recent review, Ramirez [110] attributed the success of the procedure to five principles:

1. Translation of the muscular layer of the abdominal wall to enlarge the tissue surface area.
2. Separation of muscle layers that allows for maximal individual expansion of each muscle unit.
3. Disconnection of the muscle unit from its fascial sheath envelope, which restricts horizontal motion and thereby facilitates expansion.
4. Abdominal wall musculature in approximately 70% of its surface is covering hollow viscus, which is more easily compressed than solid structures.
5. Bilateral mobilization works more efficiently than unilateral advancement by equilibrating forces of the abdominal wall and centralizing the midline.

Flap reconstruction

Local and distant flaps have been used to reconstruct hernia defects in which there is significant absolute loss of domain and in lateral defects that are not amenable to advancement techniques. Fasciocutaneous flaps may be used to reconstruct partial-thickness defects of the skin and subcutaneous tissues and full-thickness defects when used in combination with mesh. The thoracoepigastric flap is useful for defects of the upper third of the abdominal wall. The iliolumbar bipedicled flap based on the superficial circumflex iliac and lumbar perforators may be used for middle third

Table 3
Results of components separation technique

Author/year	n	Mean follow-up (mo)	Recurrence n (%)
Hultman, et al, 2005 [113]	13[a]	11.5	2 (15)
Vargo, et al, 2004 [114]	27[b]	6–27	2 (7)
Howdieshell, et al, 2004 [115]	18[c]	48	2 (11)
Lowe, et al, 2003 [116]	30	9.5	3 (10)
Lindsey, et al, 2003 [117]	10[d]	18.6	1 (10)
Jernigan, et al, 2003 [112]	73[e]	24	4 (5)
Girotto, et al, 2003 [55]	96[f]	26	21 (22)
Ewart, et al, 2003 [118]	11[g]	10	1 (9)
de vries Reilingh, et al, 2003 [119,120]	38	15.6	12 (32)
Saulis, et al, 2002 [121]	66[h]	12	3 (8)
Maas, et al, 2002 [122]	5[i]	10.6	1 (20)
Sukkar, et al, 2001 [123]	47[j]	24	1 (2)
Voigt, et al, 2001 [124]	9	14.2	0
Levine, et al, 2001 [125]	10[k]	?	0
Cohen, et al, 2001 [126]	29[l]	12–36	1 (3)
Shestak, et al, 2000 [109]	22[m]	52	1 (5)
Mathes, et al, 2000 [127]	26[n]	13.7	4 (15)
Lowe, et al, 2000 [128]	37[o]	12	4 (11)
Girotto, et al, 2000 [129]	20[p]	25.7	1 (5)
Maas, et al, 1999 [130]	4[q]	18	0
Girotto, et al, 1999 [131]	37	21	2 (5)
Kuzbari, et al, 1998 [132]	10[r]	28.8	0
Dibello, et al, 1996 [50]	35[s]	22	3 (9)
Fabian, et al, 1994 [111]	9[t]	11	1 (11)
Thomas, et al, 1993 [133]	7[u]	18	0
Ramirez, et al, 1990 [46]	11	4–12	0

[a] Component separation (CS) alone = 3, CS + mesh = 5, CS + mesh/Alloderm onlay = 5.

[b] CS = 23, CS + mesh = 2, CS + surgisis = 2.

[c] CS = 12, CS + subfascial tissue expansion (TE) = 6.

[d] Abdominal wall partitioning (accordion), staggered release of tranversalis/external oblique.

[e] Modified = internal oblique divided, approximation of medial border of posterior sheath to lateral border of anterior sheath.

[f] Mesh onlay when necessary.

[g] CS = 4, CS + TE = 3, CS + mesh onlay = 4; modified = rectus sheath incised anteriorly and/or posteriorly or flipped medially (open book) and transversalis incised.

[h] Standard CS = 25, modified (periumbilical perforator preservation) = 41.

[i] Endoscopically assisted.

[j] CS = 41, CS + fascia lata graft = 6, modified periumbilical perforator preservation.

[k] CS = 9, CS + mesh onlay = 1, modified (±) internal oblique release.

[l] CS = 24, CS + Goretex graft = 4, CS + lateral abdominal wall flap = 1.

[m] CS = 21, CS + mesh = 1.

[n] ± Mesh.

[o] CS = 20, CS + mesh = 10, endoscopically assisted = 6, endoscopically assisted + mesh = 1.

[p] CS = 8, CS + mesh onlay = 12.

[q] Modified = external oblique transected via separate lateral incision.

[r] Modified = complete rectus release from anterior and posterior sheaths.

[s] CS = 20, CS + vicryl onlay = 12, CS + Goretex onlay = 3.

[t] Modified = internal oblique divided, approximation of medial border of posterior sheath to lateral border of anterior sheath.

[u] CS = 7, CS + transversalis division = 2.

From Nguyen V, Shestak KC. Separation of anatomic components method of abdominal wall reconstruction: clinical outcome analysis and an update of surgical modifications using the technique. Clin Plastic Surg 2006;33:255; with permission.

defects. Lower third defects may be covered with a groin flap, which may reach to the umbilicus [49,127,134–137]. Superficial inferior epigastric artery and deep inferior epigastric artery flaps are useful for lower abdominal and groin defects [134,138–140].

Local muscle flaps are useful for musculofascial defects of the lateral abdominal wall (Fig. 3). The rectus abdominus is a commonly used pedicled flap based on either the superior epigastric or deep inferior epigastric arteries. The flap has a large arc of rotation capable of reaching the entire abdomen [134,135,141,142]. The rectus also may be separated completely from the posterior rectus sheath and turned medially based on a medial row of perforators to reconstruct midline defects. This technique has a reported 13% recurrence rate and a 25% incidence of local wound complications [143].

The external oblique flap based on lateral cutaneous branches of the posterior intercostal arteries has been used as a rotational flap to cover upper abdominal wall defects and as an advancement flap to cover paramedian defects. Spear and colleagues [144] reported a 3% recurrence rate at 12-month follow-up with the use of this flap.

Distant muscle flaps as either free flaps or pedicled flaps have been used for musculofascial defects not amenable to closure with local flaps or advancement techniques [145,146]. The tensor fascia lata has been used successfully as a pedicled and free flap and as an autologous fascial patch. It is based on the ascending branch of the lateral femoral circumflex artery and may be used as a muscle, fascial, or fasciocutaneous flap [145,146]. It has the advantage of being dispensable and has a good arc of rotation. It does not provide for a dynamic reconstruction, and its distal third is unreliable with a 20% to 25% rate of necrosis. Its use is complicated by a 15% to 20% incidence of donor site morbidity, including hematoma, seroma, skin

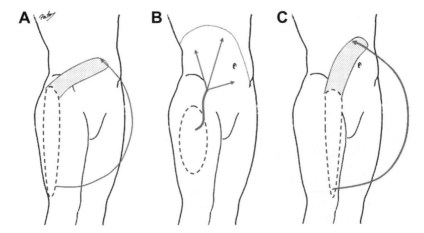

Fig. 3. Flaps in abdominal wall reconstruction. (*A*) Tensor fascia lata. (*B*) Anterolateral thigh. (*C*) Rectus femoris.

graft loss, and lateral knee instability [145,146]. Recurrence rates are also significant and range from 9% to 42% in the literature [145,146].

The anterolateral thigh flap has been used in the reconstruction of lower abdominal wall defects as either a free or pedicled flap based on septocutaneous perforating branches of the transverse and deep branches of the lateral femoral circumflex artery [147]. With the adjunctive use of mesh, this technique has demonstrated low recurrence rates in small series. It also may be used in combination with the tensor fascia lata to provide a composite graft up to 35 × 20 cm in dimension. In small series, the use of this technique has demonstrated no recurrences or flap loss in follow-up up to 24 months [134,147,148].

The rectus femoris muscle has been used successfully as either a free flap with preservation of the motor nerve or as a pedicled flap in reconstruction of the lower two thirds of the abdomen. It is a dispensable muscle with a consistent anatomy. Reports have indicated a weakness in terminal knee extension after muscle harvest, which can be minimized by approximating the vastus medialis and lateralis. It is based on the lateral femoral circumflex artery and has a large arc of superior and contralateral rotation. It can be designed as a musculofascial or musculofasciocutaneous flap based on the location and extent of the defect [149–151]. Electromyographic studies have documented motor function of the transferred muscle.

The latissimus dorsi muscle has been used as a musculocutaneous flap for defects of the upper third of the abdomen. It is based on the thoracodorsal pedicle and can be designed as either a pedicled or a free flap. As a pedicled flap, its arc of rotation is limited to coverage of upper abdominal wall defects. The area of coverage can be increased by including the pregluteal and lumbodorsal fascia. In 1979, Bostwick [152] reported the use of the latissimus as a free flap for abdominal wall reconstruction. In 1998, Ninkovic [153] reported the use of a free, innervated latissimus flap in conjunction with prolene mesh for abdominal wall reconstruction. No flap failures were reported, and electromyographic testing demonstrated reinnervation of the muscle.

The gracilis muscle has been used to reconstruct lower third abdominal wall defects. It is a thin, narrow, dispensable muscle based on the ascending branch of the medial circumflex femoral artery. It can be designed as either a muscular or musculofasciocutaneous flap and is limited to small defects because of its size and the poor reliability of its distal skin [154]. The vastus lateralis can be used as a muscular flap for reconstruction of lower third abdominal wall defects. It does not have a fascial component and its use is primarily reserved for salvage situations [155].

Tissue expansion

Tissue expansion has been used to provide well-vascularized, autologous, innervated tissue for abdominal wall reconstruction. Its use has been demonstrated in the reconstruction of congenital defects and large hernias [156–161]. Expanders may be placed in either the subcutaneous or intermuscular plane. Placement in the avascular plane between the external and internal oblique muscles allows superficial expansion of the external oblique and deep expansion of the internal oblique-tranversus abdominus musculofascial layer while preserving innervation and blood supply. Hobar and colleagues [157,158] demonstrated an approximate doubling of the layers of the anterior abdominal wall with normal function and clinically demonstrated innervated composite reconstruction of defects exceeding 50% of the abdominal surface.

Summary

Despite advances in many fields of surgery, incisional hernias still remain a significant problem. There is a lack of general consensus among surgeons regarding optimal treatment. A surgeon's approach is often based on tradition rather than clinical evidence. The surgeon's treatment plan should be comprehensive, with attention focused not merely on restoration of structural continuity. An understanding of the structural and functional anatomy of the abdominal wall and an appreciation of the importance of restoring dynamic function are necessary for the successful reconstruction of the abdominal wall.

References

[1] Bucknall TE, Cox PJ, Ellis H. Burst abdomen and incisional hernia: a prospective study of 1129 major laparotomies. Br Med J (Clin Res Ed) 1982;284(6364):519–20.
[2] George CD, Ellis H. The results of incisional hernia repair: a twelve year review. Ann R Coll Surg Engl 1986 Jul;68(4):185–7.
[3] Luijendijk RW, Hop WC, Van den Tol MP, et al. A comparison of suture repair with mesh repair for incisional hernia. N Engl J Med 2000;343(6):392–8.
[4] Burger JW, Luijendijk RW, Hop WC, et al. Long term follow up of a randomized controlled trial of suture versus mesh repair of incisonal hernia. Ann Surg 2004;240(4): 578–83 [discussion: 583–5].
[5] Mudge M, Hughes LE. Incisional hernia: a ten year prospective study of incidence and attitudes. Br J Surg 1985;72:70–1.
[6] Langer S, Christiansen J. Long-term results after incisional hernia repair. Acta Chir Scand 1985;151:217–9.
[7] Anthony T, Bergen PC, Kim LT. Factors affecting recurrence following incisional herniorrhaphy. World J Surg 2000;24(1):95–101.
[8] Leber GE, Garb JL, Alexander AJ, et al. Long term complications associated with prosthetic repair of incisional hernias. Arch Surg 1998;133(4):378–82.
[9] Read RC, Yoder G. Recent trends in management of incisional herniation. Arch Surg 1989; 124:485–8.
[10] Santora TA, Rosalyn JJ. Incisional hernia. Surg Clin North Am 1993;73:557–70.
[11] Millikan KW. Incisional hernia repair. Surg Clin North Am 2003;83:1223–34.

[12] Duepree HJ, Senagore AJ, Delaney CP, et al. Does means of access affect the incidence of small bowel obstruction and ventral hernia after bowel resection? Laparoscopy versus laparotomy. J Am Coll Surg 2003;197(2):177–81.

[13] Rutkow IM. Epidemiologic, economic and sociologic aspects of hernia surgery in the United States in the 1990s. Surg Clin North Am 1998;78:941–51.

[14] Hesselink VJ, Luijendijk RW, De Wilt JH, et al. An evaluation of risk factors in incisional hernia recurrence. Surg Gynecol Obstet 1993;176(3):228–34.

[15] Gecim IE, Kocak S, Ersoz S, et al. Recurrence after incisional hernia repair: results and risk factors. Surg Today 1996;26(8):607–9.

[16] Sorenson LT, Hemmingsen UB, Kirkeby LT, et al. Smoking is a risk factor for incisional hernia. Arch Surg 2005;140(2):119–23.

[17] Sugerman HJ, Kellum JM Jr, Reines HD, et al. Greater risk of incisional hernia with morbidly obese than steroid-dependent patients and low recurrence with prefascial polypropylene mesh. Am J Surg 1996;171(1):80–4.

[18] Koller R, Miholic J, Jakl RJ. Repair of incisional hernias with polytetrafluoroethylene. Eur J Surg 1997;163(4):261–6.

[19] Lamont PM, Ellis H. Incisional hernia in re-opened abdomens: an overlooked risk factor. Br J Surg 1988;75(4):374–6.

[20] Makela JT, Kiviniemi H, Juvonen T, et al. Factors influencing wound dehiscence after midline laparotomy. Am J Surg 1995;170(4):387–90.

[21] Carlson MA, Ludwig KA, Condon RE. Ventral hernia and other complications of 1,000 midline laparotomies. South Med J 1995;88(4):450–3.

[22] Raffetto JD, Cheung Y, Fisher JB, et al. Incision and abdominal wall hernias in patients with aneurysm or occlusive aortic disease. J Vasc Surg 2003;37:1150–4.

[23] Condon RE. Ventral abdominal hernia. In: Baker RJ, Fischer JE, editors. Mastery of surgery. 4th edition. Philadelphia: Lippincott Williams & Wilkins; 2001.

[24] Brolin RE. Prospective, randomized evaluation of midline fascial closure in gastric bypass operations. Am J Surg 1996;172(4):328–31.

[25] Thompson WR, Amaral JF, Caldwell MD, et al. Complications and weight loss in 150 consecutive gastric exclusion patients: critical review. Am J Surg 1983;146(5):602–12.

[26] Yale CE. Gastric surgery for morbid obesity: complications and long-term weight control. Arch Surg 1989;124(8):941–6.

[27] Adye B, Luna G. Incidence of abdominal wall hernia in aortic surgery. Am J Surg 1998; 175(5):400–2.

[28] Stevick CA, Long JB, Jamasbi B, et al. Ventral hernia following abdominal aortic reconstruction. Am Surg 1988;54(5):287–9.

[29] Johnson B, Sharp R, Thursby P. Incisional hernias: incidence following abdominal aortic aneurysm repair. J Cardiovasc Surg (Torino) 1995;36(5):487–90.

[30] Si Z, Bhardwaj R, Rosch R, et al. Impaired balance of type I and type III procollagen mRNA in cultured fibroblasts of patients with incisional hernia. Surgery 2002;131(3): 324–31.

[31] Playforth MJ, Sauven PD, Evans M, et al. The prediction of incisional hernia by radio-opaque markers. Ann R Coll Surg Engl 1986;68(2):82–4.

[32] Poole GV Jr. Mechanical factors in abdominal wound closure: the prevention of fascial dehiscence. Surgery 1985;97(6):631–40.

[33] Hodgson NC, Malthaner RA, Østbye T. The search for an ideal method of fascial closure: a meta-analysis. Ann Surg 2000;231(3):436–42.

[34] Jenkins TP. The burst abdominal wound: a mechanical approach. Br J Surg 1976;63(11): 873–6.

[35] Trimbos JB, van Rooij J. Amount of suture material needed for continuous or interrupted wound closure: an experimental study. Eur J Surg 1993;159(3):141–3.

[36] Cassar K, Munro A. Surgical treatment of incisional hernia. Br J Surg 2002;89:534–45.

[37] Abrahamson J, Eldar S. Abdominal incision. Lancet 1989;1(8642):847.

[38] Grevious MA, Cohen M, Shah SR, et al. Structural and functional anatomy of the abdominal wall. Clin Plast Surg 2006;33:169–79.

[39] Puckree T, Cerny F, Bishop B. Abdominal motor unit activity during respiratory and non-respiratory tasks. J Appl Physiol 1998;84(5):1707–15.

[40] Misuri G, Colagrande S, Gorini M. In vivo ultrasound assessment of respiratory function of abdominal muscles in normal subjects. Eur Respir J 1997;10(12):2861–7.

[41] Myrinkas SE, Beith ID, Harrison PJ. Stretch reflexes in the rectus abdominus muscle in man. Exp Physiol 2000;85(4):445–50.

[42] Blondeel N, Vanderstraeten GG, Monstrey SJ. The donor site morbidity of free DIEP flaps and free TRAM flaps in breast reconstruction. Br J Plast Surg 1997;50(5):322–30.

[43] Toranto IR. Resolution of back pain with wide abdominal rectus plication abdominoplasty. Plast Reconstr Surg 1990;85(4):545–55.

[44] Gracovetsky S, Farfan H, Helleur C. The abdominal mechanism. Spine 1985;10(4):317–24.

[45] Lam KS, Mehdian H. The importance of an intact abdominal musculature mechanism in maintaining spinal sagittal balance: case illustration in prune-belly syndrome. Spine 1999;24(7):712–22.

[46] Ramirez OM, Ruas E, Dellon L. "Components separation" method for closure of abdominal-wall defects: an anatomic and clinical study. Plast Reconstr Surg 1990;86(3):521–6.

[47] Wantz GE. Incisional hernia: the problem and the cure. J Am Coll Surg 1999;188(4):433–47.

[48] Core GB, Grotting JC. Reoperative surgery of the abdominal wall. In: Grotting JC, editor. Aesthetic and reconstructive plastic surgery. St Louis (MO): Quality Medical Publishing, Incorporated; 1995. p. 1327–75.

[49] Rohrich RJ, Lowe JB, Baty JD, et al. An algorithm for abdominal wall reconstruction. Plast Reconstr Surg 2000;105(1):202–16.

[50] DiBello JN Jr, Moore JH Jr. Sliding myofascial flap of rectus abdominus muscles for the closure of recurrent ventral hernias. Plast Reconstr Surg 1996;98(3):464–9.

[51] Nguyen V, Shestak KC. Separation of anatomic components method of abdominal wall reconstruction: clinical outcome analysis and an update of surgical modifications using the technique. Clin Plast Surg 2006;33:247–57.

[52] Van der Linden FT, van Vroonhoven TJ. Long term results after surgical correction of incisional hernia. Neth J Surg 1988;40:127–43.

[53] Sauerland S, Schmedt CG, Lein S, et al. Primary incisional hernia repair with or without polypropylene mesh: a report on 384 patients with 5 year follow up. Langenbecks Arch Surg 2005;390(5):408–12.

[54] Al-Salamah SM, Hussain MI, Khalid K, et al. Suture vs mesh repair for incisional hernia. Saudi Med J 2006;27(5):652–6.

[55] Girotto JA, Chiaramonte M, Menon NG, et al. Recalcitrant abdominal wall hernias: long term results of autologous tissue repair. Plast Reconstr Surg 2003;112(1):106–14.

[56] Korenkov M, Paul A, Sauerland S, et al. Classification and surgical treatment: results of an experts' meeting. Langenbecks Arch Surg 2001;386:65–73.

[57] Flum DR, Horvath K, Koepsell T. Have outcomes with incisional hernia repair improved with time? A population-based analysis. Ann Surg 2003;237(1):129–35.

[58] Voeller GR, Ramshaw B, Park AE, et al. Incisional hernia. J Am Coll Surg 1999;189(6):635–7.

[59] Grevious MA, Cohen M, Jean-Pierre F, et al. The use of prosthetics in abdominal wall reconstruction. Clin Plast Surg 2006;33:181–97.

[60] Klosterhalfen B, Rosch R, Junge K. Long term inertness of meshes. In: Schumpelick NL, editor. Meshes: benefits and risks. Berlin: Springer; 2004. p. 170–8.

[61] Cobb WS, Kercher KW, Heniford BT. The argument for lightweight polypropylene mesh in hernia repair. Surg Innov 2005;12(1):T1–7.

[62] Usher FC, Ochsner J, Tuttle Jr LL. Use of Marlex mesh in the repair of incisional hernias. Am Surg 1958;24:969–74.

[63] Stelzner F. Function of the abdominal wall and development and therapy of hernias. Langenbecks Arch Chir 1994;379(2):109–19.

[64] McCarthy JD, Twiest MW. Intraperitoneal polypropylene mesh support of incisional herniorrhaphy. Am J Surg 1981;142:707–11.

[65] Matapurkar BG, Gupta AK, Agarwal AK. A new technique of "marlex peritoneal sandwich" in the repair of large incisional hernias. World J Surg 1991;15:768–70.

[66] Temudom T, Siadati M, Sarr MG. Repair of complex giant or recurrent ventral hernias by using tension-free intraparietal prosthetic mesh (Stoppa technique): lessons learned from our initial experience (fifty patients). Surgery 1996;120:738–43.

[67] Gillion JF, Begin GF, Marecos C, et al. Expanded polytetrafluoroethylene patches used in the intraperitoneal or extraperitoneal position for repair on incisional hernias of the anterolateral abdominal wall. Am J Surg 1997;174:16–9.

[68] McLanahan D, King LT, Weems C, et al. Retrorectus prosthetic mesh repair of midline abdominal hernia. Am J Surg 1997;173:445–9.

[69] Balen EM, Diez-Caballero A, Hernandez-Lizoain JL, et al. Repair of ventral hernias using expanded polytetrafluoroethylene patch. Br J Surg 1998;85:1415–8.

[70] Turkcapar AG, Yerdel MA, Aydinuraz K, et al. Repair of midline incisional hernias using polypropylene grafts. Surg Today 1998;28:59–63.

[71] Arnaud JP, Tuech JJ, Pessaux P, et al. Surgical treatment of postoperative incisional hernia by intraperitoneal insertion of Dacron mesh and an aponeurotic graft: a report of 250 cases. Arch Surg 1999;134:1260–2.

[72] Bauer JJ, Kreel I, Gelernt IM. Twelve year experience with expanded polytetrafluoroethylene in the repair of abdominal defects. Mt Sinai Med J 1999;66(1):20–5.

[73] Utrera Gonzalez A, de la Portilla de Juan F, Carranza Albarran G. Large incisional hernia repair using intraperitoneal placement of expanded polytetrafluoroethylene. Am J Surg 1999;177:291–3.

[74] Chrysos E, Athanasakis E, Saridaki Z, et al. Surgical repair of incisional ventral hernias: tension free technique using prosthetic materials (expanded polytetrafluoroethylene Goretex dual mesh). Am Surg 2000;66:679–82.

[75] Martin-Duce A, Noguerales F, Villeta R, et al. Modifications to Rives technique for midline incisional hernia repair. Hernia 2001;5:70–2.

[76] Chevrel JP, Rath AM. The use of fibrin glues in the surgical treatment of incisional hernias. Hernia 1997;1:9–14.

[77] Larson GM. Plastic mesh repair of incisional hernias. Am J Surg 1978;135:559–63.

[78] Stoppe RE. Treatment of complicated groin and incisional hernias. World J Surg 1989;13: 545–54.

[79] Rives J, Pire JC, Flement JP, et al. Major incisional hernia. In: Chevrel JP, editor. Surgery of the abdominal wall. New York: Springer-Verlag; 1987. p. 116–44.

[80] Klinge U, Klosterhalfen B, Conze J, et al. Modified mesh for hernia repair that is adapted to the physiology of the abdominal wall. Eur J Surg 1998;164(12):951–60.

[81] Klinge U, Conze B, Klosterhalfen B, et al. Changes in abdominal wall mechanics after mesh implantation: experimental changes in mesh stability. Langenbecks Arch Chir 1996;381(6): 323–32.

[82] Millikan KW, Baptista M, Amin B, et al. Intraperitoneal underlay ventral hernia repair utilizing bilayer ePTFE and polypropylene mesh. Am Surg 2003;69:258–63.

[83] Carbajo MA, Martin del Olmo JC, Blanco JI, et al. Laparoscopic treatment versus open surgery in the solution of major incisional and abdominal wall hernias with mesh. Surg Endosc 1999;13:250–2.

[84] Ramshaw BJ, Schwab J, Mason EM, et al. Comparison of laparoscopic and open ventral herniorrhaphy. Am Surg 1999;65:827–31.

[85] Park A, Burch DW, Lovrics P. Laparoscopic and open incisional hernioplasty. Surg Endosc 1997;11:32–5.

[86] Heniford BT, Park A, Ramshaw BJ, et al. Laparoscopic ventral and incisional hernia repair in 407 patients. J Am Coll Surg 2000;190:645–50.

[87] Heniford BT, Park A, Ramshaw BJ, et al. Laparoscopic repair of ventral hernias: nine years' experience with 850 consecutive cases. Ann Surg 2003;238:391–400.

[88] Cobb W IV, Harris JB, Lokey JS, et al. Incisional herniorrhaphy with intraperitoneal composite mesh: a report of 95 cases. Am Surg 2003;69(9):784–7.

[89] Carlson G, et al. Abdominal wall reconstruction. In: Achauer BM, Eriksson E, Guturon B, editors. Plastic surgery: indications, operations, and outcomes. St Louis (MO): Mosby; 2004. p. 563–74.

[90] Jones JW, Jurkovich GJ. Polypropylene mesh closure of infected abdominal wounds. Am Surg 1989;55:73–6.

[91] Kelly ME, Behrman SW. The safety and efficacy of prosthetic hernia repair in clean-contaminated and contaminated wounds. Am Surg 2002;68(6):524–8 [discussion: 528–9].

[92] Law NW. A comparison of polypropylene mesh and expanded polytetrafluoroethylene for repair of contaminated abdominal wall defects: an experimental study. Surgery 1991; 109(5):652–5.

[93] Robertson JD, de la Torre JI, Gardner PM, et al. Abdominoplasty repair for abdominal wall hernias. Ann Plast Surg 2003;51:10–6.

[94] Badylak SF, Kokini K, Tullius B, et al. Morphologic study of small intestinal submucosa as a body wall repair device. J Surg Res 2002;103:190–202.

[95] Buinewicz B, Rosen B. Acellular cadaveric dermis (Alloderm): a new alternative for abdominal hernia repair. Ann Plast Surg 2004;52:188–94.

[96] Butler CE, Langstein HN, Kornowitz SJ. Pelvic, abdominal, and chest wall reconstruction with Alloderm in patients at increased risk for mesh-related complications. Plast Reconstr Surg 2005;116:1263–75.

[97] Espinosa-de-los-Monteros A, de la Torre JI, Marrero I, et al. Utilization of human cadaveric acellular dermis for abdominal hernia reconstruction. Ann Plast Surg 2007;58: 264–7.

[98] Adedeji OA, Bailey CA, Varma JS. Porcine dermal collagen graft in abdominal wall reconstruction. Br J Plast Surg 2002;55:85–6.

[99] Shell DH 4th, Croce MA, Cagiannos C, et al. Comparison of small-intestinal submucosa and expanded polytetrafluoroethylene as a vascular conduit in the presence of gram-positive contamination. Ann Surg 2005;241(6):995–1001 [discussion: 1001–4].

[100] Jernigan TW, Croce MA, Cagiannos C. Small intestinal submucosa for vascular reconstruction in the presence of gastrointestinal contamination. Ann Surg 2004;239(5):733–8 [discussion: 738–40].

[101] Butler CE. The role of bioprosthetics in abdominal wall reconstruction. Clin Plast Surg 2006;33:199–211.

[102] Ueno T, Pickett LC, de la Fuente SG, et al. Clinical application of porcine small intestinal submucosa in the management of infected or potentially contaminated abdominal defects. J Gastrointest Surg 2004;8:109–12.

[103] Helton WS, Fisichella PM, Berger R, et al. Short term outcomes with small intestinal submucosa for ventral abdominal hernia. Arch Surg 2005;140:549–62.

[104] Choe JM, Kothandapani R, James L, et al. Autologous, cadaveric, and synthetic materials used in sling surgery: comparative biomechanical analysis. Urology 2001;58: 482–6.

[105] Silverman RP, Li EN, Holton LH III, et al. Ventral hernia repair using allogenic acellular dermal matrix in a swine model. Hernia 2004;8:336–42.

[106] Butler CE, Prieto VG. Reduction of adhesions with composite Alloderm/polypropylene mesh implants for abdominal wall reconstruction. Plast Reconstr Surg 2004;114:464–73.

[107] Balique JG, Bouillot JL, Flament JB, et al. Intraperitoneal treatment of incisional and umbilical hernias using an innovative composite mesh: four year results of a prospective multicenter clinical trial. Hernia 2005;9:68–74.

[108] Vasconez LO, Lejour M, Gamboa-Babadilla M. Atlas of breast reconstruction. Philadelphia: JB Lippincott; 1991.

[109] Shestak KC, Edington HJ, Johnson RR. The separation of anatomic components technique for the reconstruction of massive midline abdominal wall defects: anatomy, surgical technique, applications, and limitations revisited. Plast Reconstr Surg 2000;105(2):731–8.

[110] Ramirez OM. Inception and evolution of the components separation technique: personal recollections. Clin Plast Surg 2006;33:241–6.

[111] Fabian TC, Croce MA, Pritchard FE. Planned ventral hernia: staged management for acute abdominal wall defects. Ann Surg 1994;219(6):643–50 [discussion: 651].

[112] Jernigan TW, Fabian TC, Croce MA. Staged management of giant abdominal wall defects: acute and long term results. Ann Surg 2003;238(3):349–55.

[113] Hultman CS, Pratt B, Cairns BA. Multi-disciplinary approach to abdominal wall reconstruction after decompressive laparotomy for abdominal compartment syndrome. Ann Plast Surg 2005;54(3):269–75.

[114] Vargo D. Component separation in the management of the difficult abdominal wall. Am J Surg 2004;188(6):633–7.

[115] Howdieshell TR, Proctor CD, Sternberg E. Temporary abdominal closure followed by definitive abdominal wall reconstruction of the open abdomen. Am J Surg 2004;188(3):301–6.

[116] Lowe JB III, Lowe JB, Baty JD. Risks associated with components separation for closure of complex abdominal wall defects. Plast Reconstr Surg 2003;111(3):1276–83 [discussion: 1286–8].

[117] Lindsey JT. Abdominal wall partitioning (the accordion effect) for reconstruction of major defects: a retrospective review of 10 patients. Plast Reconstr Surg 2003;112(2):477–85.

[118] Ewart CJ, Lankford AB, Gamboa MG. Successful closure of abdominal wall hernias using the components separation technique. Ann Plast Surg 2003;50(3):269–73 [discussion: 273–4]

[119] de Vries Reilegh TS. Components separation technique for the repair of large abdominal wall hernias. J Am Coll Surg 2003;196(1):32–7.

[120] Losanoff JE, Richman BW, Sauter ER. Component separation method for abdominal wall reconstruction. J Am Coll Surg 2003;196(5):825–6.

[121] Saulis AS, Dumanian GA. Periumbilical rectus abdominis perforator preservation significantly reduces superficial wound complications in separation of parts hernia repair. Plast Reconstr Surg 2002;109(7):2275–80 [discussion: 2281–2].

[122] Maas SM, van Engel M, Leeksma NG. A modification of the components separation technique for the repair of complicated ventral hernias. J Am Coll Surg 2002;194(3):388–90.

[123] Sukkar SM, Dumanian GA, Szczerba SM. Challenging abdominal wall defects. Am J Surg 2001;181(2):115–21.

[124] Voigt M, Andree C, Galla TJ. Reconstruction of abdominal wall midline defects: the abdominal wall components separation. Zentralbl Chir 2001;126(12):1000–4.

[125] Levine JP, Karp NS. Restoration of abdominal wall integrity as a salvage procedure in difficult recurrent abdominal wall hernias using a method of wide myofascial release. Plast Reconstr Surg 2001;107(3):706–17.

[126] Cohen M, Morales R Jr, Fildes J. Staged reconstruction after gunshot wounds to the abdomen. Plast Reconstr Surg 2001;108(1):83–92.

[127] Mathes SJ, Steinwald PM, Foster RD, et al. Complex abdominal wall reconstruction: a comparison of flap and mesh closure. Ann Surg 2000;232(4):586–96.

[128] Lowe JB, Garza IR, Bowman JL. Endoscopically assisted components separation technique for closure of abdominal wall defects. Plast Reconstr Surg 2000;105(2):720–9.

[129] Girotto JA, Malaisrie SC, Bulkely G. Recurrent ventral herniation in Ehlers-Danlos syndrome. Plast Reconstr Surg 2000;106(7):1520–6.

[130] Maas SM, van Engel M, Leeksma NG. A modification of the components separation technique for closure of abdominal wall defects in the presence of an enterostomy. J Am Coll Surg 1999;189(1):138–40.

[131] Girotto JA, Ko MJ, Redett R. Closure of chronic abdominal wall defects: a long term evaluation of the components separation method. Ann Plast Surg 1999;42(4):385–94.
[132] Kuzbari R, Worseg AP, Tairych G. Sliding door technique for the repair of midline incisional hernias. Plast Reconstr Surg 1998;101(5):1235–42.
[133] Thomas WO III, Parry SW, Rodning CB. Ventral/incisional abdominal herniorrhaphy by fascial partition/release. Plast Reconstr Surg 1993;91(6):1080–6.
[134] Lowe JB. Updated algorithm for abdominal wall reconstruction. Clin Plast Surg 2006;33: 225–40.
[135] Mathes SJ, Nahai F. Clinical application of muscle and musculocutaneous flaps. St Louis (MO): Mosby; 1982.
[136] Mathes SJ, Nahai F. Reconstructive surgery: principles, anatomy, and technique. New York: Churchill Livingstone; 1997.
[137] Ohtsuka H, Ochi K, Seike H. Reconstruction of a large lateral abdominal wall defect with an iliolumbar bipedicled flap. Br J Plast Surg 1984;37(3):327–9.
[138] Gottlieb ME, Chandrasekhar B, Terz JJ, et al. Clinical applications of the extended deep inferior epigastric flap. Plast Reconstr Surg 1986;78(6):782–92.
[139] Stern HS, Nahai F. The versatile superficial inferior epigastric artery free flap. Br J Plast Surg 1992;45(4):270–4.
[140] Classen D. The extended deep inferior epigastric flap: a case series. Ann Plast Surg 1999; 42(2):137–41.
[141] Parkash S, Palepu J. Rectus abdominus myocutaneous flap: clinical experience with ipsilateral and contralateral flaps. Br J Surg 1983;70(2):68–70.
[142] Mathes SJ, Bostwick J III. A rectus abdominus myocutaneous flap to reconstruct abdominal wall defects. Br J Plast Surg 1977;30(4):282–3.
[143] DeFranzo AJ, Kingman GJ, Sterchi JM, et al. Rectus turnover flaps for the reconstruction of large midline abdominal wall defects. Ann Plast Surg 1996;37(1):18–23.
[144] Spear SL, Walker RK. The external oblique flap for reconstruction of the rectus sheath. Plast Reconstr Surg 1992;90(4):608–13.
[145] Disa JJ, Goldberg NH, Carlton JM, et al. Restoring abdominal wall integrity in contaminated tissue deficient wounds using autologous fascia grafts. Plast Reconstr Surg 1988; 101(4):979–86.
[146] Williams JK, Carlson GW, deChalain T, et al. Role of tensor fascia lata in abdominal wall reconstruction. Plast Reconstr Surg 1998;101(3):802–5.
[147] Kimata Y, Uchiyama K, Sekido M, et al. Anterolateral thigh flap for abdominal wall reconstruction. Plast Reconstr Surg 1999;103(4):1191–7.
[148] Sasaki K, Nozaki M, Nakazawa H, et al. Reconstruction of a large abdominal wall defect using combined free tensor fascia latae musculocutaneous flap and anterolateral thigh flap. Plast Reconstr Surg 1998;102(6):2244–52.
[149] McCraw JB, Dibbell DG, Carraway JH. Clinical definition of independent myocutaneous vascular territories. Plast Recostr Surg 1977;60(3):341–52.
[150] Koshima I, Nanba Y, Tutsui T, et al. Dynamic reconstruction of large abdominal defects using free rectus femoris. Ann Plast Surg 2003;50(4):420–4.
[151] Caulfield WH, Curtsinger L, Powell G. Donor leg morbidity after pedicled rectus femoris muscle flap transfer for abdominal and pelvic reconstruction. Ann Plast Surg 1994;32(4): 377–982.
[152] Bostwick J 3rd, Vasconez LO, Nahai F, et al. Sixty latissimus dorsi flaps. Plast Reconstr Surg 1979;63(1):31–41.
[153] Ninkovic M, Kronberger P, Harpf C. Free innervated latissimus dorsi muscle for reconstruction of full-thickness abdominal wall defects. Plast Reconstr Surg 1998;101(4):971–8.
[154] Venugopalan S. Repair of midline abdominal incisional hernia by gracilis muscle transfer. Br J Plast Surg 1980;33(1):43–5.
[155] Dowden RV, McCraw JB. The vastus lateralis muscle flap: technique and applications. Ann Plast Surg 1980;4(5):396–404.

[156] Jacobsen WM, Petty PM, Bite U, et al. Massive abdominal wall hernia reconstruction with expanded external/internal oblique and transversalis fascia. Plast Reconstr Surg 1997; 100(2):326–35.

[157] Hobar PC, Rohrich RJ, Byrd HS. Abdominal-wall reconstruction with expanded musculofascial tissue in a posttraumatic defect. Plast Reconstr Surg 1994;94(2):379–83.

[158] Byrd HS, Hobar PC. Abdominal wall expansion in congenital defects. Plast Reconstr Surg 1989;84(2):347–52.

[159] Carlson GW, Elwood E, Losken A, et al. The role of tissue expansion in abdominal wall reconstruction. Ann Plast Surg 2000;44(2):147–53.

[160] Espinosa-de-los-Monteros A, de la Torre JI, Ahumada LA, et al. Reconstruction of the abdominal wall for incisional hernia repair. Am J Surg 2006;191:173–7.

[161] Ger R, Duboys E. The prevention and repair of large abdominal wall defects by muscle transposition: a preliminary communication. Plast Reconstr Surg 1983;72(2):170–5.

Laparoscopic Repair of Ventral Incisional Hernias: Pros and Cons

Patricia L. Turner, MD*,
Adrian E. Park, MD, FRCCS, FACS

*Division of General Surgery, Department of Surgery, University of Maryland School
of Medicine, 22 South Greene Street, Baltimore, MD 21201, USA*

Abdominal wall hernias are a familiar surgical problem. Millions of patients are affected each year, presenting most commonly with primary ventral, incisional, and inguinal hernias. Whether symptomatic or asymptomatic, hernias commonly cause pain or are aesthetically distressing to patients. These concerns, coupled with the risk of incarceration, are the most common reasons patients seek surgical repair of hernias. This article focuses on incisional hernias, reported to develop in 3% to 29% of laparotomy incisions [1].

Advances in the basic and clinical sciences have allowed a better understanding of the pathophysiology of hernia formation. It is known, for example, based on Pascal's principle of hydrostatic forces and the law of LaPlace, that a hernia will continue to enlarge over time if not treated. Increased intra-abdominal pressure will exert its greatest force on the portion of the wall that is thinnest. As the hernia enlarges, the wall thins at that point, and the diameter increases. This positive feedback loop virtually assures continued progression.

Further review of the natural history of hernias suggests that incisional hernias do not develop in the immediate postoperative period. Ongoing surveillance for 3 to 5 years post laparotomy has been shown to be necessary to identify the development and growth rate of postoperative incisional hernias [2]. Incisional hernia rates of 20% are reported with longitudinal evaluation [1]. Depending on the surgical techniques used at the time of the initial repair, recurrence rates as high as 50% have been documented for ventral and incisional hernias [3]. It also has been demonstrated that recurrences typically occur more rapidly than the initial hernia developed [4,5].

* Corresponding author.
E-mail address: pturner@smail.umaryland.edu (P.L. Turner).

0039-6109/08/$ - see front matter © 2008 Elsevier Inc. All rights reserved.
doi:10.1016/j.suc.2007.11.003
surgical.theclinics.com

The presence of a ventral hernia is, itself, an indication for repair when no substantial comorbid conditions exist. Although nonoperative management has been evaluated in a randomized trial for inguinal hernia [6], nonoperative management of ventral hernias has not yet been compared with elective repair in this way and is unlikely to be. Elective ventral and incisional hernia repair are undertaken largely to alleviate symptoms and to prevent hernia incarceration with subsequent strangulation of the intestine. It is estimated that about 10% of all ventral hernias result in incarceration, although the actual percentage is not known [7].

A common sequela of incarcerated ventral hernias is complete or partial bowel obstruction, with close to 50% of this population later developing strangulated hernias [8]. Almost 20% of those exhibiting strangulated hernias will need intestinal resection. Thus, their postoperative course will be more complicated, and the resection may preclude placement of a prosthesis at that exploration. For patients requiring repair of an incarcerated hernia, the overall rate of postoperative complications has been reported to be as high as 25%. Following incarcerated hernia repair, postoperative mortality rates of up to 5% have been reported, a rate substantially greater than that associated with elective hernia repair [9]. The repair of an incarcerated hernia in which bowel resection takes place proffers a postoperative mortality rate close to 20% [8]. Additionally, it is clear that there are patient populations who exhibit heightened susceptibility to incarcerated hernias. For patients treated with peritoneal dialysis, for example, the incidence of incisional hernia incarceration is reported to be in excess of 60% [10].

Historically, hernia repairs, performed primarily in an open fashion, were fraught with a high risk of recurrence. Luijendijk and colleagues [11] reported cumulative 5-year recurrence rates of 44% for hernias smaller than 6 cm and 73% for hernias between 6 cm and 12 cm. Others have reported recurrence rates after primary closure as high as 54% [12,13]. Tension-free repair using biomaterial or mesh placement now accounts for a substantial portion of all incisional hernia repairs. The frequency, now approaching 25%, with which incisional hernias are repaired laparoscopically contributes substantially to improved outcomes [14].

Early experience with prosthetic repairs and the initial significant drop in recurrence rates led to several randomized, controlled clinical trials [3,5]. The seminal study by Luijendijk and colleagues [15] provided compelling evidence that, in comparison with nonmesh repairs, mesh repairs of ventral hernias result in notably fewer recurrences. Others, including McCarthy and Twiest [16] and Gillion and colleagues [17], have duplicated these findings. Rudmik and colleagues [18], in a recent review article, identified 11 articles discussing open primary repair and compared them with 25 articles discussing prosthetic repair. With the exception of inlay mesh placement, for which the recurrence rates were comparable with those of primary repair, prosthetic mesh placement was uniformly more durable than primary repair when the mesh was placed in the underlay (intra or extraperitoneal) position and was somewhat more durable when the mesh was placed in the onlay position. Taken together, these studies present compelling evidence that underlay placement of prosthetic material is superior to other positions.

Factors affecting hernia occurrence

A number of patient factors are thought to predispose to hernia formation. These factors include a personal history of aneurysms, morbid obesity, the size of the defect, and, in the case of recurrent hernias, the technique used in the initial repair. Other patient-oriented factors that are relevant for both laparoscopic and open approaches include diseases of abnormal collagen synthesis, such as Marfan's syndrome, Ehlers-Danlos syndrome, and osteogenesis imperfecta. Each of these conditions is correlated with an increased incidence of hernia formation [19]. Also of interest as a factor are decreased collagen I/III ratios or varied expression profiles of matrix metalloproteinases [20].

Compelling evidence suggests that the larger the initial hernia defect, the greater is the chance for recurrence after repair. Above an approximately 4-cm threshold, the risk of recurrence has been demonstrated to be threefold higher in patients undergoing a nonmesh primary tissue repair [2]. Consequently, primary repair typically is reserved for small ventral or umbilical hernias. Because the long-term recurrence rate of small incisional hernias repaired by primary closure is approximately 50% [12,21], fewer surgeons currently attempt such repairs.

Surgical approach

With an open approach to incisional hernia repairs, the prosthetic mesh can be placed above (onlay), below (underlay), or on both sides of the fascia or directly into the defect (inlay). Laparoscopically, both the inlay and underlay techniques are feasible.

Onlay mesh repairs can be performed with or without primary closure of the fascia. The foremost reason for primary fascial closure with anterior prosthetic reinforcement is that contact between the underlying viscera and the prosthetic material is avoided or minimized. Even if the hernia recurs, the anteriorly sutured prosthetic material reinforces the repair. Onlay repair without primary closure of the hernia defect or hernia sac risks exposing the mesh directly to the intra-abdominal contents. Delayed infection, fistulization, and erosion of the prosthetic material into the gastrointestinal tract may occur as a result.

The underlay technique of prosthetic placement, although used for both open and laparoscopic incisional hernia repairs, is more common in the latter. When the prosthetic material is secured posterior to the abdominal wall musculature in the preperitoneal space or subpreperitoneal space, as described by Stoppa [22], an increase in intra-abdominal pressure buttresses rather than distracts the repair. Moreover, this configuration distributes intra-abdominal forces more evenly across the surface of the prosthetic material. This approach requires that a large prosthetic support be inserted and secured with substantial overlap around the defect. The prosthetic mesh is secured with transfixing sutures that traverse the full thickness of the anterior abdominal wall. There must be ample close approximation of the mesh to healthy fascia to facilitate abdominal wall ingrowth. Stoppa's initial report demonstrated a durable hernia repair in 85% of patients with a 1.8% mortality and sepsis rate. These results have been duplicated with variable recurrence rates, as reflected in Table 1.

A discussion of fixation techniques is necessary, because one limitation of the laparoscopic approach is that the abdomen is not opened widely, so the mesh must be secured effectively with instruments that will fit through a trocar. The most effective repairs, those reported to be favored by a majority of surgeons [23], combine the use of transfixing transabdominal sutures with circumferential tacking devices. Leading authors suggest that sutures be placed every 4 to 5 cm and tacks be placed at 1-cm intervals to avoid exposing the prosthetic mesh to the intra-abdominal contents while mesh ingrowth occurs [13,24,25]. Ingrowth into the abdominal wall provides the strength of the repair; however, if the mesh is not properly stabilized, the risks of mesh migration and hernia recurrence increase, even as this ingrowth occurs [14]. The laparoscopic repair of ventral hernias with tacks alone has been reported to be associated with a high incidence of hernia recurrence [26].

To achieve the several centimeters of overlap necessary to reduce hernia recurrence via the open approach, substantial undermining of the superficial soft tissue must occur. The dissection must be taken back to healthy fascia through which the prosthetic mesh is secured, and this undermining can create a substantial dead space superficially. The laparoscopic approach uses insufflation to create a large intraperitoneal working space into which a large prosthetic support can be placed and oriented without extensive dissection of the subcutaneous tissues. This technique, in turn, provides the additional benefit of fewer postoperative wound complications.

Accessing the abdomen, however, is more difficult laparoscopically than by laparotomy, especially in a patient who may have undergone several prior intra-abdominal procedures. The placement of the initial port varies among surgeons and may include the use of an open Hassan technique or use of an optical trocar with Veress needle before insufflation. Also, unlike the open approach, port placement is a key consideration in the laparoscopic approach. The ports should be placed as far away from the defect as possible to allow access to the anterior abdominal wall with adequate room for prosthetic overlap. Substantial laparoscopic adhesiolysis often is required to facilitate the placement of subsequent ports. Once the fascial edges are cleared and the defect is fully elucidated, a prosthetic material is chosen to

Table 1
Comparison of laparoscopic and open repairs of incisional hernias with prosthetic materials

Author	Year	Study design	Type of repair	N	Recurrence (%)	Morbidity (%)
Barbaros, et al [60]	2007	Prospective randomized	Laparoscopic	23	0	22
			Open	23	4	17
Beldi, et al [33]	2006	Retrospective and prospective	Laparoscopic	49	Not reported	14
			Open	92		27
Bencini, et al [44]	2003	Prospective	Laparoscopic	42	0	5
			Open	49	6	16
Bingener, et al [59]	2007	Prospective	Laparoscopic	127	12	9
		Cohort	Open	233	9	21
Carbajo, et al [61]	1999	Prospective randomized	Laparoscopic	30	0	7
			Open	30	7	40
Chari, et al [62]	2000	Prospective case control	Laparoscopic	14	0	14
			Open	14	0	14
DeMaria, et al [63]	2000	Prospective	Laparoscopic	21	5	62
			Open	18	0	72
Earle, et al [32]	2005	Prospective	Laparoscopic	469	Not reported	1
			Open	415		0
Holzman, et al [3]	1997	Retrospective	Laparoscopic	21	10	23
			Open	16	12	31

(continued on next page)

Table 1 (*continued*)

Author	Year	Study design	Type of repair	N	Recurrence (%)	Morbidity (%)
McGreevy, et al [64]	2003	Prospective	Laparoscopic	65	Not reported	8
			Open	71		21
Park, et al [43]	1998	Prospective	Laparoscopic	56	11	18
			Open	49	35	37
Olmi, et al [55]	2007	Case Control	Laparoscopic	85	2	16
			Open	85	1	29
Raftopoulos, et al [65]	2003	Retrospective	Laparoscopic	50	2	28
			Open	22	18	45
Ramshaw, et al [12]	1999	Retrospective	Laparoscopic	79	3	19
			Open	174	21	26
Robbins, et al [54]	2001	Prospective	Laparoscopic	36	Not reported	22
			Open	18		28
Wright, et al [67]	2002	Retrospective	Laparoscopic	90	1	22
			Open	90	6	36

cover the hernia. Table 2 summarizes published comparisons of laparoscopic and open herniorrhaphies with placement of prosthetic material.

Surgical experience

In addition to the surgical technique used, surgical experience in incisional hernia procedures is considered to be of marked importance. A retrospective study comparing simple suturing (241 repairs) with mesh implantation (180 repairs) performed at a university hospital on 348 patients over a 25-year period concluded that the recurrence rate for surgeons averaging 20 or more operations (8%) was significantly better than the recurrence rate for surgeons averaging fewer than 10 operations (33%). When only mesh implantation was considered, the same study again recorded that increased experience on the part of the surgeon equated to a decreased recurrence rate, specifically from 18% to 8%. The study concluded that 16 mesh repairs, at minimum, were requisite to achieve a recurrence rate of less than 10% [27]. Similarly, the recurrence rate is affected by learning-curve mastery, with a high recurrence rate (15.7%) related to the technical learning curve associated with initial laparoscopic incisional herniorrhaphy experience falling to 10% as the learning curve was mastered [28]. The caution has been made that mastering incisional herniorrhaphy should not be considered until a ventral hernia repair series has been undertaken successfully [29]. One recent survey suggested that, after completion of residency, fellows felt competent, based on their quantitative experience, to perform ventral herniorrhaphies, a confidence extended to only two other laparoscopic procedures—cholecystectomy and thoracoscopy [30]. In another survey, minimally invasive surgery fellows indicated that the number of ventral herniorrhaphies they expected to perform during their fellowships was comparable to the number they believed necessary to achieve optimal expertise and comfort [31].

Advantages

The popularity of laparoscopic incisional hernia repair is increasing [32]. The early postoperative adverse events, overall safety, and clinical effectiveness of laparoscopic and open repair are similar. The laparoscopic approach offers several key advantages over the open approach, including low risks of infection and shortened hospital stay in addition to reductions in complication rates, postoperative pain, and postoperative ileus. The lower recurrence rates reported with laparoscopy are convincing, although they remain to be demonstrated conclusively. Even lowered overall hospital costs have been associated with laparoscopic hernia repair [18,23,33–36].

Another advantage of the laparoscopic approach is the ability to address an enterotomy without needing to convert to an open procedure with return

Table 2
Outcomes of laparoscopic incisional hernia repairs using prosthetic materials

Author	Year	N	Mean or median follow-up	Conversion (%)	Seroma (%)	Mesh or wound infection (%)	Recurrences (%)
Aura, et al [66]	2002	86	37 months	1	2	0	7
Bageacu, et al [28]	2002	159	49 months	14	16	3	16
Ben-Haim, et al [67]	2002	100	19 months	4	11	0	2
Berger, et al [45]	2002	150	1–2 years	2	93	0	3
Birgisson, et al [68]	2001	64	9 months	0	5	3	0
Bower, et al [69]	2004	100	7 months	1	1	2	2
Carbajo, et al [29]	2003	270	44 months	< 1	12	0	4
Chowbey, et al [48]	2000	202	35 months	1	32	3	1
Eid, et al [53]	2003	79	34 months	1	4	0	5
Franklin, et al [6]	2003	384	47 months	4	3	1	3
Frantzides, et al [70]	2004	208	24 months	0	Not reported	1	1
Gillian, et al [26]	2002	100	Not reported	0	3	0	1
Heniford, et al [47]	2003	850	20 months	4	Most	2	5
Kirshtein, et al [71]	2002	103	26 months	3	Most	5	4
LeBlanc, et al [72]	2003	200	36 months	4	8	2	7
Olmi, et al [73]	2006	178	29 months	0	4	1	2
Perrone, et al [74]	2005	116	22 months	10	21	5	8
Rosen, et al [75]	2003	100	30 months	12	4	6	17
Sanchez, et al [76]	2004	90	12 months	6	9	0	3
Stickel, et al [36]	2007	62	14 months	2	Not reported	2	5
Toy, et al [77]	1998	144	7 months	0	16	3	4

to the operating theater at a later date to perform a definitive laparoscopic hernia repair with prosthetic material. A recent series described nine patients who underwent attempted laparoscopic incisional hernia repair but were deemed inappropriate for immediate mesh placement because of enterotomy, need for bowel resection, or deserosalization. In an open approach, these patients probably would have had a less durable repair performed with absorbable mesh rather than risk prosthetic infection. The laparoscopic approach allowed each patient to be monitored as an inpatient with a planned return to the operating room for placement of mesh for definitive repair without sacrificing any of the established benefits of the minimally invasive approach [37].

The use of mesh is, without doubt, the reason for the reduced recurrence associated with incisional hernia repairs. A number of different prosthetic meshes have been formulated. When mesh is used as an underlay prosthesis, a key consideration should be whether the mesh will be in direct contact with the intra-abdominal viscera. Some newer prosthetic materials, expanded polytetrafluoroethylene (ePTFE), for example, have an adhesion barrier on the intestinal side that minimizes the risk of adhesions and fistulization. The other side of the prosthetic material is in direct contact with the abdominal wall and is corrugated to promote rapid ingrowth. Other materials, however, such as polypropylene, although in common use for some time, are contraindicated for placement in direct contact with the intestine. A recent study comparing preperitoneal and intraperitoneal placement of polypropylene found significantly higher rates of small bowel resection (21% versus 0%), surgical site infection (26% versus 4%), and enterocutaneous fistula (5% versus 0%) with intraperitoneal placement of polypropylene in patients who subsequently underwent repeat laparotomy or laparoscopy [38]. Several newer materials—including hydrophilic prosthetic materials that are easily managed in the laparoscopic field—are currently in use. There were early indications that hydrophilic material might provide bowel protection [39]. One such mesh in common use is Parietex (Sofradim, Trevoux, France), whose hydrophilic absorbable film has been credited with protecting the mesh from contact with viscera during integration, thus minimizing intra-abdominal adhesions and viscera erosion [40,41]. Long-term data on these adhesion barriers are still lacking, however.

An additional benefit of the laparoscopic approach is that a single procedure allows large or multiple hernias to be repaired without extending the incision and also allows identification and repair of previously clinically silent defects. Placement of additional 5-mm trocars as necessary often is tolerated well by patients and does not contribute significantly to postoperative discomfort [42].

Another demonstrated laparoscopic advantage treated more fully elsewhere in this article is the ability to evaluate the abdominal wall fully with substantially improved visualization [43]. Laparoscopic adhesiolysis allows the abdominal wall to be inspected in a more thorough way, permitting identification of remote or "Swiss-cheese" defects that might have been missed with the less optimal visualization of the open approach.

Overall laparoscopic ventral incisional repair has been credited with lessening technical impediments and disadvantageous conditions when compared with traditional open repair. Table 2 summarizes studies of laparoscopic ventral hernia repairs with prosthetic materials, including recurrence rates and rates of mesh and wound infections. The concern that laparoscopic management of large prostheses (30 × 20 cm) presented some technical difficulty has been dispelled [44]. Use of 12-mm trocars adequately facilitates such large prostheses, as Carbajo and colleagues [29] demonstrated with no incidents of mesh sepsis. That same research demonstrated complete restoration of the abdominal wall characterized by both integrity and stability.

Disadvantages

Seromas are one of the most common postoperative findings in both laparoscopic and open incisional hernia repairs [45]. In large open hernia repairs, the resultant dead space beneath the skin flaps often is treated prophylactically by the placement of closed suction drains so that the resultant seroma is aspirated as it forms. In laparoscopy, because drains are not routinely placed, seromas are seen more often. The presence of seroma is so prevalent, in fact, that many surgeons do not consider the occurrence of routine self-limited seromas as pathologic, reserving that description for seromas that require intervention (eg, drainage), that become infected, or that persist beyond a defined amount of time, usually 6 to 8 weeks [46,47]. Common practices include placing the patient in an abdominal binder postoperatively, and research has indicated significant reduction in seroma and hematoma formation with this method [48,49]. A cogent preoperative discussion with patients, informing them of the risk of seroma formation, reduces unfounded postoperative concerns, because the seromas usually resolve spontaneously.

Consideration must be given to the use of carbon dioxide as the insufflation agent during laparoscopy. The additional carbon dioxide burden is a contraindication to laparoscopic herniorrhaphy for patients who have severe chronic obstructive pulmonary disease. Because even a relatively modest increase in afterload or decrease in preload would prove problematic, patients who have extremely poor cardiac reserve may be better served by an open approach or watchful waiting [50].

Accessing the abdomen for a laparoscopic hernia repair and performing adhesiolysis does carry a potential risk of injury to intestine, which, if missed, can lead to intra-abdominal sepsis. Itani and colleagues [51] have reported the rates of bowel injury as 7.2% in open hernia repairs and 9% in laparoscopic procedures. Others have reported that the incidence of bowel injuries differs insignificantly between laparoscopic and open approaches and is low in both approaches [52]. The bowel actually is easier to identify in laparoscopic surgery than in open surgery, because it generally hangs down, away from the abdominal wall, and insufflation permits better plane definition [53]. Additionally, intestinal injuries may not be reported as consistently in the open literature as in laparoscopic papers. It is possible that these injuries occur in much higher percentages in traditional open surgery, but, because they do not require a change in procedure, they may be underrecognized.

In any case, prompt recognition of these injuries is critical to avoid late complications. These injuries can be obvious (eg, traction or sharp dissection injuries) or can be subtle (eg, a delayed thermal injury). Careful attention to tissue handling and thorough inspection of the intestine using meticulous completion laparoscopy to assess for intestinal injuries can minimize these risks.

Bleeding from abdominal wall vessels is another complication that rarely occurs in an open approach but can cause frank hemorrhage or significant hematoma if not recognized. At times, a trocar can stem the bleeding temporarily, but the bleeding may resume in the early postoperative period.

As has been discussed, transfixing sutures typically are used to facilitate close approximation of the prosthetic material to the abdominal wall so adequate ingrowth can occur. The presence of these sutures, therefore, contributes substantially to the repair. Persistent pain at these suture sites is a problem unique to the laparoscopic approach and occurs in 1% to 3% of patients [6]. This discomfort may be caused by the sutures entrapping an intercostal nerve, or the suture itself may compress muscle significantly enough to cause persistent pain. This discomfort is often self limited, but conservative measures such as the use of nonsteroidal anti-inflammatory drugs or local injection of steroid or anesthetic may provide symptomatic relief in the interim.

As would be expected, wound complications are reduced significantly in laparoscopic ventral hernia repairs when compared with open repairs [54]. In a series by Olmi and colleagues [55], wound complications also were noted to be significantly lower in laparoscopic hernia repairs than in open repairs (1.1% versus 8.2%). The laparoscopic approach diminishes the need to raise large tissue flaps or devitalize tissues, procedures that increase the risk of mesh infection. Although mesh infection occurs less often after laparoscopic hernia repair than after an open approach, its management can require a more involved algorithm, because treatment of the infection sometimes requires removal of the prosthesis. This decision, in many cases, depends on the prosthetic material used and requires close monitoring of the patient to determine whether salvage is possible. Occasional case reports notwithstanding [56], infection of the popular two-sided prosthetic ePTFE, unlike most other formulations, often requires removal [57]. In many cases, a wound or mesh infection following an open repair with prosthetic materials other than ePTFE can be managed nonoperatively with local wound-care interventions.

The open approach does provide more opportunity for revision of the wound itself. In patients who have had multiple prior operations and for whom an unsightly scar is a significant concern, the ability to revise the scar or to perform associated procedures such as abdominoplasty concurrently is available only with the open approach.

Risk factors for recurrence of hernia include a larger hernia defect, longer operating times, previous hernia repairs, and morbid obesity [47]. In a meta-analysis comparing short- and long-term outcomes for patients undergoing laparoscopic or open incisional hernia repair, a trend toward lower hernia recurrence rates following laparoscopic repair when compared with an open repair was noted but failed to achieve statistical significance [35]. Other authors have identified defective wound healing and an impaired scarring process as equal to technical error in hernia recurrence [58].

Shorter hospital stays and significantly less major morbidity have been demonstrated recently after laparoscopic ventral hernia repairs in a 10-year institutional cohort study [59]. Cost, however, may represent a relative disadvantage to the laparoscopic approach. Operating room supply costs can be significantly greater with laparoscopic than with open repairs ($2237 versus $664). The operative time was significantly longer as well (149 versus 89 minutes) [32]. These figures probably reflect the positioning, port placement, and specialized equipment needed to perform a laparoscopic hernia repair.

Overall hospital costs for these patients, however, were slightly lower, reflecting the shorter length of stay of the laparoscopic patient (1 ± 0.2 days versus 2 ± 0.6 days). The same authors demonstrated a slightly higher rate of postoperative encounters within 30 days of laparoscopic hernia repairs, with an associated additional cost.

Summary

There has been substantial literature generated on the topic of incisional hernia repair and the laparoscopic and open approaches. Each has advantages and disadvantages. The collective results of all of these studies suggest that laparoscopic ventral hernia repairs have reduced perioperative morbidity, fewer wound complications, and lower rates of hernia recurrence. These benefits suggest that for many patients laparoscopy is an appropriate approach for the repair of incisional hernias in both straightforward and complex presentations. There is still a role for the traditional open approach, primarily in patients who have a specific contraindication to a minimally invasive approach or in whom additional procedures are planned.

Additionally, advances in the development of new prosthetic materials, new devices, and techniques for prosthetic placement may further reduce postoperative morbidity, minimize recurrences, and improve patient care.

Acknowledgment

The authors acknowledge the thoughtful editing of this article provided by Rosemary Klein.

References

[1] Mudge M, Hughes L. Incisional hernia: a 10-year prospective study of incidence and attitudes. Br J Surg 1985;72:70–1.

[2] Bucknall TE, Cox PJ, Ellis H. Burst abdomen and incisional hernia: a prospective study of 1129 major laparotomies. Br Med J 1982;284:931–3.

[3] Holzman MD, Purut CM, Reintgen K, et al. Laparoscopic ventral and incisional hernioplasty. Surg Endosc 1997;11:32–5.

[4] Langer S, Christiansen J. Long-term results after incisional hernia repair. Acta Chir Scand 1985;151:217–9.

[5] van der Linden FT, van Vroonhoven TJ. Long-term results after surgical correction of incisional hernia repair. Neth J Surg 1988;40:127–9.

[6] Franklin ME Jr, Gonzalez JJ, Glass JL, et al. Laparoscopic ventral and incisional hernia repair: an 11-year experience. Hernia 2004;8:23–7.

[7] Courtney CA, Lee AC, Wilson C, et al. Ventral hernia repair: a study of current practice. Hernia 2003;7:44–6.

[8] Kulah B, Duzgun AP, Moran M, et al. Emergency hernia repairs in elderly patients. Am J Surg 2001;182:455–9.

[9] Sowula A, Groele H. Treatment of incarcerated abdominal hernia. Wiad Lek 2003;56:40–4.

[10] Cherney DZ, Siccion Z, Chu M, et al. Natural history and outcome of incarcerated abdominal hernias in peritoneal dialysis patients. Adv Perit Dial 2004;20:86–9.

[11] Luijendijk RW, Jeekel J, Storm RK, et al. The low transverse Pfannenstiel incision and the prevalence of incisional hernia and nerve entrapment. Ann Surg 1997;225:365–9.

[12] Ramshaw BJ, Estartia P, Schwab J, et al. Comparison of laparoscopic and open ventral herniorrhaphy. Am Surg 1999;65:827–31.

[13] Larson GM. Ventral hernia repair by the laparoscopic approach. Surg Clin North Am 2000;80:1329–40.

[14] Park AE, Roth JS, Kavic SM. Abdominal wall hernia. Curr Probl Surg 2006,43:321–75.

[15] Luijendijk RW, Hop WC, van den Tol MP, et al. A comparison of suture repair with mesh repair of incisional hernia. N Engl J Med 2000;343:392–8.

[16] McCarthy JD, Twiest MW. Intraperitoneal polypropylene mesh support of incisional herniorrhaphy. Am J Surg 1982;142:707–11.

[17] Gillion JF, Begin GF, Marecos C, et al. Expanded polytetrafluoroethylene position for repair of incisional hernias of the anterolateral abdominal wall. Am J Surg 1997;177:291–3.

[18] Rudmik LR, Schieman C, Dixon E, et al. Laparoscopic hernia repair: a review of the literature. Hernia 2006;10:110–9.

[19] Liem MSL, van der Graaf Y, Beemer FA, et al. Increased risk for inguinal hernia in patients with Ehlers-Danlos syndrome. Surgery 1997;122:114–5.

[20] Klinge U, Si ZY, Zheng H, et al. Collagen I/III and matrix metalloproteinases (MMP) 1 and 13 in the fascia of patients with incisional hernias. J Invest Surg 2001;14:47–54.

[21] Burger JWA, Luijendijk RW, Hop WCJ, et al. Long-term follow-up of a randomized controlled trial of suture versus mesh repair of incisional hernia. Ann Surg 2004;240:578–85.

[22] Louis D, Stoppa R, Henry X, et al. Postoperative eventration. Apropos of 247 surgically treated cases. J Chir 1985;122:523–7.

[23] Carlson MA, Frantzides CT, Shostrom VK, et al. Minimally invasive ventral herniorrhaphy: an analysis of 6,266 published cases. Hernia.

[24] Heniford BT, Park A, Ramshaw BJ, et al. Laparoscopic ventral and incisional hernia repair in 407 patients. J Am Coll Surg 2000;190:645–50.

[25] Helton WS, Fisichella PM, Berger R, et al. Short-term outcomes with small intestinal submucosa for ventral abdominal hernia. Arch Surg 2005;140:549–62.

[26] Gillian GK, Geis WP, Grover G. Laparoscopic incisional and ventral hernia repair (LIVH): an evolving outpatient technique. Journal of the Society of Laparoendoscopic Surgeons 2002, 26:315–22.

[27] Langer C, Schaper A, Liersch T, et al. Prognosis factors in incisional hernia surgery. Hernia 2005;9:16–21.

[28] Bageacu S, Blanc P, Breton C, et al. Laparoscopic repair of incisional hernia. A retrospective study of 159 patients. Surg Endosc 2002;16:345–8.

[29] Carbajo MA, Martin del Olmo JC, Blanco JI, et al. Laparoscopic approach to incisional hernia: lessons learned from 270 patients over 8 years. Surg Endosc 2003;17:118–22.

[30] Park A, Kavic SM, Lee TH, et al. Minimally invasive surgery: the evolution of fellowship. Surgery 2007;142:505–13.

[31] Tichansky DS, Taddeucci RJ, Harper J, et al. Minimally invasive surgery fellows would perform a wider variety of cases in their "ideal" fellowship. Surg Endosc [serial online] 2007. Available at: http://www.springerlink.com/content/0466p26276411390/. Accessed October 18, 2007.

[32] Earle D, Seymour N, Fellinger E, et al. Laparoscopic versus open incisional hernia repair: a single-institution analysis of hospital resource utilization for 884 consecutive cases. Surg Endosc 2006;20:71–5.

[33] Beldi G, Ipaktchi R, Wagner M, et al. Laparoscopic ventral hernia repair is safe and cost effective. Surg Endosc 2006;20:92–5.

[34] Müller-Riemenschneider F, Roll S, Friedrich M, et al. Medical effectiveness and safety of conventional compared to laparoscopic incisional hernia repair: a systematic review. Surg Endosc

[35] Sains PS, Tilney HS, Purkayastha S, et al. Outcomes following laparoscopic versus open repair of incisional hernia. World J Surg 2006;30:2056–64.

[36] Stickel M, Rentsch M, Clevert D-A, et al. Laparoscopic mesh repair of incisional hernia: an alternative to the conventional open repair? Hernia 2007;11:217–22.

[37] Lederman AB, Ramshaw BJ. A short-term delayed approach to laparoscopic ventral hernia when injury is suspected. Surg Innov 2005;12:31–5.

[38] Halm JA, de Wall LL, Steyerberg EW, et al. Intraperitoneal polypropylene mesh hernia repair complicates subsequent abdominal surgery. World J Surg 2007;31:423–9.

[39] Mutter D, Rodeheaver GT, Diemunsch P, et al. A new composite mesh (collagen-polyester) for intra-abdominal laparoscopic hernia repair. Surg Endosc 1998;12:595.

[40] Chelala E, Gaede F, Douillez V, et al. The suturing concept for laparoscopic mesh fixation in ventral and incisional hernias: preliminary results. Hernia 2003;7:191–6.

[41] Chelala E, Thoma M, Tatete B, et al. The suturing concept for laparoscopic mesh fixation in ventral and incisional hernia repair: mid-term analysis of 400 cases. Surg Endosc 2007;21: 391–5.

[42] Kua KB, Coleman M, Martin I, et al. Laparoscopic repair of ventral incisional hernia. ANZ J Surg 2002;72:296–9.

[43] Park A, Birch DW, Lovrics P. Laparoscopic and open incisional hernia repair: a comparison study. Surgery 1998;124:816–22.

[44] Bencini L, Sanchez LJ, Boffi B, et al. Incisional hernia repair. Retrospective comparison of laparoscopic and open techniques. Surg Endosc 2003;17:1546–51.

[45] Berger D, Bientzle M, Müller A. Postoperative complications after laparoscopic incisional hernia repair. Incidence and treatment. Surg Endosc 2002;16:1720–3.

[46] Susmallian S, Gewurtz G, Ezri I, et al. Seroma after laparoscopic repair of hernia with PTFE patch: is it really a complication? Hernia 2001;5:139–41.

[47] Heniford BT, Park A, Ramshaw BJ, et al. Laparoscopic repair of ventral hernias: nine year's experience with 850 consecutive cases. Ann Surg 2003;238:391–9.

[48] Chowbey PK, Sharma A, Khullar R, et al. Laparoscopic ventral hernia repair. J Laparoendosc Adv Surg Tech A 2000;10:79–84.

[49] LeBlanc KA. Laparoscopic incisional and ventral hernia repair: complications—how to avoid and handle. Hernia 2004;8:323–31.

[50] Henny CP, Hofland J. Laparoscopic surgery: pitfalls due to anesthesia, positioning, and pneumoperitoneum. Surg Endosc 2005;19:1163–71.

[51] Itani KMF, Neumayer L, Reda D, et al. Repair of ventral incisional hernia: the design of a randomized trial to compare open and laparoscopic surgical techniques. Am J Surg 2004;188:22S–9S.

[52] Feldman LS, Wexler MJ, Fraser SA. Laparoscopic hernia repair. What's new ACS surgery. Available at: http://www.medscape.com/viewarticle/506634. Accessed November, 2007.

[53] Eid GM, Prince JM, Mattar SM, et al. Medium-term follow-up confirms the safety and durability of laparoscopic ventral hernia repair with PTFE. Surgery 2003;134:599–603, 2003.

[54] Robbins SB, Pofahl WE, Gonzalez RP. Laparoscopic ventral hernia repair reduces wound complications. Am Surg 2001;67:896–900.

[55] Olmi S, Scaini A, Cesana GC, et al. Laparoscopic versus open incisional hernia repair. Surg Endosc 2007;21:555–9.

[56] Kercher KW, Sing Rf, Matthews BD, et al. Successful salvage of infected PTFE mesh after ventral hernia repair. Ostomy Wound Manage 2002;48:40–2, 44–5.

[57] Deysine M. Pathophysiology, prevention and management of prosthetic infections in hernia surgery. Surg Clin North Am 1998;78:1105–15.

[58] Klinge U, Binnebosel M, Rosch R, et al. Hernia recurrence as a problem of biology and collagen. Journal of Minimal Access Surgery 2006;2:151–4.

[59] Bingener J, Buck L, Richards M, et al. Long-term outcomes in laparoscopic vs open ventral hernia repair. Arch Surg 2007;142:562–7.

[60] Barbaros U, Asoglu A, Seven R, et al. The comparison of laparoscopic and open ventral hernia repairs: a prospective randomized study. Hernia 2007;11:51–6.

[61] Carbajo MA, Martin del Olmo JC, Blanco JI, et al. Laparoscopic treatment vs open surgery in the solution of major incisional and abdominal wall hernias with mesh. Surg Endosc 1999;13:250–2.

[62] Chari R, Chari V, Eisenstat M, et al. A case controlled study of laparoscopic incisional hernia repair. Surg Endosc 1999;14:117–9.

[63] DeMaria EJ, Moss JM, Sugerman HJ. Laparoscopic intraperitoneal polytetrafluoroethylene (PTFE) prosthetic patch repair of ventral hernia: prospective comparison to open prefascial polypropylene mesh repair. Surg Endosc 2000,14:326–9.

[64] McGreevy JM, Goodney PP, Birkmeyer CM, et al. A prospective study comparing the complication rates between laparoscopic and open ventral hernia repairs. Surg Endosc 2003;17:1778–80.

[65] Raftopoulos I, Vanuno D, Khorsand J, et al. Comparison of open and laparoscopic prosthetic repair of large ventral hernias. J Soc Laparoendosc Surg 2003;7:227–32.

[66] Robbins Aura T, Habib E, Mekkaoui M, et al. Laparoscopic tension-free repair of anterior abdominal wall incision and ventral hernias with an intraperitoneal Gore-Tex mesh: prospective study and review of the literature. J Laparoendosc Adv Surg Tech 2002;12: 263–7.

[67] Ben-Haim M, Kuriansky J, Tal R, et al. Pitfalls and complications with laparoscopic intraperitoneal expanded polytetrafluoroethylene patch repair of postoperative ventral hernia. Surg Endosc 2002;16:785–8.

[68] Birgisson G, Park AE, Mastrangelo MJ, et al. Obesity and laparoscopic repair of ventral hernias. Surg Endosc 2001;15:1419–22.

[69] Bower CE, Reade CC, Kirby LW, et al. Complications of laparoscopic incisional-ventral hernia repair. Surg Endosc 2004;18:672–5.

[70] Frantzides CT, Carlson MA, Zografakis JG, et al. Minimally invasive incisional herniorrhaphy. A review of 208 cases. Surg Endosc 2004;18:1488–91.

[71] Kirshtein B, Lantsberg L, Avinoach E, et al. Laparoscopic repair of large incisional hernias. Surg Endosc 2002;16:1717–9.

[72] LeBlanc KA, Whitaker JM, Bellanger DE, et al. Laparoscopic incisional and ventral hernioplasty: lessons learned from 200 patients. Hernia 2003;7:118–24.

[73] Olmi S, Erba L, Magnone S, et al. Prospective clinical study of laparoscopic treatment of incisional and ventral hernia using a composite mesh: indications, complications and results. Hernia 2006;10:243–7.

[74] Perrone JM, Soper NJ, Eagon JC, et al. Perioperative outcomes and complications of laparoscopic ventral hernia repair. Surgery 2005;138:708–15 [discussion: 715–6].
[75] Rosen M, Brody F, Ponsky J, et al. Recurrence after laparoscopic ventral hernia repair. A five-year experience. Surg Endosc 2003;17:123–8.
[76] Sanchez LJ, Bencini L, Moretti R. Recurrences after laparoscopic ventral hernia repair: results and critical review. Hernia 2004;8:138–43.
[77] Toy FK, Bailey RW, Carey S, et al. Prospective multicenter study of laparoscopic ventral hernioplasty. Preliminary results. Surg Endosc 1998;12:955–9.

SURGICAL
CLINICS OF
NORTH AMERICA

Surg Clin N Am 88 (2008) 101–112

Prosthetic Material in Ventral Hernia Repair: How Do I Choose?

Sharon Bachman, MD, Bruce Ramshaw, MD*

*Department of General Surgery, One Hospital Drive, DC 075.00,
University of Missouri-Columbia, Columbia, MO 65212, USA*

The evolution of modern ventral hernia repair began in 1958 when Francis Usher [1] published the first of his many papers describing the use of polypropylene mesh for tension-free hernia repairs. This mesh was rightly recognized as a huge leap forward in the reduction of recurrence rates after hernia repairs [2,3]. However, the same properties that led to incorporation of mesh into the abdominal wall also led to adherence of bowel to mesh if the mesh was exposed to the peritoneal cavity. Mesh could then migrate through the bowel wall or incite fistula formation, with potentially disastrous infectious consequences [4–9].

This realization led to the development of "second-generation" mesh, the barrier meshes, which provide a protective layer to prevent intraperitoneal contents from adhering to the prosthetic. With the prevention of adhesions as the goal, these barrier meshes are designed to prevent ingrowth of viscera into the mesh. These meshes have been partly responsible for the popularization of the underlay technique of ventral hernia repair, primarily with the laparoscopic approach.

This article is based on the experiences and opinions of the authors' group at the Missouri Hernia Institute, University of Missouri–Columbia. The authors' evaluations of the currently available products designed and/or marketed for use in ventral hernia repair are based on currently available knowledge and concepts. The products presented are available in the United States. Products only available outside of the United States are not included in this review. Source data include published literature, official corporate literature, and personal experience and opinion. In the interest of full disclosure, Dr. Ramshaw makes known that he has or has had business relationships with the following companies: W.L. Gore, Covidien, Ethicon Endosurgery, Ethicon, Tissue Sciences Laboratory, Cook Surgical, Stryker, MTF, and Atrium. Support received from these companies includes grants, such as educational grants; honoraria; fellowship support; and royalties. Activities in connection with these companies include consulting, speaking, teaching, advising, and conducting research.

* Corresponding author.
E-mail address: ramshawb@health.missouri.edu (B. Ramshaw).

Acellular collagen scaffolds, which are biologic materials, represent so-called "third-generation" mesh. Although the long-term outcomes for primary hernia repairs with these materials are still being investigated, they have a moderately good success rate for salvaging contaminated and infected fields, especially when placed with wide overlap [10–16].

These technologic advances and the growth of the hernia repair market have led to a proliferation of materials. This article summarizes the similarities and differences of the mesh options and provides surgeons with some guidance in selecting meshes.

A brief description of abdominal wall mechanics

To understand what sort of properties a mesh should have, it is important to look at the tissues it is replacing and/or reinforcing. Klinge and colleagues [17] described a mathematical model that calculated the force of the abdominal wall to be 16 N/cm. This same group also examined the elasticity of the abdominal wall in human cadavers. They described the average male abdominal wall elasticity at 16 N to be 23 ($\pm$ 7%) and 15 ($\pm$ 5%) in the vertical direction and 15 ($\pm$ 5%) in the horizontal direction, while the average female abdominal wall elasticity at 16 N females was 32 ($\pm$ 7%) in the vertical direction and 17 ($\pm$ 5%) in the horizontal direction [18].

Cobb and colleagues [19] actually measured intra-abdominal pressure via intravesicular measurements in healthy volunteers, and documented pressures up to 252 mm Hg over a variety of maneuvers, including lifting, coughing, and jumping. This correlates to forces of up to 27 N/cm [19].

With these numbers in mind, compare a maximum force on the abdominal wall of 27 N/cm with the measured burst force of some of the more common synthetic mesh materials. Marlex has a tensile strength of 59 N/cm, Atrium mesh 56 N/cm, and Vypro (lightweight mesh) 16 N/cm [20]. This same study noted that recurrences in humans invariably occurred at the mesh margin, where the mesh interfaced with tissue [20]. The finding that recurrences occur at the mesh margin is also bolstered by Binnebosel [21] in an experimental model that simulated the abdominal wall and two types of defects. In a pressure-controlled chamber, Ultrapro mesh was place in sublay and overlay positions over two types of simulated fascial defects. As the pressure within the chamber was increased to 200 mm Hg with carbon dioxide insufflation, the mesh dislocated at the edges of the "defect" and slipped into the defect. Increasing the mesh overlap to 4 cm from the defect edges eliminated mesh disruption in three of the four models tested. The lightweight mesh remained intact in all tests [21].

The study by Klinge and colleagues [17] examined the directionality of strength, and measured tensile strength of the vertical and horizontal directions of three meshes. Marlex and Prolene were both over five times stronger than the calculated abdominal wall strength, and Mersilene was at least twice as strong. A similar trend was noted in an animal study conducted by Cobb. Mesh was implanted into swine for 5 months and then tested for burst strength. Native tissue ruptured at 232 N, lightweight polypropylene mesh burst at 576 N, midweight at 590 N, and heavyweight mesh at 1218 N [22].

These data have lent scientific support to the theory that synthetic mesh materials, especially traditional "heavyweight" polypropylene mesh, are overengineered for their purpose. This excess prosthetic can lead to more complications, including decreased mesh flexibility, loss of abdominal wall compliance, inflammation, and scarring of surrounding tissues, potentially leading to pain, a sensation of feeling the mesh in the abdominal wall, and mesh contraction and wadding, which in turn may result in a recurrent hernia [23–26]. Meanwhile, new data demonstrate that current materials are not inert. Polypropylene especially is susceptible to degradation via oxidation [27]. The chronic inflammatory response incited by the heavy foreign-body load leads to perpetual exposure of the material to powerful macrophage-produced oxidants. Over time, this markedly alters the surface appearance and properties of the material [27].

The area of heavyweight polypropylene mesh has also been shown to contract up to 54% in experimental models [28], although all mesh types contract to some degree with acute wound-healing [29,30].

Multiple studies in both animals [31] and humans demonstrate that lightweight, macroporous mesh products provide the same benefits of reducing hernia recurrence rates, potentially with fewer undesirable side effects. The overall argument for lightweight mesh is nicely summarized in several papers [31–35]. In a randomized, multicenter study from Europe, patients undergoing a Rives-type preperitoneal sublay ventral hernia repair were randomized among three standard meshes (Atruim, Marlex, and Mersilene) and one lightweight mesh (Vypro) [34]. This study was somewhat limited by some of the material property differences between Mersilene and the two polypropylene standard meshes, as well as by some of the variability in operative technique among the participating medical centers (mesh fixation with absorbable suture at three centers). The recurrence rates were not significantly different and appeared to be technique-specific (absorbable suture fixation) [34].

Another European study of patients undergoing open preperitoneal sublay procedures compared the use of Prolene (heavyweight polypropylene) mesh with Vypro (lightweight polypropylene). This study demonstrated a significant increase in long-term chronic pain and feelings of a "stiff abdomen" in patients who had heavyweight polypropylene used for their hernia repair [35].

A group of 347 explanted mesh specimens were studied for markers of biocompatibility [33]. Inflammatory infiltrate, connective-tissue formation, and immunohistochemical markers for rates of cell proliferation and apoptosis were all reduced in the one lightweight, large-pored mesh (Vypro), compared with traditional polypropylene meshes (Marlex, Prolene, Atrium, and Surgipro). The lightweight mesh had a lower rate of chronic pain and infection and no fistulization compared with the other meshes [33]. This is the largest collection of explanted mesh reported.

Mesh materials

This section describes the basic mesh materials, as well as the newer products available (Boxes 1, 2, and 3).

Uncoated mesh

The original meshes widely available were woven and knitted from either polypropylene or polyester fibers. Polypropylene consists of a carbon backbone, with alternating methyl and hydrogen groups attached to the carbon chain. These hydrogen–carbon bonds are susceptible to oxidation [27]. Polylpropylene fibers can be manipulated into weaves or knits of differing design and density. Popular variations include monofilament and dual-filament knits. Multifilament variations are also available. The trend toward lightweight mesh has led to the incorporation of absorbable strands into the weave to provide stiffness at implantation. The strands are resorbed, leading to a lighter permanent material. Lightweight mesh can have both thinner fibers and wider mesh pores.

Polyester is a carbon-based polymer that forms strong fibers. Hence, it is used in fabrics, but also has multiple other uses. Polyethylene terephthalate (PET or Dacron) is the most common polyester, although there are many other forms. This structure is hydrophilic, whereas polypropylene is

---

Box 1. Examples of nonprotected macroporous mesh for uncontaminated ventral hernia repair without exposure to viscera

Heavyweight polypropylene
    Prolene (Ethicon)
    Marlex (Bard)
Lightweight polypropylene
    Ultrapro (Ethicon)
    ProLite (Atrium)
    TiMesh (GfE)
Polyester
    Parietex: flat and three-dimensional (Covidien)
    Mersilene (Ethicon)
Expanded polyfluorotetraethylene
    MotifMesh (Proxy Biomedical)

Box 2. Examples of mesh for intraperitoneal use or when potential exposure to bowel is suspected

Expanded polyfluorotetraethylene
   DualMesh, DualMesh plus (W.L. Gore)
   Dulex (Bard/Davol)
Polypropylene–expanded polyfluorotetraethylene
   Composix (Bard/Davol)
      E/X: heavyweight polypropylene
      L/P: lightweight polypropylene
Lightweight polypropylene–carboxymethylcellulose-sodium
   hyaluronate-polyethylene glycol
   Sepramesh (Genzyme)
Lightweight polypropylene–polydioxanone–oxidized regenerated
   cellulose
   Proceed (Ethicon)
Lightweight polypropylene–omega-3 fatty acid
   C-Qur (Atrium)
Polyester–collagen-polyethylene glycol-glycerol
   Parietex Composite (Covidien)

Box 3. Examples of biologic mesh and prices[a]

Human dermis
   AlloDerm (LifeCell; $26.08/cm^2)
   AlloMax (Bard/Davol; $26.00/cm^2)
   FlexHD (MTF)
Porcine dermis
   Permacol (TSL; $8.33/cm^2)
   Collamend (Bard/Davol; $16.00/cm^2)
   Strattice (LifeCell)
   XenMatrix (Brennan Medical)
Porcine small intestine submucosa
   Surgisis (Cook; $3.40/cm^2)
Fetal bovine dermis
   SurgiMend (TEI Bioscience; $22.00/cm^2)
Bovine pericardium
   Tutopatch (Tutogen Medical)
   Veritas (Synovis; $8.60/cm^2)

———
[a] *Data from* Bellows CF, Alder A, Helton WS. Abdominal wall reconstruction using biological tissue grafts: present status and future opportunities. Expert Rev Med Devices. 2006;3(5):657–75.

hydrophobic. Polyester is resistant to oxidation, but is susceptible to hydrolysis. Knitted multifilament polyester has been available for many years (Mersilene). Examples of newer polyester mesh include a flat, screenlike two-dimensional mesh and a multifilament three-dimensional weave. A paper by Leber and colleagues [36] published in 1998 compared the use of Mersilene with Marlex, Prolene, and Gore-Tex for ventral hernia repairs, and found higher rates of infection, small-bowel obstruction, recurrence, and fistula with Mersilene placement. However, this study used a variety of repair techniques and had a high rate of complications overall. Other investigators comparing Mersilene and Prolene using the same Rives-Stoppa technique of hernia repair had a low rate of complications for both meshes, and no difference in complication rate between the two [37]. It is now recommended that bowel be separated from a macroporous mesh of any material.

Coated or barrier mesh

Tissue-separating meshes were developed in response to the challenges of placing mesh intra-abdominally. The ideal intraperitoneal prosthetic would have two sides with opposite functions: The surface exposed to viscera would completely repel any adhesions or ingrowth, while the peritoneal surface would integrate through the peritoneum and preperitoneal fat into the musculo-fascial abdominal wall. Such a mesh does not currently exist.

The first widely used prosthetic for intraperitoneal adhesion reduction was expanded polyfluorotetraethylene (ePTFE). This molecule consists of a long carbon chain with two side fluorine atoms per carbon. The first publications of the original Teflon meshes were by pediatric surgeons looking for a prosthetic they could easily remove from newborns as they grew [38]. The first series of open ePTFE mesh implants in adults was described in 1987 and the first laparoscopic repairs in 1993 [39,40]. The currently available ePTFE materials have microscopic pores on the visceral surface (3 μm wide) that make ingrowth quite difficult. At reoperation, adhesions are usually minimal or easy to lyse [41]. The abdominal wall side is engineered with wider pores (>100 μm) and ridges to encourage ingrowth of mesh into the tissue. Despite this, the ingrowth and incorporation to the peritoneal surface can be relatively easy to disrupt. Therefore, adequate fixation of the mesh is quite important [42].

The next innovation was the merging of heavyweight polypropylene mesh with a layer of ePTFE. This composite graft allows for a macroporous mesh to be exposed to the anterior abdominal wall, while the undersurface resists ingrowth. This mesh has been popular for many years. Some problems can occur when there is a differential in contraction between the polypropylene and the ePTFE layers, which leads to rolling of the mesh edges and thus exposure of the polypropylene to bowel [23,43].

A number of available meshes form a temporary composite with an absorbable material, providing a barrier between the mesh and the viscera. The mesh needs to be protected for 7 to 14 days until a neoperitoneum is created.

Polypropylene meshes that are impregnated with Seprafilm (Sepramesh), oxidized regenerated cellulose (Proceed), and omega-3 fatty acids (C-Qur) form a hydrogel barrier, which is resorbed over time. Polyester mesh coated with a collagen layer is also available (Parietex Composite). These materials are all designed for intra-abdominal use. Numerous animal studies document the antiadhesive properties of these meshes compared with bare macroporous polypropylene [30,42,44–51]. The documented literature on observations of mesh during reoperation of human subjects remains scanty [41], although we have noted in our clinical practice that adhesions to ePTFE are easily disrupted with blunt dissection. Also, on several reoperations in cases where collagen-coated polyester mesh or oxidized regenerated cellulose–coated midweight polypropylene mesh had been implanted, there were also minimal adhesions. The point fixation devices used during laparoscopic repairs serve as the nidus of the most tenacious adhesions [52–55].

Biologic mesh

Biologic mesh materials are based on collagen scaffolds derived from a donor source. Dermis from human, porcine, and fetal bovine sources are decellularized to leave only the highly organized collagen architecture with the surrounding extracellular ground tissue. Other natural collagen sources in additional to the dermal products include porcine small intestine submucosa (which is layered for strength) and bovine pericardium.

The collagen in these materials can be left in its natural state or chemically crosslinked to be more resistant to the collagenase produced in wounds. By increasing crosslinking, the persistence of the mesh is also increased. Uncrosslinked mesh can be totally incorporated and reabsorbed within 3 months, whereas a highly crosslinked mesh can persist for years. It is not yet known if outcomes are affected based on the type of biologic mesh used in various clinical scenarios.

Most of the human studies published on biologic materials are from difficult clinical situations. Because angiogenesis is a part of the remodeling of the mesh, these materials can potentially resist infection. Other findings demonstrate some resistance to adhesion formation. There are some early reports on the use of biologic mesh in humans for primary hernia repairs in the inguinal region [56–58] as well as intraperitoneally for hiatal hernia repairs [59]. There are no current published reports on the use of biologics for primary repairs of ventral hernias. Long-term studies will be necessary before these materials are widely and routinely used as a primary mesh. Genetic studies of collagen formation will also be necessary help to determine if patients who form hernias are able to lay down normal collagen as they remodel biologic mesh.

How do I choose?

A frequent question from surgeons is: "With the wide variety of mesh products to choose from, which mesh is best?" At this point, there is no "best" mesh, so the decision of which mesh to use is based on several factors: the type of procedure being done, the clinical situation, the desired handling characteristics, and the products available to the surgeon based upon hospital materials contracts and costs.

Although heavyweight polypropylene mesh is currently the most frequently used mesh in the world, no situation mandates its use. Surgeon comfort level with these thick, stiff materials is high. Heavyweight polypropylene mesh is easy to handle and gives a feeling that a satisfactorily "strong" repair will ensue. However, as discussed previously, it is clear that these materials are mechanically overengineered for their function, and the potential complications are significant [20,23]. The body of literature against the use of these materials will continue to grow. It is clear that most "lightweight" materials, whether polypropylene or polyester, are sufficiently stronger than the anterior abdominal wall tissue, while inciting less inflammation, shrinking less, and offering more compliant characteristics than "heavyweight" polypropylene.

Risk of exposure

The first step of the mesh decision tree is to consider risk of exposure of mesh to intraperitoneal contents, which is directly related to the repair technique. If there is no risk of mesh–bowel interaction (overlay technique, retro-rectus position with little tension on the posterior closure), then a lightweight, macroporous mesh made of polypropylene or polyester is appropriate.

If there is concern that the mesh may become exposed to bowel, such as in the breakdown of a posterior closure of a retro-rectus repair under great tension, or if the mesh is being placed as an underlay open or laparoscopically, then a barrier mesh that rebuffs ingrowth of adherent viscera is appropriate. ePTFE has been safely used for this purpose for many years. It is very strong and possibly more inert compared with other available prosthetic materials. However, it is hydrophobic and presents a large foreign-material load to the patient. It is also more difficult to handle compared with other tissue-separating meshes because of the lack of memory in ePTFE. There are many composite meshes available. Some of the older materials have encountered some complications, especially when heavyweight polypropylene has been combined with ePTFE (Fig. 1) [43]. Now available is a newer variation of this material that is a composite of lightweight polypropylene and ePTFE. Other newer composite barrier meshes coat lightweight mesh with substances forming a barrier that allows for regrowth of the peritoneal epithelium before absorption of the barrier material.

Clinical scenario

The choice of mesh may be directed by the clinical scenario, such as when there is contamination or infection at the site of repair. Although products

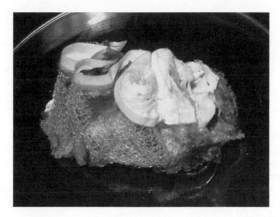

Fig. 1. An explanted mesh consisting of a heavyweight polypropylene–ePTFE composite, after cleaning. This specimen is notable for the contraction of the mesh, which led to exposure of the polypropylene to the viscera.

that contain antibacterial agents exist, the implantation of permanent synthetic mesh in infected fields is still not recommended. Absorbable synthetic mesh, such as Vicryl, does not prevent formation of future hernias [60] and, when placed in the peritoneal cavity in proximity to viscera, can result in significant adhesions and fistula formation [61,62]. We have reoperated on patients who had received Vicryl meshes for open abdomens and experienced an inflammatory reaction produced by the resorption of the Vicryl, leading to a frozen abdomen due to the extent of the adhesion formation. Biologic mesh has been touted as the solution for infected fields. Even so, certain rules still apply: The source of infection must be controlled and well drained, and the technique must be similar to a synthetic mesh repair. Wide overlap of mesh edges and placement in a retro-rectus position rather than inlay help decrease recurrence rates [10]. It is unclear how potential collagen deposition alterations in patients disposed toward hernia formation will influence long-term remodeling of these materials.

Cost

Another consideration is the cost of the material. It is difficult to obtain the true price of any mesh, as the cost to each hospital differs significantly depending on the materials contracts at that institution. Many surgeons are limited to specific brands because of these contractual arrangements, and such arrangements make it almost impossible to compare mesh costs head to head between companies. However, more highly engineered mesh is more expensive and barrier meshes are up to ten times more expensive than uncoated, macroporous mesh. Biologics are up to ten times more expensive than barrier meshes.

References

[1] Usher FC, Ochsner J, Tuttle LL Jr. Use of Marlex mesh in the repair of incisional hernias. Am Surg 1958;24(12):969–74.

[2] Burger JW, Luijendijk RW, Hop WC, et al. Long-term follow-up of a randomized controlled trial of suture versus mesh repair of incisional hernia. Ann Surg 2004;240(4):578–83 [discussion: 583–5].

[3] Luijendijk RW, Hop WC, van den Tol MP, et al. A comparison of suture repair with mesh repair for incisional hernia. N Engl J Med 2000;343(6):392–8.

[4] Amid PK, Shulman AG, Lichtenstein IL, et al. Biomaterials for abdominal wall hernia surgery and principles of their applications. Langenbecks Arch Chir 1994;379(3):168–71.

[5] Costa D, Tomas A, Lacueva J, et al. Late enterocutaneous fistula as a complication after umbilical hernioplasty. Hernia 2004;8(3):271–2.

[6] DeGuzman LJ, Nyhus LM, Yared G, et al. Colocutaneous fistula formation following polypropylene mesh placement for repair of a ventral hernia: diagnosis by colonoscopy. Endoscopy 1995;27(6):459–61.

[7] Fernandez Lobato R, Martinez Santos C, Ortega Deballon P, et al. Colocutaneous fistula due to polypropylene mesh. Hernia 2001;5(2):107–9.

[8] Losanoff JE, Richman BW, Jones JW. Entero-colocutaneous fistula: a late consequence of polypropylene mesh abdominal wall repair: case report and review of the literature. Hernia 2002;6(3):144–7.

[9] Ott V, Groebli Y, Schneider R. Late intestinal fistula formation after incisional hernia using intraperitoneal mesh. Hernia 2005;9(1):103–4.

[10] Franklin ME Jr, Gonzalez JJ Jr, Glass JL. Use of porcine small intestinal submucosa as a prosthetic device for laparoscopic repair of hernias in contaminated fields: 2-year follow-up. Hernia 2004;8(3):186–9.

[11] Franklin ME Jr, Gonzalez JJ Jr, Michaelson RP, et al. Preliminary experience with new bioactive prosthetic material for repair of hernias in infected fields. Hernia 2002;6(4): 171–4.

[12] Helton WS, Fisichella PM, Berger R, et al. Short-term outcomes with small intestinal submucosa for ventral abdominal hernia. Arch Surg 2005;140(6):549–60 [discussion: 560–2].

[13] Ueno T, Pickett LC, de la Fuente SG, et al. Clinical application of porcine small intestinal submucosa in the management of infected or potentially contaminated abdominal defects. J Gastrointest Surg 2004;8(1):109–12.

[14] Catena F, Ansaloni L, Gazzotti F, et al. Use of porcine dermal collagen graft (Permacol) for hernia repair in contaminated fields. Hernia 2007;11(1):57–60.

[15] Schuster R, Singh J, Safadi BY, et al. The use of acellular dermal matrix for contaminated abdominal wall defects: Wound status predicts success. Am J Surg 2006;192(5):594–7.

[16] Diaz JJ Jr, Guy J, Berkes MB, et al. Acellular dermal allograft for ventral hernia repair in the compromised surgical field. Am Surg 2006;72(12):1181–7 [discussion: 1187–8].

[17] Klinge U, Klosterhalfen B, Conze J, et al. Modified mesh for hernia repair that is adapted to the physiology of the abdominal wall. Eur J Surg 1998;164(12):951–60.

[18] Junge K, Klinge U, Prescher A, et al. Elasticity of the anterior abdominal wall and impact for reparation of incisional hernias using mesh implants. Hernia 2001;5(3):113–8.

[19] Cobb WS, Burns JM, Kercher KW, et al. Normal intraabdominal pressure in healthy adults. J Surg Res 2005;129(2):231–5.

[20] Welty G, Klinge U, Klosterhalfen B, et al. Functional impairment and complaints following incisional hernia repair with different polypropylene meshes. Hernia 2001;5(3):142–7.

[21] Binnebosel M, Rosch R, Junge K, et al. Biomechanical analyses of overlap and mesh dislocation in an incisional hernia model in vitro. Surgery 2007;142(3):365–71.

[22] Cobb WS, Burns JM, Peindl RD, et al. Textile analysis of heavy weight, mid-weight, and light weight polypropylene mesh in a porcine ventral hernia model. J Surg Res 2006; 136(1):1–7.

[23] Klinge U, Klosterhalfen B, Muller M, et al. Foreign body reaction to meshes used for the repair of abdominal wall hernias. Eur J Surg 1999;165(7):665–73.

[24] LeBlanc KA, Whitaker JM. Management of chronic postoperative pain following incisional hernia repair with Composix mesh: a report of two cases. Hernia 2002;6(4):194–7.

[25] Klosterhalfen B, Klinge U, Hermanns B, et al. [Pathology of traditional surgical nets for hernia repair after long-term implantation in humans]. Chirurg 2000;71(1):43–51 [German].

[26] Coda A, Bendavid R, Botto-Micca F, et al. Structural alterations of prosthetic meshes in humans. Hernia 2003;7(1):29–34.

[27] Costello CR, Bachman SL, Ramshaw BJ, et al. Materials characterization of explanted polypropylene hernia meshes. J Biomed Mater Res B Appl Biomater 2007;83B(1):44–9.

[28] Klinge U, Klosterhalfen B, Muller M, et al. Shrinking of polypropylene mesh in vivo: an experimental study in dogs. Eur J Surg 1998;164(12):965–9.

[29] Gonzalez R, Ramshaw BJ. Comparison of tissue integration between polyester and polypropylene prostheses in the preperitoneal space. Am Surg 2003;69(6):471–6 [discussion: 476–7].

[30] Harrell AG, Novitsky YW, Peindl RD, et al. Prospective evaluation of adhesion formation and shrinkage of intra-abdominal prosthetics in a rabbit model. Am Surg 2006;72(9):808–13 [discussion: 813–4].

[31] Junge K, Klinge U, Rosch R, et al. Functional and morphologic properties of a modified mesh for inguinal hernia repair. World J Surg 2002;26(12):1472–80.

[32] Cobb WS, Kercher KW, Heniford BT. The argument for lightweight polypropylene mesh in hernia repair. Surg Innov 2005;12(1):63–9.

[33] Klosterhalfen B, Junge K, Klinge U. The lightweight and large porous mesh concept for hernia repair. Expert Rev Med Devices 2005;2(1):103–17.

[34] Conze J, Kingsnorth AN, Flament JB, et al. Randomized clinical trial comparing lightweight composite mesh with polyester or polypropylene mesh for incisional hernia repair. Br J Surg 2005;92(12):1488–93.

[35] Schmidbauer S, Ladurner R, Hallfeldt KK, et al. Heavy-weight versus low-weight polypropylene meshes for open sublay mesh repair of incisional hernia. Eur J Med Res 2005;10(6):247–53.

[36] Leber GE, Garb JL, Alexander AI, et al. Long-term complications associated with prosthetic repair of incisional hernias. Arch Surg 1998;133(4):378–82.

[37] Yaghoobi Notash A, Notash AY, Farshi JS, et al. Outcomes of the Rives-Stoppa technique in incisional hernia repair: ten years of experience. Hernia 2007;11(1):25–9.

[38] Talbert JL, Rodgers BM, Moazam F. Surgical management of massive ventral hernias in children. J Pediatr Surg 1977;12(1):63–7.

[39] Bauer JJ, Salky BA, Gelernt IM, et al. Repair of large abdominal wall defects with expanded polytetrafluoroethylene (PTFE). Ann Surg 1987;206(6):765–9.

[40] LeBlanc KA, Booth WV. Laparoscopic repair of incisional abdominal hernias using expanded polytetrafluoroethylene: preliminary findings. Surg Laparosc Endosc 1993;3(1):39–41.

[41] Koehler RH, Begos D, Berger D, et al. Minimal adhesions to ePTFE mesh after laparoscopic ventral incisional hernia repair: reoperative findings in 65 cases. JSLS 2003;7(4):335–40.

[42] McGinty JJ, Hogle NJ, McCarthy H, et al. A comparative study of adhesion formation and abdominal wall ingrowth after laparoscopic ventral hernia repair in a porcine model using multiple types of mesh. Surg Endosc 2005;19(6):786–90.

[43] Saettele TM, Bachman SL, Costello CR, et al. Use of porcine dermal collagen as a prosthetic mesh in a contaminated field for ventral hernia repair: a case report. Hernia 2007;11(3):279–85.

[44] Bellon JM, Garcia-Honduvilla N, Serrano N, et al. Composite prostheses for the repair of abdominal wall defects: effect of the structure of the adhesion barrier component. Hernia 2005;9(4):338–43.

[45] Matthews BD, Pratt BL, Pollinger HS, et al. Assessment of adhesion formation to intra-abdominal polypropylene mesh and polytetrafluoroethylene mesh. J Surg Res 2003;114(2):126–32.

[46] Matthews BD, Pratt BL, Backus CL, et al. Comparison of adhesion formation to intra-abdominal mesh after laparoscopic adhesiolysis in the New Zealand white rabbit. Am Surg 2002;68(11):936–40 [discussion: 941].

[47] Matthews BD, Mostafa G, Carbonell AM, et al. Evaluation of adhesion formation and host tissue response to intra-abdominal polytetrafluoroethylene mesh and composite prosthetic mesh. J Surg Res 2005;123(2):227–34.

[48] Baptista ML, Bonsack ME, Felemovicius I, et al. Abdominal adhesions to prosthetic mesh evaluated by laparoscopy and electron microscopy. J Am Coll Surg 2000;190(3):271–80.

[49] Kayaoglu HA, Ozkan N, Hazinedaroglu SM, et al. Comparison of adhesive properties of five different prosthetic materials used in hernioplasty. J Invest Surg 2005;18(2):89–95.

[50] Bellon JM, Serrano N, Rodriguez M, et al. Composite prostheses used to repair abdominal wall defects: physical or chemical adhesion barriers? J Biomed Mater Res B Appl Biomater 2005;74(2):718–24.

[51] Borrazzo EC, Belmont MF, Boffa D, et al. Effect of prosthetic material on adhesion formation after laparoscopic ventral hernia repair in a porcine model. Hernia 2004;8(2):108–12.

[52] Karahasanoglu T, Onur E, Baca B, et al. Spiral tacks may contribute to intra-abdominal adhesion formation. Surg Today 2004;34(10):860–4.

[53] Joels CS, Matthews BD, Kercher KW, et al. Evaluation of adhesion formation, mesh fixation strength, and hydroxyproline content after intraabdominal placement of polytetrafluoroethylene mesh secured using titanium spiral tacks, nitinol anchors, and polypropylene suture or polyglactin 910 suture. Surg Endosc 2005;19(6):780–5.

[54] Duffy AJ, Hogle NJ, LaPerle KM, et al. Comparison of two composite meshes using two fixation devices in a porcine laparoscopic ventral hernia repair model. Hernia 2004;8(4):358–64.

[55] LeBlanc KA, Stout RW, Kearney MT, et al. Comparison of adhesion formation associated with Pro-Tack (US Surgical) versus a new mesh fixation device, Salute (ONUX Medical). Surg Endosc 2003;17(9):1409–17.

[56] Ridgway DM, Mahmood F, Moore L, et al. A blinded randomised controlled trial comparing porcine dermal collagen with polypropylene for primary inguinal hernia repair. J Am Coll Surg 2007;205(3s):A15.

[57] Edelman DS, Selesnick H. "Sports" hernia: treatment with biologic mesh (Surgisis): a preliminary study. Surg Endosc 2006;20(6):971–3.

[58] Edelman DS. Laparoscopic herniorrhaphy with porcine small intestinal submucosa: a preliminary study. JSLS 2002;6(3):203–5.

[59] Oelschlager BK, Carlos AP, John H, et al. Biologic prosthesis reduces recurrence after laparoscopic paraesophageal hernia repair: a multicenter, prospective, randomized trial. Ann Surg 2006;244(4):481–90.

[60] Pans A, Elen P, Dewé W, et al. Long-term results of polyglactin mesh for the prevention of incisional hernias in obese patients. World J Surg 1998;22(5):479–82 [discussion: 482–3].

[61] de Vries Reilingh TS, van Goor H, Koppe MJ, et al. Interposition of polyglactin mesh does not prevent adhesion formation between viscera and polypropylene mesh. J Surg Res 2007; 140(1):27–30.

[62] Vrijland WW, Bonthuis F, Steyerberg EW, et al. Peritoneal adhesions to prosthetic materials: choice of mesh for incisional hernia repair. Surg Endosc 2000;14(10):960–3.

SURGICAL
CLINICS OF
NORTH AMERICA

Surg Clin N Am 88 (2008) 113–125

Parastomal Hernias

Leif A. Israelsson, MD, PhD[a,b,*]

[a]*Department of Surgery and Perioperative Science, Umeå University, Umeå, Sweden*
[b]*Kirurgkliniken, Sundsvalls Sjukhus, SE-851 86 Sundsvall, Sweden*

Although he never performed the procedure, Littre, in 1710, introduced the concept of a colostomy as a medically useful procedure. In 1793 the first successful colostomy was performed by Duret on an infant who suffered colonic obstruction due to an imperforate anus. Although ostomies have existed since that time, knowledge in this field derives mainly from retrospective clinical reports. Parastomal hernia seems to be a frequent occurrence, to the point where some degree of parastomal herniation has even been considered to be an almost inevitable complication of colostomy formation [1].

Several surgical techniques have been attempted to prevent parastomal hernia; despite these efforts, herniation remains a major surgical problem [2]. Parastomal hernia is difficult to treat with open or laparoscopic techniques, and high recurrence rates have been reported after repair [2].

Definition of parastomal hernia

A parastomal hernia is an incisional hernia related to an abdominal wall stoma [3]. Parastomal hernia has been classified into four subtypes: (1) the subcutaneous type with a subcutaneous hernia sac, (2) the interstitial type with a hernia sac within the muscle/aponeurotic layers of the abdomen, (3) the perstomal type with the bowel prolapsing through a circumferential hernia sac enclosing the stoma, and (4) the intrastomal type in ileostomies with a hernia sac between the intestinal wall and the everted intestinal layer [4]. This classification has not been used in clinical studies, as it is difficult to distinguish these types of parastomal hernias during physical examination.

The definition of parastomal hernia used at follow-up is seldom present in clinical reports. In two clinical reports, herniation was defined as a palpable

* Kirurgkliniken, Sundsvalls Sjukhus, SE-851 86 Sundsvall, Sweden.
E-mail address: leif.israelsson@lvn.se

0039-6109/08/$ - see front matter
doi:10.1016/j.suc.2007.10.003 *surgical.theclinics.com*

defect or bulge adjacent to the stoma [5–7]. In one study, herniation was defined as a palpable "cough impulse" at the ostomy site [8]. In another study, adding a CT scan resulted in a radiological definition of any intra-abdominal content protruding along the ostomy [5]. In all other available clinical reports, the definition of parastomal hernia used at follow-up was not given.

In some studies, a distinction has been made between parastomal hernia and stoma prolapse [9–15]. However, neither parastomal hernia nor stoma prolapse was defined in these presentations. In a recent Cochrane report on loop stomas, parastomal hernia was defined as the formation of a hernia beside the stoma; stoma prolapse was defined as eversion of the stoma through the abdominal wall [16]. Guidance on how to differentiate between them at clinical examination and then exclude the presence of a concomitant herniation when prolapse is present was not given. As prolapse is an undesired complication of stoma formation, which is not readily differentiated from herniation, many authors have probably considered both as parastomal hernias.

The lack of a proper definition of parastomal hernia in reported cases makes it difficult to compare rates of parastomal hernia between different series and to estimate the true rate of herniation. Similar to ventral incisional hernia, recurrence rate of parastomal hernias increases with time [17]. It is generally agreed that follow-up should be no less than 12 months after the index operation to detect a ventral incisional hernia [18].

In future studies, the definition of parastomal hernia should be included at a follow-up that is no less than 12 months after the index operation. The present author proposes that parastomal hernia be defined as any palpable defect or bulge adjacent to the stoma detected when the patient is supine with legs elevated or while coughing or straining when the patient is erect [2,19,20]. If a CT scan is added to the clinical examination, parastomal hernia should probably be defined as any intra-abdominal content protruding along the ostomy Table 1 [5].

Incidence of parastomal hernia

The rate of parastomal hernia varies between 5% and 52%. This wide variation is probably due to the different definitions of hernia used at follow-up and its timing [5–8,11–15,17,21–34]. The use of a CT scan may

Table 1
Suggested strategy at follow up for parastomal hernia

Follow-up	12 months at least
Clinical examination	Any palpable defect or bulge adjacent to the stoma with the patient supine and legs elevated or erect and coughing or straining
CT scan	Any intra-abdominal content protruding along the ostomy

have contributed to the high hernia rates reported during the last decade as it allows detection of small parastomal hernias [5,8,23–25]. It seems that with a CT scan, more parastomal hernias can be detected than perceived by clinical examination alone [5,8]. Follow-up time varies considerably in clinical reports, and only a few studies have followed patients for at least 1 year or longer and then reported a herniation rate of 11% to 50% [7,12,14,24,25,35]. Experiences from studies on the rate of incisional hernia indicate that the highest hernia rates reported are the most accurate [36]. Considering that no uniform definition of parastomal hernia has been used in these reports and the variability of follow-up time, the true rate of parastomal hernia is very difficult to estimate, but it is probably between 30% and 50% in general surgical practice.

With ileostomies after a Bricker diversion, parastomal herniation seems to occur with similar frequency as with other ostomies (5%–65%) [35, 37–42]. The rate of parastomal hernia has been suggested to be lower after an ileostomy than after a colostomy, but this is rather doubtful as it has not been the case in a number of studies [8,14,38]. The rate of herniation is probably similar with loop ileostomies as with loop colostomies [16,43,44]. Hernia rates are difficult to compare between end stomas and loop stomas, as with the latter, bowel continuity is often restored and follow-up time is therefore different for the two groups [2].

Surgical considerations in stoma formation

Several retrospective reports have illustrated the results of various surgical techniques used in the construction of a stoma. There seems to be great variation among surgeons on how to bring out a stoma [3]. An enterostoma should never be brought out through the laparotomy wound as this has produced disastrous results in terms of infection, wound dehiscence, and herniation [1,45–47]. In two retrospective studies, an extraperitoneal construction of the stoma has been associated with a lower rate of parastomal herniation than an intraperitoneal route [1,24]. This technique has therefore been advocated by some surgeons but has also been challenged by others [48,49].

With stomas brought through the rectus abdominis muscle, a lower rate of parastomal hernia will be encountered than if brought out lateral to the muscle; in a retrospective study of 130 patients, the hernia rate was lower with enterostomas formed through the rectus muscle (3%) than lateral to the muscle (22%) [30]. In another study, of 93 patients, the rates were similar at 1% and 19%, respectively [22]. Four other retrospective studies did not confirm these findings, and there are no randomized studies available in this field [8,23,24,50]. It is nonetheless probably wise to bring out enterostomas through the rectus abdominis muscle as this is not associated with any disadvantages [49].

It has been recommended that the enterostomal opening in the abdominal wall should not be too large, as larger openings may be associated with an increased risk of parastomal herniation [1,12,29,47,49,51]. However, no evidence exists as to what is "too large" of an opening. It has been suggested that the opening should be made large enough to allow the bowel to pass and that the diameter of the opening should be around 2.5 cm [2,49]. There is no need to fixate the mesentery or suture the bowel to the aponeurosis as this has not reduced the rate of herniation [2,14,24,25].

Some surgeons have advocated laparoscopic surgery for the construction of stomas for fecal diversion [52]. In 263 patients with stomas created laparoscopically, the rate of parastomal hernia was reported to be between 0% and 12%, but follow-up time was less than 12 months [53]. Trephine devices have been tried for the formation of stomas, and in one clinical series no complication was discovered in 18 patients within 24 months [54]. In another study, two prolapses and two parastomal hernias were found in 17 patients within 2 to 48 months [55]. Other nontechnical risk factors for parastomal hernia formation that should be taken into consideration include obesity, wound infection, old age, corticosteroid use, chronic respiratory disorders, and malnutrition [1,4,50,56,57].

Surgical treatment of parastomal hernia

Surgical repair is indicated in 11% to 70% of patients with a parastomal hernia [8,12,15,30,35]. Local aponeurotic repair is not an acceptable mode of treatment because it results in an unacceptable recurrence rate within the range of 50% to 76% [1,4,49,57–61].

Relocation of the stoma into another quadrant of the abdominal wall is another way of addressing a parastomal hernia. This usually requires a formal celiotomy, but lesser means have been tried in small numbers of patients [62–65]. After relocation, the risk of a recurrent parastomal hernia at the new site is at least as high as after the primary enterostomy, and recurrence rates of 24% to 86% are reported [4,57,58,60,62,66]. If the stoma is relocated a second time, recurrence rates are further increased [57]. The stoma should not be relocated into a quadrant on the same side of the abdominal wall as this seems to be associated with an increased risk of recurrence [60].

The often large defect in the abdominal wall at the parastomal hernia site is in effect an incisional hernia and requires repair as such [67]. When the defect at the original stoma site is sutured, a recurrent hernia is very frequent and was present in 6 of 23 (26%) patients on physical exam and in 11 of 23 (48%) when a CT scan was used for follow-up [5]. In another study of 8 patients, the stoma was relocated to the same side of the abdominal wall and an inlay mesh repair of the abdominal wall defect was performed; no complications were reported within 15 months [68]. This technique violates the principle that relocation should be to the contralateral side of the abdomen. Moreover, the inlay mesh technique has been abandoned for incisional hernia repair owing to unfavorable outcome. As recurrence rates are high with these methods, other ways have been developed for parastomal hernia repair.

The strategy that has been chosen is based on the similarities between incisional hernia and parastomal hernia [69]. Mesh repair is a well-established method for repairing incisional hernias [67,70]. Meshes can be placed in an onlay, an inlay, a sublay, or an intraperitoneal onlay position (IPOM) [51,56,68,69,71–77]. With an onlay technique, the mesh is placed on the anterior aponeurosis. With a sublay technique, it is placed dorsal to the rectus muscle, anterior to the posterior rectus sheath. With the IPOM technique, the mesh is placed intra-abdominally on the peritoneum. These techniques all demand that the mesh be placed with considerable overlap and in all directions extend 5 to 10 cm beyond the edge of the defect. With an inlay technique, the mesh is cut to the size of the abdominal wall defect and sutured to wound edges Fig. 1.

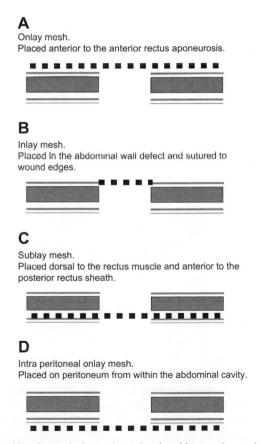

A
Onlay mesh.
Placed anterior to the anterior rectus aponeurosis.

B
Inlay mesh.
Placed in the abdominal wall defect and sutured to wound edges.

C
Sublay mesh.
Placed dorsal to the rectus muscle and anterior to the posterior rectus sheath.

D
Intra peritoneal onlay mesh.
Placed on peritoneum from within the abdominal cavity.

Fig. 1. In parastomal hernia repair the mesh can be placed in an onlay, an inlay, a sublay, or an intraperitoneal onlay (IPOM) position. (A) Onlay mesh—placed anterior to the anterior rectus aponeurosis. (B) Inlay mesh—placed in the abdominal wall defect and sutured to wound edges. (C) Sublay mesh—placed dorsal to the rectus muscle and anterior to the posterior rectus sheath. (D) Intraperitoneal onlay mesh—placed on peritoneum from within the abdominal cavity.

The inlay mesh technique has largely been abandoned in incisional hernia surgery because of the high recurrence rates with this technique. The IPOM technique can be employed with both open and laparoscopic techniques. With prosthetic mesh repair of parastomal hernia, lower recurrence rates have been reported compared with suture repair or relocation of the stoma, but large studies with sufficient length of follow-up or randomized studies are not available [49,57,68,69,78].

There are several types of meshes available. These consist of nonabsorbable, absorbable [69], partly absorbable [69], and acellular collagen matrix [79] meshes, all of which have been used for parastomal hernia repair. Polypropylene meshes and low-weight meshes can be placed in a contaminated environment without major complications [6,80,81]. There are potential dangers associated with the use of meshes though, such as fistula formation, adhesions, septic complications, and seroma formation [10,81,82]. Meshes that induce an inflammatory tissue response cannot be placed in contact with abdominal contents without a high risk of fistula formation, adhesions, and septic complications [83]. A mesh constructed of two layers is therefore usually used with the IPOM technique. The mesh surface facing the abdominal wall is usually of a nonabsorbable material inducing tissue response and allowing for integration of the mesh within the abdominal wall. The mesh surface facing abdominal contents is a nonreactive material causing a low or negligible inflammatory response so that adhesions are not formed. The most common mesh used is expanded polytetrafluoroethylene (ePTFE). A drawback of ePTFE is that the mesh is prone to develop infection in contaminated areas; if an infection occurs, the mesh must be removed.

Incisional hernia repair with a sublay mesh technique produces good results and has been proposed as the most advantageous technique for mesh repair of parastomal hernias [4,69,71–73]. It is theoretically attractive as it allows good anatomical preparation and the intra-abdominal pressure does not displace the mesh easily. With this technique polypropylene meshes are frequently used. Few nonrandomized reports are available on the outcome after sublay mesh repair of parastomal hernia [69,84–86]. They include only between 1 and 10 patients each and in only one study, follow-up time exceeds 12 months. When results from these studies are pooled together, the incidence of recurrence is 2 in 27 repairs (7%).

Parastomal hernia repair with an onlay mesh technique was described in 1981 [87]. Theoretically, the intra-abdominal pressure tends to displace the mesh that therefore must be anchored to the anterior rectus aponeurosis, and this demands extensive flap mobilization. Only a few nonrandomized reports are available on this technique [76,78,79,88–90]. They each report on three to nine patients, and in no more than three studies does follow-up time exceed 12 months. When results from these reports are pooled together, the incidence of recurrence is 2 in 35 repairs (6%). In a number of other reports, a mixture of various mesh techniques has been employed for parastomal hernia repair [10,51,57,58,81,91–97].

Thus, there are retrospective studies available indicating that onlay and sublay mesh repair produces better results than suture repair or relocation of the stoma, but the clinical evidence is not particularly strong as randomized studies are lacking, as is long-term follow-up.

Repairing parastomal hernia with the IPOM technique with an open surgical technique has been presented in two case reports [98,99]. The open IPOM technique was also used in two nonrandomized studies, and when these results are pooled together show 4 recurrences out of 36 repairs (11%) [100,101]. There are a few case reports presenting the laparoscopic IPOM technique [102–104]. The laparoscopic IPOM technique has also been reported in four nonrandomized studies that, when pooled together, resulted in 7 recurrences out of 72 repairs (10%) [105–108]. The laparoscopic technique is not feasible in all patients, and in one study the laparoscopic procedure had to be converted into open surgery in 8 out of 55 patients (15%) [107]. Bowel injury is also a problem in laparoscopic surgery and occurred in 13 of 59 operations (22%) in two studies [105,107]. Infection of an ePTFE mesh requires the mesh to be removed as reported in one study in 4 of 47 (9%) patients undergoing ePTFE laparoscopic mesh repair [107].

Thus, all studies looking at the IPOM technique are retrospective with no long-term follow-up. When performed laparoscopically, the incidences of bowel injury and mesh infection are high. ePTFE mesh, which is used in these cases, is prone to infection and its use should be carefully considered. Consequences of an ePTFE mesh present at subsequent contaminated surgery are not known Table 2.

Prevention

Prosthetic meshes with a large pore size of about 5 mm with a reduced polypropylene content and a high proportion of absorbable material have been available for several years (Vypro, Ultrapro, Ethicon, Norderstedt, Germany). With a low-weight mesh the degree of inflammation in the vicinity of the mesh is diminished [109], which may reduce the risk of the mesh eroding into the bowel [69]. In a prospective randomized study, 27 patients were randomized to a conventional enterostomy through the rectus abdominis muscle and 27 patients to the same procedure with the addition of a low-weight mesh placed in a sublay position. The mesh was not associated with infection or other early complications [6]. At 12-month follow-up, the rate of parastomal hernia was significantly lower with the mesh (5% versus 50%) [6,7]. Long-term follow-up is not yet available from this trial [110]. In a nonrandomized study, a prophylactic mesh in a sublay position was used in 18 patients, and no recurrence was noted within 6 to 28 months [111]. Parastomal hernia occurred within 2 to 26 months in 2 of 24 patients receiving a prophylactic mesh in an onlay position [112].

Placing a large-pore mesh with a reduced polypropylene content and a high proportion of absorbable material in a sublay position at the primary

Table 2
Methods used for repair of parastomal hernia

Suture repair	Very high recurrence rates
Relocation of the stoma	Very high recurrence rates—extremely high if the stoma is not moved to the other side of the abdominal wall
	A high risk of incisional hernia at the primary hernia site
	A prophylactic mesh might improve results
Onlay/sublay mesh repair	Has produced lower recurrence rates than suture repair or relocation has
	No randomized study is available—only small clinical series
	Long-term follow-up is lacking
IPOM; open surgery	Has produced recurrence rates similar to other mesh repairs
	No randomized study is available—only small clinical series
	Long-term follow-up is lacking
	Infection of the mesh is a problem
	Re-entering the abdomen is possibly a problem
IPOM; laparoscopic surgery	Has produced recurrence rates similar to other mesh repairs
	No randomized study is available—only small clinical series
	Long-term follow-up is lacking
	Bowel injury is a risk
	Infection of the mesh is a problem
	Re-entering the abdomen is possibly a problem

Abbreviation: IPOM, intraperitoneal onlay position.

operation is as yet the only method that has reduced the rate of parastomal hernia in a randomized study [113]. No adverse effects have been detected so far, but adverse late effects cannot be ruled out before long-term follow-up is completed.

The prophylactic mesh technique offers a novel way of treating parastomal hernia. Relocating the stoma into another quadrant with a prophylactic mesh at the new site, in combination with a sublay mesh repair of the abdominal wall defect at the primary stoma site, may have the potential of decreasing recurrence rates [110]. The defect in the abdominal wall is then repaired in a standardized way [20]. The prophylactic mesh has the potential of producing a low risk of herniation at the new site [7]. Only a small non-randomized series of 13 patients with no recurrence detected at 12-month follow-up has been reported so far [110].

Summary

Parastomal hernia represents a major surgical problem, and the incidence is probably 30% to 50%. Several surgical techniques have been tried to prevent parastomal hernias from developing. A large-pore mesh with a reduced polypropylene content and a high proportion of absorbable material placed in a sublay position at the primary operation is so far the only method that has reduced the rate of parastomal hernia in a randomized study.

For parastomal hernia repair, several surgical techniques have been attempted and small clinical series reported with short follow-up time. Recurrence rates are high with suture repair and relocation of the stoma; recurrence rates have been lower with mesh repairs. Several mesh repair techniques are used in open and laparoscopic surgery. Randomized trials with long-term follow-up are needed for better evidence.

References

[1] Goligher JC. Surgery of the anus, colon and rectum. 5th edition. London: Baillière Tindall; 1984. p. 894.
[2] Carne PW, Robertson GM, Frizelle FA. Parastomal hernia. Br J Surg 2003;90(7):784–93.
[3] Pearl RK. Parastomal hernias. World J Surg 1989;13:569–72.
[4] Devlin HB, Kingsnorth A. Parastomal hernia. In: Devlin A, Kingsnorth A, editors. Management of abdominal hernias. 2nd edition. London: Butterworths; 1998. p. 257–66.
[5] Cingi A, Cakir T, Sever A, et al. Enterostomy site hernias: a clinical and computerized tomographic evaluation. Dis Colon Rectum 2006;49(10):1559–63.
[6] Jänes A, Cengiz Y, Israelsson LA. Randomized clinical trial of the use of a prosthetic mesh to prevent parastomal hernia. Br J Surg 2004;91:280–2.
[7] Jänes A, Cengiz Y, Israelsson LA. Preventing parastomal hernia with a prosthetic mesh: a randomized study. Arch Surg 2004;139:1356–8.
[8] Williams JG, Etherington R, Hayward MW, et al. Paraileostomy hernia: a clinical and radiological study. Br J Surg 1990;77(12):1355–7.
[9] Hasegawa H, Yoshioka K, Keighley MR. Randomized trial of fecal diversion for sphincter repair. Dis Colon Rectum 2000;43(7):961–4.
[10] Steele SR, Lee P, Martin MJ, et al. Is parastomal hernia repair with polypropylene mesh safe? Am J Surg 2003;185(5):436–40.
[11] Arumugam PJ, Bevan L, Macdonald L, et al. A prospective audit of stomas–analysis of risk factors and complications and their management. Colorectal Dis 2003;5(1):49–52.
[12] Kronborg O, Kramhohft J, Backer O, et al. Late complications following operations for cancer of the rectum and anus. Dis Colon Rectum 1974;17:750–3.
[13] Abrams BL, Alsikafi FH, Waterman NG. Colostomy: a new look at morbidity and mortality. Am Surg 1979;45(7):462–4.
[14] Makela JT, Turko PH, Laitenen ST. Analysis of late stomal complications following ostomy surgery. Ann Chir Gynaecol 1997;86(4):305–10.
[15] Burns FJ. Complications of colostomy. Dis Colon Rectum 1970;13(6):448–50.
[16] Guenaga KF, Lustosa SA, Saad SS, et al. Ileostomy or colostomy for temporary decompression of colorectal anastomosis. Cochrane Database Syst Rev 2007;1:CD004647.
[17] Scarpa M, Barollo M, Keighley MR. Ileostomy for constipation: long-term postoperative outcome. Colorectal Dis 2005;7(3):224–7.
[18] Ellis H, Gajraj H, George CD. Incisional hernias: when do they occur? Br J Surg 1983;70(5): 290–1.
[19] Abcarian H. Peristomal hernias. New York: Igaku-Shoin; 1995.
[20] Cengiz Y, Israelsson LA. Parastomal hernia. European Surgery 2003;35:28–31.
[21] Burgess P, Matthew VV, Devlin HB. A review of terminal colostomy complications following abdominoperineal resection for carcinoma. Br J Surg 1984;71:1004.
[22] Eldrup J, Wied U, Bishoff N, et al. Parakolostomihernier. Incidens og relation till stomiens placering. Ugeskr Laeger 1982;144:3742–3.
[23] Ortiz H, Sara MJ, Armendariz P, et al. Does the frequency of paracolostomy hernias depend on the position of the colostomy in the abdominal wall? Int J Colorectal Dis 1994;9(2):65–7.
[24] Londono-Schimmer EE, Leong AP, Phillips RK. Life table analysis of stomal complications following colostomy. Dis Colon Rectum 1994;37(9):916–20.

[25] Leong AP, Londono-Schimmer EE, Phillips RK. Life-table analysis of stomal complications following ileostomy. Br J Surg 1994;81(5):727–9.

[26] Birnbaum W, Ferrier P. Complications of abdominal colostomy. Am J Surg 1952;83:64–7.

[27] Cevese PG, D'Amico DF, Biasiato R, et al. Peristomal hernia following end-colostomy: a conservative approach. Ital J Surg Sci 1984;14(3):207–9.

[28] Cheung MT. Complications of an abdominal stoma: an analysis of 322 stomas. Aust N Z J Surg 1995;65(11):808–11.

[29] Pearl RK, Prasad ML, Orsay CP, et al. Early local complications from intestinal stomas. Arch Surg 1985;120(10):1145–7.

[30] Sjodahl R, Anderberg B, Bolin T. Parastomal hernia in relation to site of the abdominal stoma. Br J Surg 1988;75(4):339–41.

[31] Baslev A. Kolostomitilvaerelse. Ugeskr Laeger 1973;135:2799–804.

[32] Stelzner S, Hellmich G, Ludwig K. Die versorgong der Parakolostomiehernie nach Sugarbaker. Zentralbl Chir 1999;124(Suppl 2):13–7.

[33] Everingham L. The parastomal hernia dilemma. World Council of Enterostomal Therapists Journal 1998;18:32–4.

[34] Tretbar L. Kirurgi vid stomikomplikationer. Stomijournalen: nordisk tidskrift för stomi vård 1988;2(4):10–1.

[35] Singh G, Wilkinson JM, Thomas DG. Supravesical diversion for incontinence: a long-term follow-up. Br J Urol 1997;79(3):348–53.

[36] Cengiz Y, Israelsson LA. Incisional hernias in midline incisions: an eight-year follow up. Hernia 1998;2:175–7.

[37] Ho KM, Fawcett DP. Parastomal hernia repair using the lateral approach. BJU Int 2004; 94(4):598–602.

[38] Marshall FF, Leadbetter WF, Dretler SP. Ileal conduit parastomal hernias. J Urol 1975; 114(1):40–2.

[39] Bloom DA, Grossman HB, Konnak JW. Stomal construction and reconstruction. Urol Clin North Am 1986;13(2):275–83.

[40] Fontaine E, Barthelemy Y, Houlgatte A, et al. Twenty-year experience with jejunal conduits. Urology 1997;50(2):207–13.

[41] Farnham SB, Cookson MS. Surgical complications of urinary diversion. World J Urol 2004;22(3):157–67.

[42] Wood DN, Allen SE, Hussain M, et al. Stomal complications of ileal conduits are significantly higher when formed in women with intractable urinary incontinence. J Urol 2004; 172(6 Pt 1):2300–3.

[43] Tilney W, Sains P, Lovegrove R, et al. Comparison of outcomes following ileostomy versus colostomy for defuntioning colorectal anastomoses. World J Surg 2007;31:1142–51.

[44] Edwards DP, Leppington-Clarke A, Sexton R, et al. Stoma-related complications are more frequent after transverse colostomy than loop ileostomy: a prospective randomized clinical trial. Br J Surg 2001;88(3):360–3.

[45] Hulten L, Kewenter J, Kock NG. [Complications of ileostomy and colostomy and their treatment]. Chirurg 1976;47(1):16–21 [in German].

[46] Pearl RK, Prasad ML, Orsay CP, et al. A survey of technical considerations in the construction of intestinal stomas. Ann Surg 1988;51:462–5.

[47] Todd IP. Intestinal stomas. London: Heinemann Medical Books; 1978.

[48] Devlin H. Management of of abdominal hernias. London: Butterworths; 1988.

[49] Martin L, Foster G. Parastomal hernia. Ann R Coll Surg Engl 1996;78(2):81–4.

[50] Marks CG, Ritchie JK. The complications of synchronous combined excision for adenocarcinoma of the rectum at St Mark's Hospital. Br J Surg 1975;62(11):901–5.

[51] de Ruiter P, Bijnen AB. Successful local repair of paracolostomy hernia with a newly developed prosthetic device. Int J Colorectal Dis 1992;7(3):132–4.

[52] Liu J, Bruch HP, Farke S, et al. Stoma formation for fecal diversion: a plea for the laparoscopic approach. Tech Coloproctol 2005;9(1):9–14 [discussion: 14].

[53] Carne PW, Frye JN, Robertson GM, et al. Parastomal hernia following minimally invasive stoma formation. ANZ J Surg 2003;73(10):843–5.

[54] Resnick S. New method of bowel stoma formation. Am J Surg 1986;152(5):545–8.

[55] Anderson ID, Hill J, Vohra R, et al. An improved means of faecal diversion: the trephine stoma. Br J Surg 1992;79(10):1080–1.

[56] Leslie D. The parastomal hernia. Surg Clin North Am 1984;64(2):407–15.

[57] Rubin MS, Schoetz DJ Jr, Matthews JB. Parastomal hernia. Is stoma relocation superior to fascial repair? Arch Surg 1994;129(4).413–8.

[58] Rieger N, Moore J, Hewett P, et al. Parastomal hernia repair. Colorectal Dis 2004;6(3): 203–5.

[59] Cheung MT, Chia NH, Chiu WY. Surgical treatment of parastomal hernia complicating sigmoid colostomies. Dis Colon Rectum 2001;44(2):266–70.

[60] Allen-Mersh TG, Thomson JP. Surgical treatment of colostomy complications. Br J Surg 1988;75(5):416–8.

[61] Horgan K, Hughes LE. Para-ileostomy hernia: failure of a local repair technique. Br J Surg 1986;73(6):439–40.

[62] Baig MK, Larach JA, Chang S, et al. Outcome of parastomal hernia repair with and without midline laparotomy. Tech Coloproctol 2006;10(4):282–6.

[63] Botet X, Boldo E, Llaurado JM. Colonic parastomal hernia repair by translocation without formal laparotomy. Br J Surg 1996;83(7):981.

[64] Nomura T, Mimata H, Yamasaki M, et al. Repair of ileal conduit parastomal hernia by translocation of the stoma. Int J Urol 2003;10(12):680–2.

[65] Kaufman JJ. Repair of parastomal hernia by translocation of the stoma without laparotomy. J Urol 1983;129(2):278–9.

[66] Pearl RK, Sone JH. Management of peristomal hernia: techniques of repair. In: Greenburg AG, editor. Nyhus and Condon's Hernia. 5th edition. Philadelphia: Lippincott Williams & Wilkins; 2002. p. 415–22.

[67] Cassar K, Munro A. Surgical treatment of incisional hernia. Br J Surg 2002;89:534–45.

[68] Stephenson BM, Phillips RK. Parastomal hernia: local resiting and mesh repair. Br J Surg 1995;82(10):1395–6.

[69] Kasperk R, Klinge U, Schumpelick V. The repair of large parastomal hernias using a midline approach and a prosthetic mesh in the sublay position. Am J Surg 2000;179(3):186–8.

[70] Schumpelick V, Klinge U. Incisional abdominal hernia: the open mesh repair. Langenbecks Arch Surg 2004;389:1–5.

[71] Rives J, Lardennois B, Flament JB, et al. [The utilisation of a dacron material in the treatment of hernias of the groin]. Acta Chir Belg 1971;70(3):284–6 [in French].

[72] Rives J, Pire JC, Flament JB, et al. [Treatment of large eventrations. New therapeutic indications apropos of 322 cases]. Chirurgie 1985;111(3):215–25 [in French].

[73] Stoppa R, Petit J, Abourachid H, et al. [Original procedure of groin hernia repair: interposition without fixation of Dacron tulle prosthesis by subperitoneal median approach]. Chirurgie 1973;99(2):119–23 [in French].

[74] Rosin JD, Bonardi RA. Paracolostomy hernia repair with Marlex mesh: a new technique. Dis Colon Rectum 1977;20(4):299–302.

[75] Abdu RA. Repair of paracolostomy hernias with Marlex mesh. Dis Colon Rectum 1982; 25(6):529–31.

[76] Venditti D, Gargiani M, Milito G. Parastomal hernia surgery: personal experience with use of polypropylene mesh. Tech Coloproctol 2001;5(2):85–8.

[77] Bayer I, Kyzer S, Chaimoff C. A new approach to primary strengthening of colostomy with Marlex mesh to prevent paracolostomy hernia. Surg Gynecol Obstet 1986;163(6):579–80.

[78] Amin SN, Armitage NC, Abercrombie JF, et al. Lateral repair of parastomal hernia. Ann R Coll Surg Engl 2001;83(3):206–8.

[79] Kish KJ, Buinewicz BR, Morris JB. Acellular dermal matrix (AlloDerm): new material in the repair of stoma site hernias. Am Surg 2005;71(12):1047–50.

[80] Kelly ME, Behrman SW. The safety and efficacy of prosthetic hernia repair in clean-contaminated and contaminated wounds. Am Surg 2002;68(6):524–8.

[81] Geisler DJ, Reilly JC, Vaughan SG, et al. Safety and outcome of use of nonabsorbable mesh for repair of fascial defects in the presence of open bowel. Dis Colon Rectum 2003;46(8): 1118–23.

[82] Aldridge AJ, Simson JN. Erosion and perforation of colon by synthetic mesh in a recurrent paracolostomy hernia. Hernia 2001;5(2):110–2.

[83] Morris-Stiff G, Hughes LE. The continuing challenge of parastomal hernia: failure of a novel polypropylene mesh repair. Ann R Coll Surg Engl 1998;80(3):184–7.

[84] Hopkins TB, Trento A. Parastomal ileal loop hernia repair with marlex mesh. J Urol 1982; 128(4):811–2.

[85] Egun A, Hill J, MacLennan I, et al. Preperitoneal approach to parastomal hernia with coexistent large incisional hernia. Colorectal Dis 2002;4(2):132–4.

[86] Longman RJ, Thomson WH. Mesh repair of parastomal hernias–a safety modification. Colorectal Dis 2005;7(3):292–4.

[87] Leslie D. The parastomal hernia. Aust N Z J Surg 1981;51(5):485–6.

[88] Franks ME, Hrebinko RL Jr. Technique of parastomal hernia repair using synthetic mesh. Urology 2001;57(3):551–3.

[89] Kanellos I, Vasiliadis K, Angelopoulos S, et al. Repair of parastomal hernia with the use of polypropylene mesh extraperitoneally. Tech Coloproctol 2004;8(Suppl 1):s158–60.

[90] Kald A, Landin S, Masreliez C, et al. Mesh repair of parastomal hernias: new aspects of the Onlay technique. Tech Coloproctol 2001;5(3):169–71.

[91] Helal M, Austin P, Spyropoulos E, et al. Evaluation and management of parastomal hernia in association with continent urinary diversion. J Urol 1997;157(5):1630–2.

[92] de Ruiter P, Bijnen AB. Ring-reinforced prosthesis for paracolostomy hernia. Dig Surg 2005;22(3):152–6.

[93] Tekkis PP, Kocher HM, Payne JG. Parastomal hernia repair: modified thorlakson technique, reinforced by polypropylene mesh. Dis Colon Rectum 1999;42(11):1505–8.

[94] Tekkis PP, Kocher HM, Payne JG. The continuing challenge of parastomal hernia: failure of a novel polypropylene mesh repair. Ann R Coll Surg Engl 1999;81(2):140–1.

[95] Byers JM, Steinberg JB, Postier RG. Repair of parastomal hernias using polypropylene mesh. Arch Surg 1992;127(10):1246–7.

[96] Saclarides TJ, Hsu A, Quiros R. In situ mesh repair of parastomal hernias. Am Surg 2004; 70(8):701–5.

[97] Devalia K, Devalia H, Elzayat A. Parastomal hernia repair: a new technique. Ann R Coll Surg Engl 2005;87(1):65.

[98] Abaza R, Perring P, Sferra JJ. Novel parastomal hernia repair using a modified polypropylene and PTFE mesh. J Am Coll Surg 2005;201(2):316–7.

[99] Ballas KD, Rafailidis SF, Marakis GN, et al. Intraperitoneal ePTFE mesh repair of parastomal hernias. Hernia 2006;10(4):350–3.

[100] van Sprundel TC, Gerritsen van der Hoop A. Modified technique for parastomal hernia repair in patients with intractable stoma-care problems. Colorectal Dis 2005;7(5):445–9.

[101] Stelzner S, Hellmich G, Ludwig K. Repair of paracolostomy hernias with a prosthetic mesh in the intraperitoneal onlay position: modified Sugarbaker technique. Dis Colon Rectum 2004;47(2):185–91.

[102] Gould JC, Ellison EC. Laparoscopic parastomal hernia repair. Surg Laparosc Endosc Percutan Tech 2003;13(1):51–4.

[103] Dunet F, Pfister C, Denis R, et al. Laparoscopic management of parastomal hernia in transileal urinary diversion. J Urol 2002;167(1):236–7.

[104] Deol ZK, Shayani V. Laparoscopic parastomal hernia repair. Arch Surg 2003;138(2): 203–5.

[105] LeBlanc KA, Bellanger DE, Whitaker JM, et al. Laparoscopic parastomal hernia repair. Hernia 2005;9(2):140–4.

[106] Kozlowski PM, Wang PC, Winfield HN. Laparoscopic repair of incisional and parastomal hernias after major genitourinary or abdominal surgery. J Endourol 2001;15(2):175–9.

[107] Hansson BM, de Hingh IH, Bleichrodt RP. Laparoscopic parastomal hernia repair is feasible and safe: early results of a prospective clinical study including 55 consecutive patients. Surg Endosc 2007;21:989–93.

[108] Safadi B. Laparoscopic repair of parastomal hernias: early results. Surg Endosc 2004;18(4): 676–80.

[109] Schumpelick V, Klosterhafen B, Muller M, et al. Minimized polypropylene meshes for preperitoneal mesh plasty in incisional hernia. Chirurg 1999;70:422–30.

[110] Israelsson LA. Preventing and treating parastomal hernia. World J Surg 2005;29:1086–9.

[111] Marimuthu K, Vijayasekar C, Ghosh D, et al. Prevention of parastomal hernia using preperitoneal mesh: a prospective observational study. Colorectal Dis 2006;8(8):672–5.

[112] Gogenur I, Mortensen J, Harvald T, et al. Prevention of parastomal hernia by placement of a polypropylene mesh at the primary operation. Dis Colon Rectum 2006;49(8):1131–5.

[113] McGrath A, Porrett T, Heyman B. Parastomal hernia: an exploration of the risk factors and the implications. Br J Nurs 2006;15(6):317–21.

ELSEVIER
SAUNDERS

SURGICAL
CLINICS OF
NORTH AMERICA

Surg Clin N Am 88 (2008) 127–138

Inguinal Hernias: Should We Repair?

Kiran Turaga, MBBS, MPH,
Robert J. Fitzgibbons, Jr, MD, FACS*,
Varun Puri, MBBS, MS

Department of Surgery, Creighton University School of Medicine, 601 North 30th Street, Suite 3700, Omaha, NE 68131, USA

Inguinal herniorrhaphies have a low recurrence rate, which makes them effective at preventing life-threatening complications such as bowel obstruction or strangulation. They can be performed in an outpatient setting under local anesthesia and are associated with an uneventful recovery in most patients. For these reasons, surgeons are taught that all inguinal hernias should be repaired at diagnosis. Many surgeons perceive that bowel obstruction or incarceration with strangulation is associated with an unacceptable mortality. In addition, it is commonly believed that progression of a hernia is inevitable, and that operation becomes more difficult the longer a hernia is left unrepaired. This belief is reflected in recent recommendations by the Society for Surgery of the Alimentary Tract concerning hernia management [1] (Box 1). This attitude is also reflected by the fact that the incidence of inguinal herniorrhaphy is much higher in the United States than other countries. For example, 2800 herniorrhaphies per 1 million population are performed per year in the United States compared with 1000 per million in the United Kingdom [2].

The socioeconomic implications of this thinking are significant. Inguinal hernias are one of the most common afflictions of adults, especially men [3]. Approximately 770,000 inguinal herniorrhaphies are performed in the United States each year [4–7]. This procedure was the most common surgical operation performed by general surgeons in the United States in 1991 according to data from the National Center for Health Statistics [8]. The results are large direct costs for the surgical procedure and significant indirect costs because of time away from normal activities. The costs would even be greater if the large number of patients per annum who choose not to have their inguinal hernias repaired heeded their surgeon's recommendation [9].

---

* Corresponding author.

E-mail address: fitzjr@creighton.edu (R.J. Fitzgibbons, Jr).

0039-6109/08/$ - see front matter © 2008 Elsevier Inc. All rights reserved.
doi:10.1016/j.suc.2007.11.004   *surgical.theclinics.com*

Box 1. Recommendations of the Society of Surgery for the Alimentary Tract regarding hernia management

1. Repair of almost all groin hernias is recommended.
2. Inguinal hernias should be repaired because they enlarge over time, leading to a more difficult repair and higher risk of complications or recurrence.
3. Patients with groin hernias should undergo surgical evaluation within a month after detection.

The purpose of this review is to examine available data concerning the natural history of treated and untreated inguinal hernias. The incidence of complications with either treatment strategy is discussed using historical information from a time before herniorrhaphy became routine and contemporary data from two recently completed randomized controlled trials comparing routine repair using a tension-free technique with watchful waiting.

Natural history

The natural history of an untreated inguinal hernia is poorly understood, and until recently there were almost no contemporary data available. Published figures are based more on speculation than on scientific facts given the difficulty in finding whole groups of populations in whom no one has a hernia repaired so that a proper population-based study to determine the risk rate can be done. The most important question is the incidence of the potentially life-threatening complication of a hernia accident defined as either bowel obstruction or strangulation. Hair and colleagues [10] looked at a consecutive series of 699 patients admitted to two university departments of surgery for scheduled operations for an inguinal hernia. The median duration a patient had a hernia before presentation was only 7 months; however, 206 patients (29%) had their hernia for between 1 and 5 years, and 61 (8.8%) had their hernia for 5 years or longer. The delay allowed the calculation of Kaplan-Meier estimates to determine the cumulative probability of pain or irreducibility. The probability of a hernia becoming painful rose to 90% by 10 years; however, leisure activity was affected in only 29%, and only 13% of the employed patients had to take time off from work because of hernia-related symptoms. The cumulative probability of irreducibility increased from 6.5% at 12 months to 30% at 10 years; however, only ten of the patients required an emergency operation, and only two had infarcted hernial contents that required resection. The findings would seem to imply that the effects of delay had minimal clinical significance in this series of hernia patients. Gallegos looked at a group of patients and determined that the cumulative probability of strangulation was 2.8% at 3 months and 4.5% at

21 months [11]. Both of these studies as well as similar ones in the literature must be interpreted cautiously because of the selection bias caused by the fact that these patients choose to attend the researchers' clinics rather than being selected randomly.

Neuhauser found two groups of patients who were better suited for this analysis because they avoided some of the confounding variables, allowing a better estimation of the actual risk of a hernia complication. The first group consisted of 8633 patients enrolled in Paul Berger's truss clinic in Paris which was described in an 1896 publication [12]. This group was an important database for a study of natural history because Bassini's method had yet to be widely adopted, and elective herniorrhaphy was rarely done. Fortunately, Berger kept records on his truss patients and enumerated untoward events. There were a total of 242 bowel obstruction or strangulation accidents that translated into a yearly risk of 0.0037. Neuhauser's second group came from Cali, Colombia. Data on this group are available for 1 year (1965–1966) owing to a government initiative to aggressively examine a stratified random sample of its civilian population to determine the frequency of common conditions such as inguinal hernia. By reviewing records years later from the hospitals in the city of Cali where the population was required to be cared for, the probability of bowel obstruction or strangulation was found to be 0.0038 per year. Using the average of these two probabilities, the lifetime risk for bowel obstruction or strangulation for an 18-year-old man has been calculated using life-table analysis. Table 1 shows this probability using 1980 and 2001 life tables [13]. An often quoted publication (including the study by O'Dwyer and colleagues discussed later) from our group states that the lifetime risk for an 18-year-old man is 0.272% or 1/368 patients and for a 75-year-old 0.034% or 1/2941. This estimate was subsequently retracted because it was based on erroneous methodology [12]. The risk for bowel obstruction and strangulation is less than previously appreciated, and the mortality associated with such a major complication is probably lower than the 10% to 20% risk often quoted in older text books (Table 2).

To address this question, Neuhauser looked at Medicare discharge data on 84,995 patients from 1971, specifically examining the International

Table 1
Comparison showing increased lifetime incidence of accident in a hernia patient from 1980 due to increase in the life expectancy

Age (years)	Overall		Males		90% Males	
	1980	2001	1980	2001	1980	2001
18	1/5.18	1/4.95	1/5.49	1/5.15	1/5.4	1/5.13
72	1/22.72	1/20.41	1/27.03	1/22.73	1/25.64	1/22.22

All values expressed as "one accident per x number of patients," where x is the value shown in the table.

Table 2
Operative mortality for patients with obstructed inguinal hernias

Study	Mortality rate
Beller and Colp (1926)	0.109
Frankau (1931)	0.197
Guillen and Aldrete (1970)	0.132
Anderson and Ostberg (1972)	0.138

Classification of Disease (ICD) code 550 (inguinal hernia without obstruction) and code 552 (inguinal hernia with obstruction). He found the mortality rate at operation to be 5 per 1000 in patients without obstruction and 46.9 per 1000 in patients with obstruction, respectively [14]. In Hair's study of 699 inguinal herniorrhaphies, only 10 emergency operations were performed of which two had infarcted material that required resection. There were no deaths or serious complications in any of the patients. One of the obvious reasons for the improvement in the mortality from major hernia-related complications is better postoperative care compared with that in the early part of the twentieth century. Furthermore, access to such care is much more rapid, with almost anyone experiencing a complication having the possibility of emergency treatment within hours.

Randomized control trials

Two randomized controlled trials have recently been published that were designed to test the hypothesis that a strategy of watchful waiting is an acceptable alternative to routine operation in men with asymptomatic inguinal hernias [15,16]. The design provides valuable information about natural history. In both studies the incidence of hernia accident was acceptably low.

In the first study sponsored by the American College of Surgeons and published by the Fitzgibbons group, 720 men with inguinal hernias who did not have pain limiting usual activities and did not have new difficulty reducing their hernias within 6 weeks of screening were randomized to watchful waiting or a Lichtenstein tension-free repair using mesh. All of the men were followed up for at least 2 years, and some were observed for as long as 4.5 years depending on the date of enrollment, averaging 3.2 years. Follow-up was complete in approximately 90% of patients.

The primary outcomes were (1) pain or discomfort interfering with usual activities 2 years after enrollment, and (2) a change in the Physical Component Score (PCS) of the Short Form-36 Version 2 (SF-36V2) health-related quality of life survey from baseline at 2 years. Pain interfering with activities was defined as the selection of a level 3 or 4 response to questions with these choices: (1) no pain or discomfort due to the hernia or hernia operation; (2) mild pain that does not interfere with activities; (3) moderate pain; or (4) severe levels of pain that interfere with usual activities. These variables were measured at baseline and at the 6-month and annual visits.

Postoperative complications after a tension-free repair were assessed at the 2-week visit and as needed for 3 months. Long-term complications, including hernia recurrence, were assessed at the 6-month and annual visits [17]. Life-threatening complications were defined before the start of the study and were assessed up to 30 days after the tension-free technique.

Secondary outcomes included complications and patient-reported outcomes of pain, functional status, activity levels, and satisfaction with care. These outcomes were assessed at baseline, 6 months, and annually. Pain was also assessed at the time of crossover in watchful waiting patients who underwent the tension-free technique. Four 150-mm visual analogue surgical pain scales (SPS) were used to assess sensory and emotional aspects of hernia-related pain [18,19]. Functional status was evaluated using the SF-36V2 questionnaire and an activities assessment scale developed and validated specifically for this trial and a companion study comparing the tension-free technique with laparoscopic herniorrhaphy [20–23]. Satisfaction with care was assessed using 5-point Likert scales.

In the intention-to-treat analysis, no significant difference was found in pain limiting usual activities or the PCS of the SF-36 quality of life measurement tool at 2 years after randomization. The SPS and activities assessments were also similar between the groups. A substantial number of men crossed over to the other treatment. At the 2-year point from enrollment, nearly one quarter of the men assigned to watchful waiting requested and received an operation, most commonly because of increasing pain, whereas 17% of the men assigned to operation for a variety of reasons never had an operation and were followed with watchful waiting. The as-treated analysis was not substantially different from the intention-to-treat analysis except for the fact that patients who crossed over reported a much improved PCS of the SF-36V2.

Contrary to popular belief, there did not appear to be a penalty for delaying operation when the delayed patients were compared with the immediate operation group. The two groups were similar at baseline with respect to age, American Society of Anesthesiology (ASA) classification, preexisting conditions, hernia type, and hernia characteristics. No statistically significant differences were found between the patients in operative time, complications, recurrence rates, and satisfaction with the results of the operation. Multivariate analyses found no relation between the duration until hernia repair and operative time, the incidence of complications, long-term pain, or functional status [24].

Differences in baseline characteristics may have predicted the men who crossed over. Men who were assigned to operation and who refused seemed not as fit as those who remained in the operation group. Men who crossed over from watchful waiting to operation had more SPS-measured pain (pain when performing certain activities such as work or exercise) and perceived more unpleasantness from their pain at enrollment than those remaining in watchful waiting. Operation was remarkably effective in improving pain and the ability to undertake activities, although both intention-to-treat groups improved somewhat during the course of the study (Fig. 1).

By the end of the trial with a maximum follow-up of 4.5 years and an average of 3.2 years, the crossover rate from watchful waiting to operation had risen to one third. Recurrent hernias occurred in five patients or 1.5%. Only 2% of patients sustained long-term post herniorrhaphy pain, a rate lower than expected. Two patients experienced an acute hernia incarceration over the 5 years of the study. One was successfully reduced and repaired electively; the other required an emergency procedure and return to the operating room for hematoma evacuation. Strangulation was not present in either patient, and recovery was uneventful. These results translate into a hernia accident rate of less than 2 events per 1000 patients per year or about 0.002% per year.

Observation or operation for patients with an asymptomatic inguinal hernia

A second trial performed in Glasgow in the United Kingdom also addressed the question of watchful waiting for minimally symptomatic hernias. The study was restricted to males over the age of 55 years with an asymptomatic inguinal hernia with a visible bulge. Pain scores were measured with a Visual Analogue Scale (VAS), and the SF-36 was used to measure the general health status. Follow-up for the asymptomatic patients was at 6 months, a year, and then annually afterward.

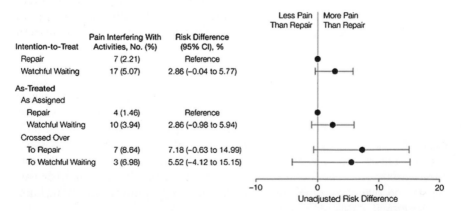

Fig. 1. Pain interfering with activities: group differences at 2 years in the Fitzgibbons study. Reference group for intention-to-treat is tension-free repair (score = 0); reference group for as-treated is patients randomized to and received tension-free repair (score = 0). (*From* Fitzgibbons RJ Jr, Giobbie-Hurder A, Gibbs JO, et al. Watchful waiting vs repair of inguinal hernia in minimally symptomatic men: a randomized clinical trial. JAMA 2006;295(3):285–92; with permission.)

The primary outcome of the study was pain measured at 1 year by the VAS. The study was adequately powered for this measurement; however, revised calculations were undertaken due to slow accrual of the study. The percentage of asymptomatic patients who were expected to develop pain was changed from 15% to 20%, which allowed the study a power of 80%.

The study recruited 160 patients with 80 in each arm. Patients who refused surgery were excluded from the study. The mean waiting period for surgery was 103 ± 97 days in the group who underwent surgery. At baseline, the patients who underwent surgery had somewhat worse general health status as measured by the SF-36, but this difference was not statistically significant. Interestingly, the pain scores between the two groups were comparable at 6 months and 12 months in the study, with no statistical significance. Among the patients who were in the observation group, 44% recorded pain at rest at 6 months which decreased to 28% at 1 year without any interventions recorded. The mean duration of the hernias before enrollment in the study was 3.04 years (2.58 years, standard deviation). There was a trend toward improvement in the SF-36 general health status and its components in the patients who underwent surgery, which was consistent in both the "treatment-received" analysis and the "intention-to-treat" analysis, but there was no statistical significance.

Twenty three patients (28.7%) crossed over from the watchful waiting to the surgery group for a variety of reasons including pain (n = 11) and an increase in size of the hernia (n = 8). A Cox proportional hazards regression model to study the influence of baseline characteristics on crossover indicated that the degree of protrusion was the only predictive factor. Three patients in the observation group were reported to have serious adverse events, whereas none were noted in the operative group, causing the researchers to conclude that early operation "may reduce serious morbidity"; however, one could argue whether these were truly adverse events of an observation strategy. One of the three patients presented with an acute incarceration which was reduced and then repaired electively. The reader must make his or her own conclusion as to whether this should be considered a complication of observation or simply a demonstration that even acute incarceration does not detract from the watchful waiting strategy because, even in the acute setting, the situation can sometimes be corrected without emergency operation. The other two serious adverse events were cardiovascular, consisting of a cerebral vascular accident in one patient and a fatal myocardial infarction in another after they crossed over from watchful waiting to the tension-free technique. The researchers stated that the medical conditions in these patients deteriorated over the observation period and suggested that if they had been operated sooner, they may not have suffered these complications. The actual length of time the patients were observed was not provided nor were any details of the medical deterioration. One could just as easily argue that the patients were given a reprieve corresponding to the length of the observation period. This group was older and therefore sicker, supported by the fact that nine patients (four in the observation group and five in the operation group) died during the relatively short median follow-up of 574 days, 6 from cardiovascular disease and 3 from cancer.

Differences between the two trials

There are some important differences between the two randomized controlled trials. The Fitzgibbons study was a multicenter trial conducted at five community and academic centers, whereas the O'Dwyer study was performed at a single hospital that was a tertiary facility for hernia surgery. The duration of follow-up was significantly longer in the Fitzgibbons study, with a median follow-up of 3.2 years compared with 1 year in the O' Dwyer study. The age of inclusion was also different in the two studies. The Fitzgibbons study included patients of all ages 18 years and over, whereas the O'Dwyer study enrolled only patients aged 55 years or older. This difference resulted in a higher overall mortality rate; nine patients died by the time the follow-up was completed (five in the surgery group and four in the observation group). The Fitzgibbons study should be considered more representative of the entire adult population because the O'Dwyer study included only older men.

The study outcome of pain was assessed using a VAS at 1 year in the O'Dwyer study and at 2 years in Fitzgibbons trial. This measure was not different between the two groups over time in either of the studies; however, the single most common reason for crossover from the observation to the surgery group was increasing pain. The change in quality of life seen in the O'Dwyer study was not similarly demonstrated in the Fitzgibbons trial, which had a longer follow-up. The individual component scores did not show a significant improvement even in the O'Dwyer study, and only the change in general health at 12 months had statistical significance (mean difference, 7.0 (95% CI, 0.2–13.7); $P = .045$). The differences at longer periods of follow-up were not reported, but it is possible that this difference may narrow between the two groups at longer follow-up as suggested by the Fitzgibbons study.

The study power was estimated at 90% to detect a difference of 10% between the two groups in the Fitzgibbons study, whereas the O'Dwyer study used a power estimate of 80% based on a difference of 15% which was later re-adjusted to 20% based on slow accrual. In addition, perceptions of quality of life may be different across different societies, and these transcontinental differences may have a role in the outcome measures recorded.

Over 40% of the study population in the clinical trial performed by Fitzgibbons and colleagues (2006) had the diagnosis of a hernia based on a cough impulse only. In contrast, O'Dwyer and colleagues (2006) only included patients if there was a visible swelling on standing. This difference may contribute to the improved health-related quality of life in the operation group at 12 months in the O'Dwyer study, which may not have been as evident in the Fitzgibbons study because many of the subjects had occult hernias. This difference also is the most likely explanation for the higher rate of crossover from observation to operation in the O'Dwyer study. Patients with chronically incarcerated hernias at baseline were excluded in the O'Dwyer trial but allowed by Fitzgibbons.

The 22% incidence of complications in the tension-free group in the Fitzgibbons trial was similar to what has previously been published in the literature. These complications included wound hematomas (6.1%), scrotal hematomas (4.5%), and wound infections (1.8%) among others. The O'Dwyer study did not note any significant postoperative complications, which may be a function of the excellent results of this specialized hernia center and not representative of the results across many centers or in a population-based setting, eliminating some of the loss of quality of life characteristics after surgery (Table 3).

Economic analysis of the O'Dwyer study showed that the cost to the health service was £401.9 ($806) higher for the surgical group at a follow-up of over 1 year. There were no significant quality of life years gained between the two groups. The Fitzgibbons study similarly demonstrated an increased cost of $1831 for patients with surgery; however, it determined that the cost per quality-adjusted life year gained from assignment to the surgical treatment group was $57,679 (95% CI, $1358–$322,765). This cost is generally considered a reasonable cutoff for a publicly funded medical procedure; hence, both watchful waiting and surgery appear to be equally cost-effective measures from an economic standpoint.

Although it is true that inguinal hernias will progress over time to incarceration, this does not seem to be associated with an appreciable increase in morbidity or mortality or even emergency surgery. The concern that a hernia may be more difficult to repair the longer it goes untreated was an issue when tissue repairs were popular, because the integrity of the musculofascial elements of the patient's groin were crucial to a successful operation. This concern has now largely been eliminated with the widespread adoption of the tension-free prosthetic approach with a recurrence rate of less than 1% regardless of the stage of the hernia.

The appreciation that the complication rate for an inguinal herniorrhaphy is more significant than surgeons would have expected has led to some rethinking. Poobalan and colleagues [25] published a critical review of inguinal herniorrhaphy studies between 1987 and 2000. The frequency of at least some long-term groin pain was as high as 53% at 1 year (range, 0%–53%). How much good do we do for a completely asymptomatic patient who undergoes a "successful" inguinal herniorrhaphy but ends up with lifestyle changes due to chronic groin pain (success meaning the lack of recurrence)? Despite popular wisdom to the contrary, it may be that patients with inguinal hernias can safely delay surgical treatment in favor of careful watchful waiting as the method of management for their hernia.

Table 3
Comparison of the Fitzgibbons and O'Dwyer studies based on baseline characteristics and study outcomes

Parameter	Fitzgibbons, et al, 2 year follow-up			O'Dwyer, et al, 1 year follow-up		
	Watchful waiting	Operation	P value	Observation	Operation	P value
Number of patients	354	356		80	80	
Mean age (years)	57.5	57.5		71.9	70.9	
Follow-up (%)	94.2	92.1		93.8	98.9	
Crossover	85/364 (23%)	62/356 (17%)		15/80 (19%)	—	
Reasons for crossover	86% Pain/ discomfort 47% Pain interfering with activity at crossover	Not stated		Pain and increase in hernia size Pain Increase in hernia size affecting work/leisure activities Acute hernia		
Outcome of pain	Pain interfering with activities, 5.1% Change from baseline pain at rest and activity Reduction in perception of pain unpleasantness on 150-mm VAS, −2.3 mm	2.2% −6.2 mm	P = NS P = NS P = .01	100-mm VAS At rest, 3.7 mm On movement, 7.6 mm	5.2 mm 5.7 mm	P = NS P = NS
Outcome SF-36	Change from baseline PCS, improvement by 0.29 points of 100	0.13 points of 100	P = NS	Perceived change in health compared with previous 12 months, −0.3 points All other components SF-36	8.5 points	P = .045 P = NS
Acute hernia events	One acute incarceration 4 months after enrolment, −0.3% at 2 years One acute incarceration and bowel obstruction at 4 years			One acute hernia		

Abbreviations: PCS, Physical Component Score of the Short Form-36, Version 2 Questionnaire; SF-36, Short Form-36 Quality of Life Questionnaire; VAS, Visual Analogue Scale.

From Chung L, O'Dwyer P. Treatment of asymptomatic inguinal hernias. The Surgeon 2007;5(2):95–100; with permission.

Although the question is moot in the symptomatic patient because the indication for surgery is discomfort and not the prevention of complications, what about the patient with either an asymptomatic or minimally symptomatic hernia?

The data confirm that a strategy of watchful waiting is a safe and acceptable option for men with minimally symptomatic (or asymptomatic) inguinal hernias. Hernia accidents occur rarely and can be treated with anticipation of a good outcome. Deferring an operation until symptoms worsen carries no penalty of increased complications and can be recommended. In specialized centers with good outcomes, operating on asymptomatic hernias may improve quality of life.

References

[1] Society for Surgery of the Alimentary Tract. Patient Care Guidelines 2000. Available at: www.ssat.com/cgi-bin/hernia6.cgi.

[2] Page B, Paterson C, Young D, et al. Pain from primary inguinal hernia and the effect of repair on pain. Br J Surg 2002;89:1315–8.

[3] Shackelford RT. Hernia of the gastrointestinal tract. In: Shackelford RT, editor. Surgery of the alimentary tract. Philadelphia: WB Saunders; 1955. p. 2222.

[4] Nyhus LM, Klein MS, Rogers FB. Inguinal hernia. Curr Probl Surg 1991;28:401–50.

[5] Rutkow IM. Demographic and socioeconomic aspects of hernia repair in the United States in 2003. Surg Clin North Am 2003;83:1045–51.

[6] Berliner SD. An approach to groin hernia. Surg Clin North Am 1984;64:197–213.

[7] Deysine M, Grimson RC, Soroff HS. Inguinal herniorrhaphy: reduced morbidity by service standardization. Arch Surg 1991;126:628–30.

[8] Rutkow IM, Robbins AW. Demographic, classificatory, and socioeconomic aspects of hernia repair in the United States. Surg Clin North Am 1993;73:413–26.

[9] Abramson JH, Gofin J, Hopp C, et al. The epidemiology of inguinal hernia: a survey in western Jerusalem. J Epidemiol Community Health 1978;32(1):59–67.

[10] Hair A, Paterson C, Wright D, et al. What effect does the duration of an inguinal hernia have on patient symptoms? J Am Coll Surg 2001;193(2):125–9.

[11] Gallegos NC, Dawson J, Jarvis M, et al. Risk of strangulation in groin hernias. Br J Surg 1991;78(10):1171–3.

[12] Neuhauser D. Elective inguinal herniorrhaphy versus truss in the elderly. In: Bunker JP, Barnes BA, Mosteller F, editors. Costs, risks, and benefits of surgery. New York: Oxford University Press; 1977. p. 223–39.

[13] Fitzgibbons RJ, Jonasson O, Gibbs J, et al. The development of a clinical trial to determine if watchful waiting is an acceptable alternative to routine herniorrhaphy for patients with minimal or no hernia symptoms. J Am Coll Surg 2003;196:737–42.

[14] Metropolitan Life Insurance Company. Expectation of life and mortality rates at single years of age, by race and sex. United States, 1991. Statist Bull 1996;75:16.

[15] Fitzgibbons RJ Jr, Giobbie-Hurder A, Gibbs JO, et al. Watchful waiting vs repair of inguinal hernia in minimally symptomatic men: a randomized clinical trial. JAMA 2006;295(3): 285–92.

[16] O'Dwyer PJ, Norrie J, Alani A, et al. Observation or operation for patients with an asymptomatic inguinal hernia: a randomized clinical trial. Ann Surg 2006;244(2):167–73.

[17] Ware JE Jr, Kosinski M, Keller SD. SF-36 Physical and Mental Health Summary Scales. a user's manual. Boston: The Health Institute, New England Medical Center; 1994.

[18] Thompson JS, Gibbs JO, Reda DJ, et al. Does delaying repair of an asymptomatic hernia have a penalty? Am J Surg 2008;195(1):89–93.

[19] Agency for Health Care Policy and Research. Acute Pain Management Guideline Panel. Acute pain management: operative or medical procedures and trauma. 1. Rockville (MD): US Department of Health and Human Services, Public Health Service. Clinical Practice Guideline; 1992.
[20] McCarthy M Jr, Chang CH, Pickard AS, et al. Visual analog scales for assessing surgical pain. J Am Coll Surg 2005;201:246–50.
[21] Ware JE Jr, Kosinski M, Gandek B. SF-36 Health Survey Manual and Interpretation Guide. Boston: The Health Institute, New England Medical Center; 1993.
[22] McCarthy M Jr, Jonasson O, Chang CH, et al. Assessment of patient functional status after surgery. J Am Coll Surg 2005;201:171–9.
[23] Neumayer L, Giobbie-Harder A, Jonasson O, et al. Open mesh versus laparoscopic mesh repair of inguinal hernia. N Engl J Med 2004;350:1819–27.
[24] Thompson, et al. Does delaying repair of an asymptomatic hernia have a penalty? Am J Surg, in press.
[25] Poobalan AS, Bruce J, Smith WC, et al. A review of chronic pain after inguinal herniorrhaphy. Clin J Pain 2003;19(1):48–54.

ELSEVIER
SAUNDERS

SURGICAL
CLINICS OF
NORTH AMERICA

Surg Clin N Am 88 (2008) 139–155

Open Repair of Inguinal Hernia: An Evidence-Based Review

Benjamin Woods, BS, MS[a],
Leigh Neumayer, MD, MS[a,b,*]

[a]Department of Surgery, University of Utah, 50 North Medical Drive,
Salt Lake City, UT 84132, USA
[b]Huntsman Cancer Hospital, Salt Lake VA Healthcare System, 1950 Circle of Hope,
Salt Lake City, UT 84112, USA

In 1960, Ravitch and Hitzrot [1] wrote the following in the preface of their book, *The Operations for Inguinal Hernia and a Current Recommendation*:

> This work arose from a discussion of the hernia repair during surgical house staff rounds at the Baltimore City Hospitals. It was apparent then, as it had often been during the past, and with other house staffs, that there was no uniformity of opinion as to the proper attribution of the various steps in any given repair of groin hernias. Frequently, there was a strong divergence of opinion as to what was meant by a "Halsted" or "Bassini" or "Ferguson" repair. The position taken by participants in the discussion was more likely to be influenced by chauvinistic attitudes, derived from the locus of their basic surgical training, than by precise historical and surgical information.

Although the repairs of today carry different eponyms (Lichtenstein, Kugel), the techniques have similar objectives. As more repairs have been added to the armamentarium, there has arisen a "strong divergence of opinion" on the approach (laparoscopic or open) and the type of mesh prosthesis (patch, patch and plug, Kugel). Who would have imagined that the treatment of inguinal hernia would continue to be such a controversial topic in the twenty-first century. For many surgeons in the middle to late part of the last century, inguinal hernia repair was a common procedure learned early in one's training, and there was a clear gold standard for repair (at least within an institution). In the last decade or so of the twentieth century, surgeons began repairing even primary inguinal hernias with mesh,

* Corresponding author. University of Utah School of Medicine and Huntsman Cancer Hospital, 1950 Circle of Hope, Salt Lake City, UT 84112.

E-mail address: leigh.neumayer@hsc.utah.edu (L. Neumayer).

0039-6109/08/$ - see front matter. Published by Elsevier Inc.
doi:10.1016/j.suc.2007.11.005

surgical.theclinics.com

something that was viewed before this time as sacrilege or, perhaps, a commentary on one's technical abilities, anatomic knowledge, or lack thereof.

Fortunately, the widespread adoption of mesh for the primary repair of an inguinal hernia was mostly driven by data suggesting that the rates of recurrence were high without it, and that if the mesh was correctly placed, the rates of recurrence seemed significantly less. As mesh for primary hernia repair became the standard, laparoscopic techniques for inguinal hernia repair were developed and refined.

Within this article, many aspects of open inguinal hernia repair and the data available to guide the surgeon's choice of technique are reviewed. Inguinal hernias are a common condition, especially in men; therefore, the majority of the literature available includes either mostly or all men. At the end of this article, the topic of groin hernias in women is briefly addressed. This review does not include the treatment of hernias in children. Additionally, although sometimes there is confusion, this article addresses inguinal and not femoral hernias. Femoral hernias are frequently treated in a similar fashion, but because of their higher rates of incarceration and strangulation and the fact that several major studies have excluded them, they are not included in this review. From here on, the term *hernia* when used without qualifiers refers to an inguinal hernia.

In recent years the literature has exploded with case reports (usually of bad outcomes), case series (usually of excellent outcomes), and randomized trials (with intermediate but probably more generalizable outcomes) on the subject of inguinal hernia repair using many different outcome measures. To the extent possible, this review uses available data from randomized multicenter trials because these most likely represent the practice of inguinal hernia treatment as experienced by most patients.

To fix or not to fix

Surgical textbooks have long advocated that the presence of an inguinal hernia is sufficient indication to repair it. Until recently, no randomized data existed to either support or refute this practice; however, within the last 2 years, two randomized trials have been published comparing watchful waiting with open mesh repair of inguinal hernias. One trial was a five-site multicenter study in the United States and Canada [2]; the other was a randomized trial conducted in England [3]. As elaborated below the results of these two trials are similar, the conclusions drawn by the investigators are quite different.

Combining the observation arms of both the North American and British trials yields nearly 400 men with at least 1.5 years of observation of their minimally symptomatic hernias. Clearly, the rate of incarceration is less than 1%, and it appears there is no increase in complications associated with waiting until symptoms worsen to repair the hernia. The data do not refute that the presence of an inguinal hernia is an indication for repair;

rather, they give reassurance to patients and their surgeons that watchful waiting is an acceptable alternative for minimally symptomatic inguinal hernias in men.

Perioperative preparation and care

Prophylactic antibiotics

Prior to the routine use of mesh, prophylactic antibiotics were rarely used because the rate of infection was low and the consequences of infection seemingly lower. Placement of a permanent prosthesis (eg, a prosthetic joint or heart valve) is frequently an indication for antibiotic prophylaxis, especially when the consequences of a surgical site infection are significant. Other considerations in the decision making for prophylactic antibiotics include whether the procedure is classified as clean or not, with clean low complexity procedures demonstrating minimal benefit from prophylactic antibiotics. Although inguinal hernia repair is classified as a clean procedure, a surgical site infection, in particular one that complicates a mesh repair, frequently requires removal of the mesh. Although the frequency of surgical site infection after groin hernia repair is low, most surgeons believe the use of prophylactic antibiotics is warranted. Only a few trials have addressed this question. In a Cochrane Database Systematic Review published in 2004 [4], eight randomized trials addressing the question of prophylactic antibiotics were identified. Only three of the eight used prosthetic mesh for the repair; the other five trials did not. There was no statistical difference in infection rates among the total patient population or the subpopulation of patients undergoing mesh repair. More recently, in a meta-analysis of 2507 patients from six randomized trials designed to assess the benefits of antibiotic prophylaxis in mesh repair of inguinal hernia published in 2007, the surgical site infection rate was 1.38% in those receiving antibiotics versus 2.89% in those not receiving antibiotics [5]. This difference translated into an odds ratio of 0.48 with a 95% CI, of 0.27 to 0.85. With the currently available data, administration of prophylactic antibiotics is recommended for mesh repair of inguinal hernias.

Perioperative patient instructions

Postoperative patient instructions should include warning signs of a complication such as a hematoma or wound infection, as well as a discussion of what can be expected regarding normal postoperative pain and activity. A frequently measured outcome in clinical trials comparing techniques of inguinal hernia repair is the time necessary for the patient to be able to return to work or normal activities; however, this return may be limited by other factors such as physician instructions to the patient and work situations. In the VA trial [6,7], both open and laparoscopic patients were given identical preoperative education and postoperative instructions. Patients were informed preoperatively that "most patients return to normal activities within 2 weeks." Postoperative instructions included no lifting restrictions and no activity restrictions. In an interesting double-blind study of the economic impact of hernia repair, Butler and colleagues [8] randomized patients to transabdominal preperitoneal polypropylene (TAPP), total extraperitoneal (TEP), or Lichtenstein repairs. The postoperative care team and the patients were blinded to the repair by a large dressing that covered the abdomen until postoperative day 3. The average number of lost work days was 12 and did not differ among the three groups. In the VA trial [7], the median time to return to normal activities was 4 days in the laparoscopic group and 5 days in the open group, a significant difference statistically, but the difference between the VA groups was small overall, especially considering that most trials have recorded a longer time period (akin to the findings of Butler and colleagues) for return to work. These larger differences may be attributable, in part, to patient expectations, work conditions (eg, the availability of workman's compensation or sick leave), and physician postoperative instructions.

The anatomy of a hernia

Thorough knowledge of inguinal anatomy is a key to performing an adequate repair. Surgeons must understand the anatomy from front to back and back to front, literally. Perhaps one of the most creative ways to teach and learn the complex three-dimensional groin anatomy is using the inguinal hernia origami developed a decade ago by Mann [9]. With proper folding of the preprinted double-sided paper, the student can "dissect" through the layers and better understand in three dimensions the relationships of the structures in the groin. Any student struggling with the anatomy is directed to this creative learning tool.

To mesh or not to mesh

In a Cochrane Database System Review in 2001 of open mesh versus open non-mesh repair [10], the researchers concluded, "There is evidence that the use of open mesh repair is associated with a reduction in the risk of recurrence of between 50% and 75%. Although the trials were heterogeneous there is also some evidence of quicker return to work and of lower rates of persisting pain following mesh repair." There was no evidence that there was a difference in the frequency of other postoperative complications including numbness, and the data were too limited to detect differential effects in patients with bilateral, femoral, or recurrent hernias. At that point in time, they also found two studies comparing flat mesh with plug and mesh and did not find any significant differences between the two techniques.

Another argument for routine placement of mesh in primary inguinal hernia repair comes from the Cochrane review of open versus laparoscopic inguinal hernia repairs published in 2003 [11]. The review included data from 41 trials including 7161 patients published before 2003 and concluded, "The review showed that laparoscopic repair takes longer and has a more serious complication rate with respect to visceral (especially bladder) and vascular injuries, but recovery is quicker with less persisting pain and numbness. Reduced hernia recurrence of around 30-50% was related to the use of mesh rather than the method of mesh placement."

These two large systematic reviews provide ample evidence for the use of mesh in all adult male inguinal hernia repairs. The next question is what configuration of the mesh to use and by which approach.

Techniques: open non-mesh and open mesh repairs

When comparing techniques of hernia repair (tissue versus mesh, laparoscopic versus open), surgeons rely first on "surgeon-centered" outcomes such as recurrence, complications, and death (Table 1). For each of the surgeon-centered outcomes, the rates depend heavily on how closely and for how long the patients are followed, on how meticulously complications are searched for and documented, and on how hernia recurrences are determined. There are also "patient-centered" outcomes which, when all else is equal, may sway a surgeon (or a patient) toward or away from a particular technique. The argument to mesh or not to mesh in open repair has been addressed previously. Postoperative pain (in particular pain lasting beyond 3 months) has been recognized in the last 10 years as a significant side effect of hernia repair. Although the incidence appears to be lower with mesh repair than with non-mesh repair [10], it is still common enough that patients should be informed of this potential complication when consent for the procedure is obtained in the clinic. In most studies with long-term follow-up, the incidence of chronic pain is approximately 6% to 13%. The recognition of this problem has led to several studies evaluating techniques to manage the ilioinguinal and genitofemoral nerves at the time of repair. Several of these studies are reviewed in the following sections, followed by a discussion of the techniques for open non-mesh repairs and several of the mesh options that have been developed over the last few decades.

Management of the nerves

When studies about the incidence of chronic pain after inguinal hernia pegged the rate at a substantial 6% to 13%, surgeons began to evaluate management of the sensory nerves during hernia repair. Several studies have compared in a randomized fashion the outcomes of pain and numbness with routine sectioning of the ilioinguinal nerves versus leaving the nerves intact. Although one study found that a prophylactic ilioinguinal

Table 1
Comparison of open techniques

Repair	Type	Recurrence rate for primary repairs	Postoperative pain	Reported advantages/disadvantages
Tissue repairs		May be as high as 17% at 10 years [14]	Many reports of pain higher than with mesh repairs	Need to understand groin anatomy for tissue repairs
Bassini	Conjoined tendon to inguinal ligament	5%–15%		
McVay	Conjoined tendon to Cooper's ligament	5%–15%		Repairs sufficient for inguinal and femoral hernias
Shouldice [12–15]	Triple layer tissue repair	<1%–7%		
Mesh repairs [16]			Chronic pain reported by as many as 20% of patients at 3 years	All mesh repairs are tension free
Lichtenstein [7,16,17]	Onlay patch	<1%–5%		Easy technique to learn, long-term experience in most institutions
Kugel [17,18]	Preperitoneal patch with spring	4%		Reported low operative times (around 35 min in some reports)
PerFix plug [19,20]	Plug and patch	4%		Fast/mesh plug migration
Prolene Hernia System [21–26]	Preperitoneal and onlay	<1%–3%		Fast (around 35 min in experienced hands) [21,24]
Stoppa [27]	Large preperitoneal mesh	<1%		Supplies laparoscopic view, mesh placed behind abdominal wall

neurectomy was associated with less chronic groin pain and a similar frequency of numbness [28], another found the opposite and suggested that preservation of the nerves reduced chronic pain [29]. The most recent meta-analysis suggests that the nerves should probably be identified during open hernia repair. Division of and preservation of the ilioinguinal nerve show similar results [30]. Although it seems intuitive that a suture tied down on a nerve would cause pain, this has not been studied in any scientific manner (and probably never will be). Sometimes a clue to the etiology of pain is to evaluate effective methods of pain control. For postherniorrhaphy chronic groin pain, there is not yet a treatment of choice, although case series of triple neurectomy seem to demonstrate success with this technique [31].

Open non-mesh techniques

Although open mesh techniques are superior to non-mesh techniques, the non-mesh repairs are described in this section as they might be used in instances when mesh placement is contraindicated, such as with contamination. The choice of a non-mesh repair is dependant on the surgeon's experience with a given technique as well as the quality of tissues available for the repair. When a pure tissue repair is not possible because of tension on the repair, a biologic graft such as acellular dermal matrix can also be considered.

Bassini repair

The Bassini repair [1] was developed in the late nineteenth century and was revolutionary at the time for low recurrence rates when compared with the previous standard of care procedures; however, recent studies comparing the Bassini repair and the closely related Shouldice repair show that the Shouldice repair is superior where recurrence rates are concerned.

The Bassini repair involves exposing the preperitoneal fat by opening the transversalis fascia from the internal inguinal ring to the pubic tubercle, followed by reconstruction of the abdominal wall. This reconstruction is performed by suturing Bassini's triple layer (includes the internal oblique, the transversus abdominus muscle, and the transversalis fascia) to the iliopubic tract/inguinal ligament with interrupted permanent sutures.

McVay's repair

Hernia treatment via the McVay repair [1] is similar to the Bassini repair with the exception that the triple layer superiorly is approximated to Cooper's ligament, not the inguinal ligament. This repair is composed of interrupted stitches that begin at the pubic tubercle and follow posteriorly along Cooper's ligament, narrowing the femoral ring and obliterating the "empty" space between the inguinal ligament and Cooper's ligament. A "transition" stitch is then placed to transition back up to the inguinal ligament at the level where the iliac vein crosses Cooper's ligament to finish the repair.

A relaxing incision in the anterior rectus fascia is usually included as part of this repair. Although in past decades this repair was chosen by many surgeons as their gold standard, currently, the primary use of this repair technique is for femoral hernias in contaminated fields.

Shouldice repair

The Shouldice repair originated when E.E. Shouldice sought more efficiency in preventing World War II recruits from being rejected from the Army due to inguinal hernias [1]. Through this effort and that of his surgical hospital following the war, recurrence rates with this technique were reduced from 20% to below 2% between 1945 and 1953.

Dissection involves exposing the crura of the external ring following exploration to the level of the external oblique, followed by incision of the external oblique in the direction of its fibers and with care not to damage the ilioinguinal nerve which is found just beneath the external oblique. The spermatic cord is then mobilized followed by ligation of the cremasteric muscle for necessary exposure and visualization of the incisional area on the transversalis fascia. The spermatic cord is reflected laterally, and the transversalis fascia is split from the internal inguinal ring as far down as necessary. The transversalis can be trimmed at this point, followed by freeing this fascia from preperitoneal fat to expose the edge of the posterior internal oblique and transversalis fascia.

Repair of the defect by the Shouldice method involves use of continuous nonabsorbable suture allowing for even distribution of tension and preventing interruption sites which could result in recurrence. The first suture line begins at the pubic tubercle, tracking laterally and approximating the iliopubic tract and the medial flap (transversalis fascia, internal oblique muscle, transversus abduminus muscle). This line continues as far as and including the stump of the cremaster muscle and then is reversed without interruption to begin the second suture line which tracks medially and approximates the internal oblique and transversalis muscles to the inguinal ligament. The third suture line is begun with a new suture and starts close to the internal ring. This line approximates the external oblique aponeurosis to the medial flap and ends at the pubic crest. The last suture line is begun by reversing the third suture line and as a more superficial reinforcing line over the top of the third line (Fig. 1).

Mesh repairs

The mesh used for noncomplicated (that is noncontaminated) inguinal hernia repairs should be a permanent material generally made out of polypropylene or mersilene. In general, polytetrafluoroethylene prostheses have not been used routinely in open repairs. An important aspect of mesh hernia repair is to understand the characteristics of the mesh. When studied in animals and humans, most of the permanent meshes used for inguinal hernia repair undergo shrinkage of between 30% and 50% over time [32,33]. This

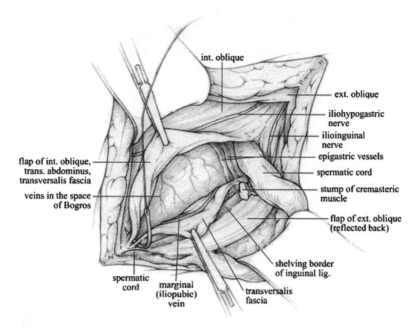

Fig. 1. Dissection completed and initial suture placement near the pubic bone. (*From* Shouldice EB. The Shouldice repair for groin hernias. Surg Clin N Am 2003;83:1173; with permission).

property makes it imperative to have mesh overlapping good fascia by at least 2 cm. In many laparoscopic hernia repair trials, using too small a piece of mesh has been associated with an increased risk of recurrence. The current size of mesh recommended for the Lichtenstein open repair is 3 by 6 in (7.5 by 15 cm).

As noted previously, in the situation of a contaminated field (eg, with strangulated bowel), if a primary tissue repair cannot be accomplished, a temporary mesh may be used (synthetic such as Vicryl or allogeneic such as Alloderm or Dermamatrix) with the assumption that there is a high likelihood of recurrence of the hernia as the temporary mesh is reabsorbed; however, by this time, the wound should have healed, and the case should once again be clean.

Lichtenstein

The Lichtenstein technique [34] of onlay mesh hernia repair was first popularized by Lichtenstein in 1984. The routine use of mesh, coined the "tension-free repair," took some time (about 10 years) to be universally adopted for primary hernia repair. The technique has undergone modifications over the years and is relatively easy to describe and teach. For both the VA laparoscopic versus open trial and the American Watchful Waiting trial, the Lichtenstein technique as described in a video made in 1997 was used

[35]. When local anesthetic was used in the trial, the authors recommended using the anesthetic technique of Lichtenstein as well. This practice results in a more uniformly anesthetized operative field independent of the operator when compared with other techniques including ilioinguinal nerve blocks. Both techniques are briefly described in the following section.

Anesthetic technique. After usual preparation and draping of the groin, 3 to 5 mL of local anesthetic (the authors used a 1:1 mixture of 1% lidocaine and 0.5% bupivacaine for the hernia trial) is infiltrated in the subcutaneous tissue along the planned incision site. Without withdrawing the needle from the skin, another 2 to 3 mL is used in the dermis to create a skin wheal along the planned incision. Starting just lateral to the lateral edge of the incision and at 2 cm intervals along the incision for a total of five injections, 2 mL of the mixture is injected below the external oblique fascia by directing the needle perpendicular to the skin and inserting until the "pop" of piercing the external oblique fascia is felt. The procedure then commences. Once the external oblique fascia is identified, another 8 to 10 mL of the mixture is injected laterally just beneath this fascia. A few milliliters may be infiltrated at the pubic tubercle, around the neck, and inside the indirect hernia sac.

Repair method. A 5-cm skin incision is made starting at the pubic tubercle and extending laterally along Langer's lines. The external oblique aponeurosis is opened including the external ring. If an indirect hernia is found, after dissecting it from the other cord structures to at least the level of the internal ring, the sac is either inverted without division when possible or divided leaving the distal portion in situ and closing the proximal sac. If a direct hernia is identified, the sac is simply inverted using an absorbable purse-string suture.

A prosthesis measuring approximately 8 × 16 cm is used. The lower edge of the prosthesis is fixed using a continuous suture to Poupart's ligament beginning medially and overlapping 2 cm onto the pubic tubercle and proceeding laterally along the ligament beyond the internal ring using three to four bites of 2.0 Prolene, ending just lateral to the internal ring. If a femoral defect is suspected, the inferior edge of the prosthesis is sutured to Cooper's ligament, beginning near the area of the pubic tubercle and continuing laterally along Cooper's ligament. A transition stitch is then accomplished between the prosthesis, Cooper's ligament, the femoral sheath, and Poupart's ligament, and the repair is then continued laterally along Poupart's ligament to just lateral to the internal ring. The superior medial border of the prosthesis is secured to the rectus sheath with an interrupted 2.0 Prolene suture, creating a wrinkle in the mesh. The superior border of the mesh is tacked to the internal oblique with an interrupted 2.0 Prolene suture. A slit is made transversely in the mesh from the lateral aspect to the location of the internal ring. The slit should be made such that the lower portion is one-third the width of the mesh. The upper and lower portions of the mesh are brought around the cord. The lower border of the upper portion and the lower border of the lower portion are then tacked to the inguinal ligament just lateral to the internal ring with an interrupted 2.0 Prolene suture, recreating the shutter mechanism of the internal ring. The tails of the mesh are placed laterally under the external oblique. Management of the cremasteric muscles (split versus divided) is at the discretion of the surgeon and frequently depends on the characteristics of the hernia and the condition of the muscle. Additional analgesia (30 mL of dilute Marcaine [10 mL of 0.5% Marcaine mixed with 20 mL of saline]) may be instilled into the operative site. The external oblique fascia is then closed, and the skin is closed with a running subcuticular suture.

Other mesh repairs

Kugel repair

The Kugel repair is considered a simple and minimally invasive repair, but its success is dependant on the experience and training of the surgeon. The Kugel repair was detailed in a recent issue of *Surgical Clinics of North America* [36]. The Kugel repair combines the ease of an anterior approach with mesh placed in the preperitoneal position. The mesh is designed to expand into its full dimensions after being rolled or folded and placed in the preperitoneal space through a relatively small opening. A 2- to 3-cm incision is located halfway between the superior iliac spine and the pubic tubercle delving through the external oblique, internal oblique, and transversalis fascia. Any indirect sac is ligated or inverted. The inferior epigastric vessels are identified and should remain attached to the transversalis fascia while the peritoneum is freed from the posterior aspect of the transversalis fascia, creating a preperitoneal pocket in which to place the Kugel patch. The Kugel patch, typically a standard size of 8 × 12 cm, is inserted into the preperitoneal space and allowed to expand. The patch is secured with a single stitch and allowed to cover the defect. The suture holds it in place along with the pressure from the peritoneum as the patient stands and proceeds with normal activities.

Plug and patch

The plug and patch or PerFix repair [37] uses a cone-shaped plug made of two layers of polypropylene mesh that is inserted into the inguinal canal in an indirect hernia, followed by the placement of a mesh patch which is sewn around the spermatic cord and laid on top of the posterior wall. Repair of a direct hernia is accomplished with this method by likewise placing the plug into the defect, followed by placement of patch around the spermatic cord in the same fashion. This repair can be used in large or small defects by employing larger or smaller sizes of premanufactured plugs, or by the construction of the required size of plug in the operating room. The utility of this patch is based on its versatility for repairing various sizes of defects and its lesser dependence on user experience and training. This technique was fully elucidated in a previous issue of *Surgical Clinics of North America* [37]. The reader is directed there for further details on the technique and its outcomes.

Migration or erosion of the plug has been infrequently reported. The plug has been associated with small bowel volvulus and diverticulitis in case reports. A review of the available reports of migration or erosion showed this complication to be rare and associated with technical error at the time of operation.

Prolene Hernia System

The Prolene Hernia System (PHS) was developed as an option inguinal hernia repair that combined the benefits of anterior and posterior mesh components. It was introduced in 1998 and since then has been studied in retrospective chart reviews [21] and randomized trials [22–26]; however, none of these studies provide long-term data (beyond 1.5 years) for recurrence.

In the procedure for using this system [21], the inguinal canal is approached anteriorly as described for the Lichtenstein repair. If present, the indirect sac is dissected and inverted, and a preperitoneal pocket is created through the internal ring using a Raytec sponge. The posterior portion of the PHS is then deployed in the preperitoneal space. The anterior portion is positioned and sutured much like the onlay patch in the Lichtenstein repair. A lateral slit is made in the PHS mesh to accommodate the cord and relocate the internal ring, usually a bit laterally. The lateral anterior portion of the PHS is then deployed under the external oblique aponeurosis laterally (Fig. 2).

The advertised advantages of the PHS in comparison with an onlay mesh or mesh plug include reduced pain and reduced recurrence rates. Only one study found a reduction in immediate postoperative pain [26]. PHS was associated with a shortened operative time by 4 to 5 minutes in two of the randomized trials [25,26] but not in the third [24]. The studies have not

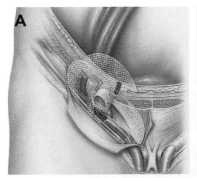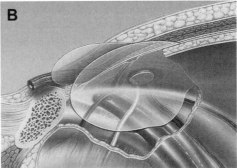

Fig. 2. (*A*) Prolene hernia system anterior view. (*B*) Prolene hernia system posterior view. (*Courtesy of* Ethicon, Inc., Somerville, NJ; with permission).

shown a difference in long-term pain. The lack of evidence supporting the advertised claims may be responsible for the low use of this system.

Stoppa

The Stoppa repair involves reinforcement of the visceral sac by a preperitoneal bilateral mesh prosthesis [27]. The technique, recommended for large, complex, or bilateral hernias, is performed using one of two standard incisions—a vertical midline subumbilical or a low horizontal skin incision. The midline fascial layers are divided, providing access to the preperitoneal space. This space is further opened with blunt dissection, much like that used for a laparoscopic approach. The hernia sacs are reduced using gentle traction. Indirect sacs should be opened and explored with the finger to simplify their dissection from the other cord structures and to ensure evacuation of their contents. Large sacs can be transected and closed proximally. A large piece of mesh (Stoppa recommended Dacron) is then prepared in a chevron shape with a dimension of 24 × 18 cm. Using clamps, the mesh is then placed into the preperitoneal space being sure to pull the cephalad lateral clamp as far as possible laterally and posteriorly, and the lower lateral clamp as far as possible behind the corresponding obturator wall. No attempt is made to secure the mesh with clips or sutures. Several variations on this repair have been reported and are outlined in available textbooks. This repair is similar in many ways to the laparoscopic repair, and familiarity with the anatomy from the "inside" is helpful when approaching hernias laparoscopically.

Teaching and learning the repair

The VA hernia trial provided a large database with which to examine some questions about the impact of resident participation in hernia repair and, to a lesser extent, the impact of surgeon experience on outcomes. To address the latter, the authors examined the impact of resident training level on outcomes such as recurrence and complications [38]. The results differed based on technique. Although there did not appear to be a significant impact of resident level of training on the outcomes of laparoscopic repair, there was a significant impact of resident level on recurrence in open repair (Fig. 3). There were no differences in complication rates, but as might be expected, operative times were significantly shorter for senior (postgraduate year [PGY] 4+) residents when compared with junior (PGY 1-2) residents (76.3 minutes and 71.6 minutes, respectively).

Although it has never been adequately studied, it appears that surgeons receive adequate training during residency in hernia repair which translates into continued reasonable results as far as recurrence rates beyond training. In the VA trial, the authors could find no relationship of volume and outcome for the attending surgeons in the open repair [39], but that finding was likely because all of the participating surgeons had passed the volume threshold for open hernia repair during their residencies. In the Watchful

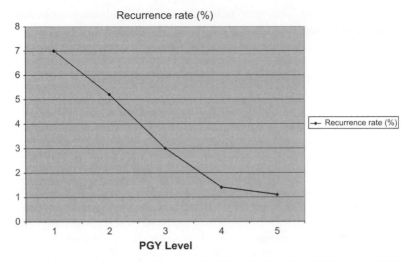

Fig. 3. Recurrence rate by postgraduate year (PGY) level. (*Data from* Wilkiemeyer M, Pappas TN, Giobbie-Hurder A, et al. Does resident post graduate year influence the outcomes of inguinal hernia repair? Ann Surg 2005;241(6):879–84.)

Waiting trial, the recurrence rate in the open repair group was lower than in the VA trial. This finding could have been due to many factors, including patient and hernia characteristics, but could also be accounted for, in part, by site or surgeon selection. In the Watchful Waiting trial, sites and surgeons with proven interest and expertise in hernia repair participated. In the VA trial, there was a less subspecialized group of surgeons participating because the structure of the VA at the time was such that nearly all general surgeons at each site qualified (by having previously performed >25 open mesh repairs) for performing repairs in the open group.

Inguinal hernias in women

In 2005, Koch and colleagues [40] published the largest series of groin hernia repairs in women. They used data from the prospectively collected Swedish Hernia Register between 1992 and 2003 to provide excellent information about the outcomes of hernia repair in women. Important points from this landmark study are as follows:

- Women undergo a higher proportion of emergency hernia repair than men (16.9% versus 5.0%).
- Women who are originally diagnosed with an indirect or direct hernia at primary repair are likely to have a femoral hernia found at reoperation for a recurrence (41.6% versus a corresponding 4.6% of men).
- Nearly 40% of women did not undergo a standard (Shouldice, Lichtenstein, plug/mesh, TAPP/TEP) repair.

- Women had a higher risk for reoperation for recurrence (relative risk, 2.61 [95% CI, 1.89–3.61] for women versus 1.92 [95% CI, 1.74–2.12] for men).
- Techniques associated with the lowest risk for reoperation in men were associated with the highest risk in women.

Using the reoperation rates after the Lichtenstein repair as reference, women had the lowest risk of reoperation after laparoscopic repairs, whereas Lichtenstein repair provided the lowest risk of reoperation in men. Given the high proportion of femoral hernias found in women at reoperation for recurrence, primary repair laparoscopically may benefit the patient in avoiding a missed femoral hernia.

Recommendations

Groin hernia continues to be a common diagnosis. In men who need repair of their hernia because of symptoms, open repair with mesh continues to be an excellent option for a first time hernia repair in adults. If a non-mesh repair is offered, it should be the Shouldice repair because, at least in experienced hands, it has been shown to have outcomes similar to open mesh repairs. For most surgeons, a Lichtenstein onlay repair is easy to learn and easily applied in most settings. It has been studied more than the other open mesh repairs in randomized trials across multiple institutions such that the results from these large studies can be generalized to both the general population and the typical general surgeon. The uniform adoption of other open mesh techniques should require further study and long-term follow-up to show that they are at a minimum equivalent to the well-studied Lichtenstein repair in terms of recurrence and long-term chronic pain, the two most significant adverse outcomes for patients.

References

[1] Ravitch MM, Hitzrot JM. The operations for inguinal hernia. St. Louis (MO): CV Mosby-Company; 1960.
[2] Fitzgibbons RJ Jr, Giobbie-Hurder A, Gibbs JO, et al. Watchful waiting vs repair of inguinal hernia in minimally symptomatic men: a randomized clinical trial. JAMA 2006;295(3): 285–92.
[3] O'Dwyer PJ, Norrie J, Alani A, et al. Observation or operation for patients with an asymptomatic inguinal hernia: a randomized clinical trial. Ann Surg 2006;244(2):167–73.
[4] Sanchez-Manuel FJ, Seco-Gil JL. Antibiotic prophylaxis for hernia repair. Cochrane Database Syst Rev 2004;18(4):CD003769.
[5] Sanabria A, Dominguez LC, Faldivieso E, et al. Prophylactic antibiotics for mesh inguinal hernioplasty: a meta-analysis. Ann Surg 2007;245(3):392–6.
[6] Neumayer L, Jonasson O, Fitzgibbons R, et al. Tension-free inguinal hernia repair: the design of a trial to compare open and laparoscopic surgical techniques. J Am Coll Surg 2003; 196(5):743–52.

[7] Neumayer L, Giobbie-Hurder A, Jonasson O, et al. Open mesh versus laparoscopic mesh repair of inguinal hernia. N Engl J Med 2004;350(18):1819–27.

[8] Butler RE, Burke R, Schneider JJ, et al. The economic impact of laparoscopic inguinal hernia repair: results of a double-blinded, prospective, randomized trial. Surg Endosc 2007; 21(3):387–90.

[9] Mann BD, Seidman A, Haley T, et al. Teaching three-dimensional surgical concepts of inguinal hernia in a time-effective manner using a two dimensional paper-cut. Am J Surg 1997;173(6):542–5.

[10] Scott N, Go PM, Graham P, et al. Open mesh versus non-mesh for groin hernia repair [review]. Cochrane Database Syst Rev 2001;(3):CD002197.

[11] McCormack K, Scott NW, Go PM, et al, The EU Hernia Trialists Collaboration. Laparoscopic techniques versus open techniques for inguinal hernia repair. Cochrane Database Syst Rev 2003;(1):CD001785. 10.1002/14651858.

[12] Butters M, Redecke J, Koninger J. Long-term results of a randomized clinical trial of Shouldice, Lichtenstein and transabdominal preperitoneal hernia repairs. Br J Surg 2007;94(5): 562–5.

[13] Arvidsson D, Berndsen FH, Larsson LG, et al. Randomized clinical trial comparing 5-year recurrence rate after laparoscopic versus Shouldice repair of primary inguinal hernia. Br J Surg 2005;92(9):1085–91.

[14] van Veen RN, Wijsmuller AR, Vrijland WW, et al. Long-term follow-up of a randomized clinical trial of non-mesh versus mesh repair of primary inguinal hernia. Br J Surg 2007; 94(4):506–10.

[15] Bay-Nielsen M, Nilsson E, Nordin P, et al. Chronic pain after open mesh and sutured repair of indirect inguinal hernia in young males. Br J Surg 2004;91(10):1372–6.

[16] Muldoon RL, Marchant K, Johnson DD, et al. Lichtenstein vs anterior preperitoneal prosthetic mesh placement in open inguinal hernia repair: a prospective, randomized trial. Hernia 2004;8(2):98–103.

[17] Dogru O, Girgin M, Bulbuller N, et al. Comparison of Kugel and Lichtenstein operations for inguinal hernia repair: results of a prospective randomized study. World J Surg 2006;30(3): 346–50.

[18] Reddy KM, Humphreys W, Chew A, et al. Inguinal hernia repair with the Kugel patch. ANZ J Surg 2005;75(1–2):43–7.

[19] Frey DM, Wildisen A, Hamel CT, et al. Randomized clinical trial of Lichtenstein's operation versus mesh plug for inguinal hernia repair. Br J Surg 2007;94(1):36–41.

[20] Adamonis W, Witkowski P, Smietanski M, et al. Is there a need for a mesh plug in inguinal hernia repair? Randomized, prospective study of the use of Hertra 1 mesh compared to PerFix plug. Hernia 2006;10(3):223–8.

[21] Awad SS, Yallalampalli S, Srour AM, et al. Improved outcomes with the Prolene Hernia System mesh compared with the time-honored Lichtenstein onlay mesh repair for inguinal hernia repair. Am J Surg 2007;193:697–701.

[22] Chauhan A, Tiwari S, Gupta A. Study of efficacy of bilayer mesh device versus conventional polypropylene hernia system in inguinal hernia repair: early results. World J Surg 2007;31(6): 1356–9.

[23] Vironen J, Nieminen J, Eklund A, et al. Randomized clinical trial of Lichtenstein patch or Prolene Hernia System for inguinal hernia repair. Br J Surg 2006;93(1):33–9.

[24] Sanjay P, Harris D, Jones P, et al. Randomized controlled trial comparing Prolene hernia system and Lichtenstein method for inguinal hernia repair. ANZ J Surg 2006;76(7):548–52.

[25] Nienhuijs SW, van Oort I, Keemers-Gels ME, et al. Randomized trial comparing the Prolene Hernia System, mesh plug repair and Lichtenstein method for open inguinal hernia repair. Br J Surg 2005;92(1):33–8.

[26] Kingsnorth AN, Wright D, Porter CS, et al. Prolene Hernia System compared with Lichtenstein patch: a randomized double blind study of short-term and medium-term outcomes in primary inguinal hernia repair. Hernia 2002;6(3):113–9.

[27] Stoppa R, et al. Reinforcement of the visceral sac by a preperitoneal bilateral mesh prosthesis in groin hernia repair. In: Bendavid R, Abrahamson J, Arregui MM, editors. Abdominal wall hernias: principles and management. New York: Springer-Verlag; 2001. p. 428–30.

[28] Mui WL, Ng CS, Fung TM, et al. Prophylactic ilioinguinal neurectomy in open inguinal hernia repair: a double blind randomized trial. Ann Surg 2006;244(1):27–33.

[29] Altieri S, Rotondi F, Di Giorgio A, et al. Influence of preservation versus division of ilioinguinal, iliohypogastric and genital nerves during open mesh herniorrhaphy: prospective multicentric study of chronic groin pain. Ann Surg 2006;243(4):553–8.

[30] Wijsmuller AR, Van Veen RN, Bosch JL, et al. Nerve management during open hernia repair. Br J Surg 2007;94(1):17–22.

[31] Aasvang E, Kehlet H. Surgical management of chronic pain after inguinal hernia repair. Br J Surg 2005;92(7):795–801.

[32] Cobb WS, Burns JM, Peindl RC, et al. Textile analysis of heavy weight, mid-weight, and light weight polypropylene mesh in a porcine ventral hernia model. J Surg Res 2006;136:1–7.

[33] Coda A, Bendavid R, Botto-Micca F, et al. Structural alterations of prosthetic mesh in humans. Hernia 2003;7:29–34.

[34] Amid PK, et al. Lichtenstein tension free hernioplasty for the repair of primary and recurrent inguinal hernias. In: Bendavid R, Abrahamson J, Arregui MM, editors. Abdominal wall hernias: principles and management. New York: Springer-Verlag; 2001. p. 423–6.

[35] Amid PZ. Lichtenstein open tension-free hernioplasty. 1997 video in Am Coll Surg Educational Library CC-1869.

[36] Kugel RD. The Kugel repair for groin hernias. Surg Clin North Am 2003;83(5):1119–39.

[37] Rutkow IM. The PerFix plug repair for groin hernias. Surg Clin North Am 2003;83(5):1079–98, vi [review] [Erratum in: Surg Clin North Am 2003;83(6)xiii].

[38] Wilkicmeyer M, Pappas TN, Giobbie-Hurder A, et al. Does resident post graduate year influence the outcomes of inguinal hernia repair? Ann Surg 2005;241(6):879–84.

[39] Neumayer LA, Gawande AA, Wang J, et al. CSP #456 Investigators. Proficiency of surgeons in inguinal hernia repair: effect of experience and age. Ann Surg 2005;242(3):344–8, [discussion: 348–52].

[40] Koch A, Edwards A, Haapaniemi S, et al. Prospective evaluation of 6895 groin hernia repairs in women. Br J Surg 2005;92:1553–8.

ELSEVIER
SAUNDERS

SURGICAL
CLINICS OF
NORTH AMERICA

Surg Clin N Am 88 (2008) 157–178

Laparoscopic Inguinal Hernia Repair

Mark C. Takata, MD[a], Quan-Yang Duh, MD[b,c,*]

[a]Division of General Surgery, Scripps Clinic, La Jolla, CA, USA
[b]Surgical Services, Veterans Affairs Medical Center, 4150 Clement Street,
San Francisco, CA 94121, USA
[c]Department of Surgery, University of California San Francisco, Parnassus Avenue,
San Francisco, CA 94143, USA

Since the early 1990s, laparoscopy has provided surgeons with new and innovative ways to treat various surgical problems. Many of these minimally invasive techniques have gained universal acceptance by demonstrating improved patient outcomes. This technology has been applied to the treatment of inguinal hernias, and many laparoscopic techniques for repair have been described.

In 1990, Ger and colleagues [1] performed the first laparoscopic inguinal hernia repair in dogs by stapling the abdominal opening of the patent processus vaginalis. Other minimally invasive techniques were later developed, including a plug and patch repair [2] and an intraperitoneal onlay mesh repair [3]. The plug and patch repair was not widely accepted because of high recurrence rates coupled with small bowel obstructions related to adhesions [4]. The intraperitoneal onlay mesh repair involved placing mesh over the inguinal hernia defect intra-abdominally without performing a preperitoneal dissection. Although this operation was relatively simple, it was abandoned because of the risk of mesh erosion into bowel [4].

Today, most laparoscopic inguinal hernia repairs are performed with placement of a synthetic mesh into the preperitoneal space, which can be accomplished in one of two ways: the transabdominal preperitoneal (TAPP) approach or the totally extraperitoneal (TEP) approach. The TAPP approach, first described by Arregui and colleagues [5] in 1992, requires laparoscopic access into the peritoneal cavity and placement of mesh in the preperitoneal space after reducing the hernia sac. The first TEP inguinal hernia repair was described by McKernan and Laws [6] in 1993. This approach involves preperitoneal dissection and mesh placement without entering into the abdominal cavity.

---

* Corresponding author. Surgical Services, Veterans Affairs Medical Center, 4150 Clement Street, San Francisco, CA 94121.

E-mail address: quan-yang.duh@med.va.gov (Q-Y. Duh).

0039-6109/08/$ - see front matter © 2008 Elsevier Inc. All rights reserved.
doi:10.1016/j.suc.2007.10.005   *surgical.theclinics.com*

Before laparoscopic techniques were applied to inguinal hernias, recurrence rates from open hernia repair significantly decreased after the replacement of sutured repair with prosthetic material for tension-free tissue reinforcement. Stoppa [7] introduced the posterior approach to the inguinal hernia in 1975. The hallmarks of this approach included complete dissection of the preperitoneal space, identification of all myopectineal orifices, and placement of mesh over the entire inguinal-femoral region. The anterior open inguinal hernia repair with mesh was described by Lichtenstein [8] in 1989. This tension-free operation gained enormous popularity in the early 1990s after it proved to be simple, safe, effective, and easily reproducible [9,10].

The introduction of laparoscopic and open tension-free hernia repair in the 1990s created enormous interest in the study of outcomes following the many different surgical options. In the last 17 years, many articles, co-operative study groups, meetings, and societies have been devoted to hernia repair. By the end of the 1990s, it had been shown that the open or laparoscopic placement of mesh improved recurrence rates and reduced the chance of persistent pain, compared with the conventional sutured repairs [11,12]. As mesh proved beneficial, attention appropriately shifted away from comparing mesh with sutured repair to open mesh with laparoscopic repair. Despite intense study devoted to laparoscopic inguinal hernia repair, acceptance of this procedure has been slow. It is usually reserved for specific indications and performed by surgeons specializing in this technique. The purpose of this article is to describe the TAPP and TEP techniques for inguinal hernia repair, provide indications and contraindications for laparoscopic repair, discuss the advantages and disadvantages of each technique, and provide an overview of the vast amount of literature comparing tension-free open and laparoscopic inguinal hernia repair.

Operative procedure

Positioning for transabdominal preperitoneal repair and totally extraperitoneal repair

The patient is supine with both arms tucked, and general anesthesia is used. The monitor is placed at the foot of the operating bed, with the surgeon standing by the patient's shoulder on the opposite side of the hernia. If bilateral inguinal hernias are present, the surgeon starts opposite the side of the larger, more symptomatic hernia. The patient needs to be paralyzed to allow for insufflation of the peritoneal (TAPP) or preperitoneal (TEP) space. After pneumoperitoneum is established and the trocars are inserted, the patient is placed in the Trendelenburg's position.

Operative steps for transabdominal preperitoneal repair

This operation is performed using three trocars: one 10-mm subumbilical port and two 5-mm ports, one in the right lower quadrant and one in the left lower quadrant in the same axial plane as the subumbilical port approximately 5 to 7 cm away. Using a 10-mm, 30°-angled laparoscope, the groin anatomy is inspected. The inferior epigastric vessels, the internal inguinal ring with the spermatic vessels, and the vas deferens should be identified. These three structures form the so-called "Mercedes-Benz" sign (Fig. 1). The peritoneum is incised several centimeters above the peritoneal defect, from the edge of the median umbilical ligament laterally toward the anterior superior iliac spine. Dissection is performed in the preperitoneal avascular plane between the peritoneum and the transversalis fascia to provide visualization of the myopectineal orifices.

For an indirect hernia, the cord structures are isolated and dissected free from the surrounding tissues. In the process, the indirect hernia sac is identified, usually found on the anterolateral side of the cord and adherent to it. When separating the sac from the cord, it is important to handle the vas deferens and the spermatic vessels with care to minimize trauma. If the sac is sufficiently small, it should be completely dissected free from the cord and returned to the peritoneal cavity. Occasionally, a large sac will be encountered, in which case it should be dissected and divided beyond the internal ring, and the subsequent peritoneal defect closed with an endoloop suture. The distal end of the transected sac should be left open to avoid formation of a hydrocele.

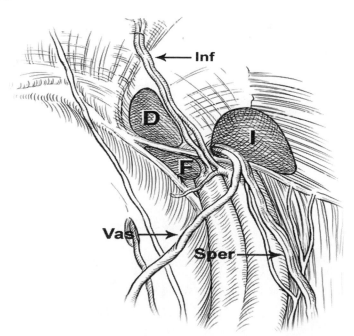

Fig. 1. Right groin anatomy. The intersection of these three structures forms the "Mercedes-Benz" sign. D, direct hernia; F, femoral hernia; I, indirect hernia; Inf, inferior epigastric vessels; Sper, spermatic vessels; Vas, vas deferens.

Direct hernia sacs are typically easier to reduce than indirect sacs. Once the preperitoneal space has been dissected out laterally, the direct hernia defect is addressed by separating the peritoneum from the overlying myopectineal orifice. When reducing the direct hernia sac, a "pseudosac" may be present, which is transversalis fascia that overlies and adheres to the peritoneum and invaginates into the preperitoneal space during the dissection. This layer must be separated from the true hernia sac in order for the peritoneum to be released back fully into the peritoneal cavity. Once the pseudosac is freed, it will typically retract anteriorly into the direct hernia defect.

Prosthetic mesh is required for TAPP repairs, and a large piece of polypropylene mesh (16 × 12 cm) is used to cover the myopectineal orifices, including the direct, indirect, and femoral hernia spaces. For direct hernias, a preformed, contoured mesh (Bard 3D Max Mesh) can be used for coverage (Fig. 2). For indirect hernias, the authors prefer to use a trimmed piece of flat mesh slit medially with the tails wrapped around the cord structures. The tails are placed around the cord in a lateral-to-medial fashion and fixed to Cooper's ligament (Fig. 3). The slit in the mesh allows it to lie flat in the preperitoneal space while still providing complete coverage of the indirect hernia defect. However, some surgeons use the same preformed mesh for direct and indirect hernias. It is important that the preperitoneal space is completely dissected out so that the edge of the mesh does not fold within this space and compromise the repair. The mesh should be fixed medially at

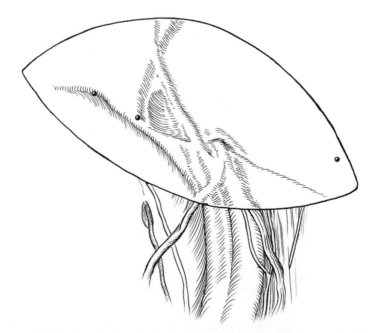

Fig. 2. Repair of right direct or femoral hernia with preformed, contoured mesh (Bard 3D Max Mesh).

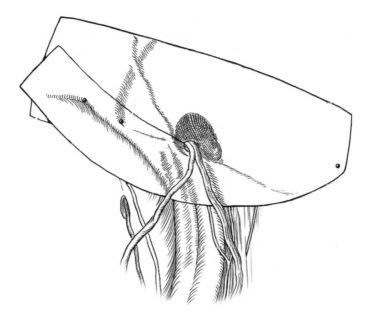

Fig. 3. Repair of right indirect hernia with a large (16 cm × 12 cm) piece of flat mesh that is slit medially, passing the lower tail around the spermatic cord structures. The two tails are then overlapped and fixed to Cooper's ligament medially.

Cooper's ligament and laterally above the iliopubic tract to prevent movement of the mesh. When fixing the mesh laterally with tacks or staples, it is important to feel the tip of the device on the outside of the abdomen with the opposite hand to ensure that fixation occurs above the inguinal ligament. This technique will avoid nerve injury. In addition, the mesh should be placed with a slight overlap of the midline to ensure adequate coverage of the entire posterior floor of the groin. Finally, the mesh is covered by securing the peritoneal flap back to its original position.

Operative steps for totally extraperitoneal repair

This operation is performed using three trocars: one 10-mm subumbilical port with an attached structural balloon and two 5-mm ports, one in the right lower quadrant and one in the left lower quadrant in the same axial plane as the subumbilical port approximately 5 to 7 cm away. All ports are placed within the preperitoneal space. The first trocar placed is the 10-mm subumbilical port, using an open technique. Once through the subumbilical skin incision, this port is positioned slightly off the midline to stay in the space behind the rectus muscle and in front of the posterior rectus sheath. If it is placed in the midline, where the anterior and posterior rectus sheaths merge, it will enter the peritoneal cavity. Following this port placement, a 10-mm, 30°-angled laparoscope is inserted and used to dissect bluntly the areolar tissue in the preperitoneal space, using a gentle sweeping motion. The preperitoneal space is cleared out laterally toward the anterior superior iliac spine to provide enough space for the other ports. Alternatively, a balloon dissector can be used instead of manual dissection, although it is more expensive.

After the two 5-mm ports are placed, the inferior epigastric vessels, the pubic bone, and Cooper's ligament are identified. Cooper's ligament is found just lateral and slightly cephalad to the pubic bone and is where the mesh will be anchored medially. This dissection should be done under direct vision to avoid injury to the small veins that overlie the pubic bone and the bladder, which is anterior.

As Cooper's ligament is exposed, a direct hernia, if present, will generally be reduced. If it is not, gentle traction on the peritoneal attachments should provide enough force to reduce the sac. Occasionally, in chronic direct hernias, a "pseudosac" may be present. The pseudosac is a posterior invagination of the transversalis fascia and should be distinguished from the direct hernia sac, which is continuous with the peritoneum.

The indirect hernia sac is found along the spermatic cord and just cephalad to it. Within the spermatic cord, the vas deferens and the spermatic vessels are located medially and laterally, respectively, merging through the internal ring. The intersection of the inferior epigastric vessels, the vas deferens, and the spermatic vessels forms the Mercedes-Benz sign (see Fig. 1). Cord lipomas, if identified, are usually found laterally along the spermatic vessels.

Usually, the indirect hernia sac is reduced from the internal ring by gentle traction and dissection. If the sac is too long or too large, it can be isolated, divided just beyond the internal ring, and closed with an endoloop. The distal end of the transected sac should be left open to avoid formation of a hydrocele. The sac, which is continuous with the peritoneum, is reduced by dissecting it off the cord structures.

When repairing direct hernias, preformed, contoured mesh (Bard 3D Max Mesh) can be used. The contoured surface and stiffness of the mesh make it easy to manipulate, and it tends not to move within the preperitoneal space (see Fig. 2). For an indirect hernia, however, the authors use a large (16 cm × 12 cm) piece of flat mesh that is slit medially, passing the lower tail around the spermatic cord structures. The two tails are then overlapped and fixed to Cooper's ligament medially (see Fig. 3). Slitting the mesh medially and placing the lower tail below the cord structures ensures complete coverage of the indirect inguinal hernia site without having to add additional points of fixation of the mesh. The lateral edge of the mesh should be fixed to the anterior abdominal wall while palpating from outside the abdomen with the opposite hand to ensure that fixation does not occur below the iliopubic tract where the nerves are.

Indications and contraindications

In some specific situations, a laparoscopic repair of an inguinal hernia works better than open repair. A recurrence from a prior open inguinal hernia repair is best repaired laparoscopically. In this situation, the surgeon avoids dissecting through scar tissue and can avoid missing additional defects by assessing the entire myopectineal orifice. The advantages to the patient include less postoperative pain, shorter convalescence, and similar or improved recurrence rates, compared with reoperative open mesh repair [13–16].

Bilateral inguinal hernias are also good indications for the laparoscopic approach, which has been nicely demonstrated by two prospective randomized trials comparing the TAPP repair with the open mesh repair [14,17]. Both studies showed a significant advantage of the laparoscopic repair over the open repair in terms of less postoperative pain and an earlier return to work, without finding any difference in recurrence rates or complications.

When the diagnosis of an inguinal hernia is uncertain, diagnostic laparoscopy provides a definitive diagnosis and an opportunity to repair the hernia using the same approach. However, establishing a diagnosis of an inguinal hernia in obese patients is often difficult. In this group of patients, laparoscopy will establish the diagnosis and provide a method of repair that avoids a large groin incision in patients who are susceptible to wound complications.

Lastly, patients who are eager to return to normal physical activity are good candidates for the laparoscopic approach. In contrast to the anterior repair, the mesh is placed posterior during laparoscopic repair and any increase in intra-abdominal pressure will push the mesh in position against the abdominal wall. Therefore, the authors do not limit physical activity after a laparoscopic inguinal hernia repair. It usually takes patients about 2 to 3 weeks to return comfortably to their normal activity.

Specific contraindications also exist for a laparoscopic inguinal hernia repair. Because general anesthesia is necessary for the laparoscopic approach, an open approach should be performed when the patient's medical condition makes general anesthesia more risky. These cases include elderly patients and anyone who has significant cardiac or pulmonary comorbidities. In addition, patients who have had prior or who have planned pelvic or extraperitoneal operations (eg, radical prostatectomy) or who have had a recurrence from a prior laparoscopic repair, should have an open inguinal hernia repair. Lastly, patients who have a strangulated hernia should have an open repair. In this situation, laparoscopic repair is much more difficult and dangerous and it may be necessary to perform a primary sutured repair if the field is contaminated. Although incarceration is not a contraindication, it makes the operation more difficult and should be performed by an experienced laparoscopic hernia surgeon.

Literature review

The use of mesh, regardless of approach, has proved to produce results superior to those of conventional sutured inguinal hernia repair [11,12]. Since the early 1990s, the rise in popularity of open mesh and laparoscopic inguinal hernia repairs has provided an abundance of investigation comparing these two techniques. The retrospective reviews and small randomized controlled trials that were first published uncovered valuable information but they lacked standardization and were limited by recruitment of sufficient numbers of patients for the desired statistical power. These studies eventually led to large multicenter prospective randomized controlled trials and meta-analyses. The result is a wealth of information that answers some questions and leaves others in need of more research.

The objectives of this section are to summarize the literature and provide evidence-based conclusions by reviewing the single-institution and multicenter randomized trials and the major meta-analyses that compare laparoscopic with open mesh inguinal hernia repairs (Tables 1–4). Systematic reviews are not included because they report on results from a heterogeneous group of studies looking at similar outcomes. They provide an overview of the literature without engaging in statistical analysis. Meta-analyses were included if they used and presented rigorous statistical analysis to form conclusions about data grouped together from individual randomized series. Interpretation of these results should be made with caution because the methodologies and populations differ from one study to the next. However, the value of data obtained from a large number of patients should not be underestimated and many of the conclusions are validated by solid statistical methods.

Table 1
Single-institution prospective randomized trials comparing transabdominal preperitoneal and open mesh inguinal hernia repair

Investigator	Year	Type of operation	n	Follow up (months)
Payne, et al [18]	1994	Open (Lichtenstein)	52	10.0
		TAPP	48	—
Filipi, et al [19]	1996	Open (Lichtenstein)	29	11.0
		TAPP	24	—
Heikkinen, et al [20]	1997	Open (Lichtenstein)	18	10.0
		TAPP	20	—
Aitola, et al [21]	1998	Open (Stoppa)	25	18.0
		TAPP	24	—
Heikkinen, et al [22]	1998	Open (Lichtenstein)	20	17.0
		TAPP	18	—
Paganini, et al [23]	1998	Open (Lichtenstein)	56	28.0
		TAPP	52	—
Wellwood, et al [24]	1998	Open (Lichtenstein)	200	—
		TAPP	200	—
Picchio, et al [25]	1999	Open (Lichtenstein)	52	2.0
		TAPP	53	—
Douek, et al [26]	2003	Open (Lichtenstein)	120	69.0
		TAPP	122	—
Anadol, et al [27]	2004	Open (Lichtenstein)	25	13.5
		TAPP	25	—

Table 2
Single-institution prospective randomized trials comparing totally extraperitoneal repair and open mesh inguinal hernia repair

Investigator	Year	Type of operation	n	Follow up (months)
Wright, et al [28]	1996	Open (Lichtenstein)	60	1
		TEP	60	—
Champault, et al [29]	1997	Open (Stoppa)	49	20
		TEP	51	—
Heikkinen, et al [30]	1998	Open (Lichtenstein)	23	10
		TEP	22	—
Khoury, et al [31]	1998	Open (plug and patch)	142	17
		TEP	150	—
Andersson, et al [32]	2003	Open (Lichtenstein)	87	12
		TEP	81	—
Bringman, et al [33]	2003	Open (plug and patch, Lichtenstein)	103	20
		TEP	92	—
Colak, et al [34]	2003	Open (Lichtenstein)	67	11
		TEP	67	—
Lal, et al [35]	2003	Open (Lichtenstein)	25	13
		TEP	25	—
Eklund, et al [36]	2006	Open (Lichtenstein)	706	3
		TEP	665	—

The main outcomes of interest are operative time, complications, postoperative pain, return to activities, recurrence rates, and cost. According to Hawn and colleagues [45], the two most important indicators of an effective inguinal herniorrhaphy are recurrence and neuralgia. Using data from the Veterans Affairs (VA) Cooperative Study [40], patient-reported outcomes and satisfaction were most negatively impacted by postoperative neuralgia and hernia recurrence, which emphasizes the importance of interpreting and understanding the data so preoperative discussions with the patient address these important outcomes.

The emphasis in this article is placed on the specific comparison of the TAPP and TEP repairs with the open mesh repairs. Results from one study to the next often have wide variation and are largely a reflection of different methods of obtaining data and different patterns of reporting subjective information. An attempt is made to clarify these differences. In addition, results that are included in many of the meta-analyses that compare laparoscopic with conventional open sutured hernia repair are excluded from this article.

Operative time

Laparoscopic repair takes longer than open mesh repair (Table 5). Only one single-institution trial demonstrated a nonsignificant shorter operative time in the laparoscopic group [22]. Two of the three multicenter randomized trials collected operative time data and reported operative times that

Table 3
Multicenter prospective randomized trials comparing laparoscopic and open mesh inguinal hernia repair

Study group	Year	Type of operation	n	Follow up (months)
MRC Laparoscopic Groin	1999/2001	Open (89% Lichtenstein)	453	12
Hernia Group [37,38]		Lap (TAPP and TEP)	462	12
SCUR Hernia Repair	1999	Open (Stoppa)	200	12
Study Group [39]		Lap (TAPP)	200	12
VA Cooperative Study [40]	2004	Open (Lichtenstein)	994	24
		Lap (90% TEP and 10% TAPP)	989	24

Abbreviations: Lap, Laparoscopic; MRC, Medical Research Council; VA, Veterans Affairs.

were 15 and 27 minutes longer in the laparoscopic group. The three meta-analyses [41,42,44] that reviewed this subject had similar results.

The important issues regarding operative time center on surgeon experience, clinical relevance, and cost. Operative times decrease after approximately 30 to 50 cases [46,47]. It is unlikely that a decrease in operative time of 15 to 30 minutes will have any measurable clinical benefit. However, in terms of cost, the effect could be important. One of the main reasons laparoscopic repair is more expensive than open repair is operative time. One potential way to decrease operative time and assist the surgeon along the learning curve is to use the balloon dissector for TEP repairs [48,49]. However, many surgeons think the cost of using the balloon, especially when the dissection can be performed well with a reusable instrument, does not justify the minimal decrease in operative time. The issue of cost is discussed in a separate section.

Complications

Complications after laparoscopic and open hernia repair are not uniformly reported in the literature. This lack of standardization plays a large role in the variability seen in Table 6. Some investigators report everything from constipation to urinary retention and combine perioperative with

Table 4
Meta-analyses comparing laparoscopic and open inguinal hernia repair

Investigator	Year	Number of trials	Types of operation with mesh
Chung, et al [41]	1999	14 randomized trials	6 TAPP versus open mesh
Grant (European Union) [42]	2002	41 randomized trials	13 TAPP versus open mesh, 6 TEP versus open mesh
Memon, et al [43]	2003	29 randomized trials	10 TAPP versus open mesh, 5 TEP versus open mesh
Stengel, et al [44]	2004	41 randomized trials	13 TAPP versus open mesh, 6 TEP versus open mesh

Table 5

Comparison of operative time between laparoscopic (transabdominal preperitoneal and totally extraperitoneal) and open mesh repair

	Operative time (min)	
Investigator	Laparoscopic	Open
TAPP versus open mesh		
Payne, et al [18]	68	56
Filipi, et al [19]	109	87
Heikkinen, et al [20]	72	45
Aitola, et al [21]	66	55
Heikkinen, et al [22]	62	65
Paganini [23]	67	48
Wellwood, et al [24]	45	45
Picchio, et al [25]	50	34
Anadol, et al [27]	57	54
TEP versus open mesh		
Wright, et al [28]	38	45
Heikkinen, et al [30]	68	53
Khoury, et al [31]	32	31
Andersson, et al [32]	81	59
Bringman, et al [33]	50	45
Colak, et al [34]	57	50
Lal, et al [35]	76	54
Eklund, et al [36]	55	55
Multicenter prospective randomized trials		
MRC [37]	58	43
SCUR [39]	65	38

Abbreviations: MRC, Medical Research Council; SCUR, SCUR Hernia Repair Study Group.

long-term follow-up complications. Others only include perioperative events and are less liberal with the labeling of a complication.

Laparoscopic hernia repair has a history of unique and potentially serious intraoperative complications not seen with open hernia repair. Most of these complications were encountered when the techniques of laparoscopy were still relatively new and experience was minimal. The Medical Research Council (MRC) Laparoscopic Groin Hernia Group [37] reported three major complications during TAPP repairs: one bladder injury, one common iliac artery injury, and one injury to the lateral femoral cutaneous nerve. The SCUR Hernia Repair Study Group (SCUR) [39] reported two bladder injuries that occurred during TAPP repairs. The laparoscopic groups of the European Union Hernia Trialists Collaboration reported 15 visceral or vascular injuries [42], mainly in TAPP repairs. Finally, small bowel obstruction after TAPP repair from herniation of the intestine through the peritoneal opening was a complication that occurred before the importance of complete peritoneal closure was understood [50]. The incidence of these injuries has substantially decreased as experience has grown and as many centers changed to the TEP repair [51].

Table 6
Comparison of complication rates between laparoscopic (transabdominal preperitoneal and totally extraperitoneal) and open mesh repair

	Complication rate	
Investigator	Laparoscopic	Open
TAPP versus open mesh		
Payne, et al [18]	6 (12%)	9 (18%)
Filipi, et al [19]	3 (13%)	3 (10%)
Heikkinen, et al [20]	4 (20%)	16 (89%)
Aitola, et al [21]	5 (21%)	2 (8%)
Heikkinen, et al [22]	5 (28%)	8 (40%)
Paganini, et al [23]	14 (27%)	15 (27%)
Picchio, et al [25]	14 (26%)	13 (25%)
Douek, et al [26]	13 (11%)	52 (43%)
Anadol, et al [27]	2 (8%)	2 (8%)
TEP versus open mesh		
Wright, et al [28]	15 (25%)	50 (83%)
Champault, et al [29]	2 (4%)	11 (30%)
Khoury, et al [31]	20 (13%)	33 (23%)
Andersson, et al [32]	7 (9%)	4 (5%)
Bringman, et al [33]	9 (10%)	21 (20%)
Colak, et al [34]	10 (13%)	11 (16%)
Lal, et al [35]	6 (24%)	3 (12%)
Eklund, et al [36]	83 (14%)	101 (16%)
Multicenter prospective randomized trials		
MRC [37]	29.9%	43.5%
SCUR [39]	31%	24%
VA [40]	39%	33%

Other complications unique to laparoscopic hernia repair are trocar site hemorrhage, trocar site herniation, and injury to the epigastric or gonadal vessels. Other, less serious, complications associated more with the use of laparoscopy and less to surgeon technique are hypotension secondary to elevated intra-abdominal pressure, hypercapnia, subcutaneous emphysema, pneumothorax, and increased peak airway pressures. Most of the time, these are minor problems correctable by lowering the intra-abdominal pressure or completely evacuating the intra-abdominal carbon dioxide. However, if improvement is not achieved, it may be necessary to delay repair.

The same postoperative complications may occur after laparoscopic and open repair. These include urinary retention, groin hematoma, neuralgia, groin pain, testicular problems, wound infection, and mesh complications. Fitzgibbons and colleagues [52] found a significant decrease (7.0%–1.8%) in postoperative neuralgia manifested by leg pain after surgeons performed 30 laparoscopic cases. This finding reflects a better understanding of the nerve anatomy from the intra-abdominal or preperitoneal perspective as experience increases. In addition, if mesh fixation is desired, it is important to secure the mesh cephalad to the inguinal ligament to avoid nerve entrapment.

Table 6 demonstrates that complication rates after laparoscopic repair are similar or better than open mesh repair for most of the randomized trials. Although the VA Cooperative Study [40] concluded that the rate of complications was higher in the laparoscopic group (39%) compared with the open group (33%), it did not separate complications according to TAPP or TEP repair. The MRC trial [37] found a higher rate of complications in the open group (43.5%) compared with the laparoscopic group (29.9%). Similarly, the meta-analysis by Memon and colleagues [43] reported a statistically significant reduction of 38% in the relative odds of complications after laparoscopic repair. The European Union meta-analysis [42] found no difference in the complication rate. Overall, as the major complications have declined and our familiarity with the technique has increased, it has become clear that laparoscopic inguinal hernia repair performed by experienced surgeons is safe.

Postoperative pain

Two issues regarding postoperative pain after inguinal hernia repair should be addressed. First, pain experienced in the first few weeks should be differentiated from the low risk of chronic pain that may persist months to years after inguinal hernia repair. Second, when reviewing the large amount of information in the literature about this subject it becomes clear that pain may be reported in multiple ways, which makes it difficult to quantify and compare accurately postoperative pain from one study to the next.

Most studies comparing TAPP and TEP to open mesh repair found that pain in the perioperative period is significantly less after laparoscopic inguinal hernia repair (Table 7), which is one of the major advantages of most laparoscopic operations. The SCUR trial [39] found no significant difference in graded pain scores on the 7-day postoperative visit. During this visit, 70.5% of patients in the laparoscopic group, compared with 59.8% in the open mesh group, reported no pain but at the 8-week visit, patients in the open mesh group reported significantly more pain. Using the mean score on a visual analog scale, the VA trial [40] found significantly less pain in the laparoscopic group on the day of the operation and at 2 weeks.

Chronic pain is arguably a more important determinant of a successful inguinal hernia repair than perioperative pain. The spectrum of severity is wide. It is sometimes a debilitating complication for the patient and a difficult problem for the surgeon to treat. However, the incidence is too low to demonstrate differences by small single-institution randomized studies. At 1 year after the operation, the laparoscopic group in the MRC trial [37] had a significantly lower rate of persistent groin pain than those who had had open mesh repair (28.7% versus 36.7%). Similarly, the incidence of neuralgia or other pain at 2 years after the operation was 9.8% in the laparoscopic group, compared with 14.3% in the open mesh group, in the VA trial [40]. The SCUR trial [39] did not find any difference in persistent pain at 1 year. The European Union meta-analysis [42] found significantly fewer cases of

Table 7
Comparison of postoperative pain between laparoscopic (transabdominal preperitoneal and totally extraperitoneal) and open mesh repair

Investigator	In favor of laparoscopy or open
TAPP versus open mesh	
Filipi, et al [19]	Laparoscopy
Heikkinen, et al [20]	Laparoscopy
Aitola, et al [21]	Laparoscopy
Heikkinen, et al [22]	No difference
Paganini, et al [23]	No difference
Wellwood, et al [24]	Laparoscopy
Picchio, et al [25]	No difference
Anadol, et al [27]	Laparoscopy
TEP versus open mesh	
Wright, et al [28]	Laparoscopy
Champault, et al [29]	Laparoscopy
Heikkinen, et al [30]	Laparoscopy
Khoury, et al [31]	Laparoscopy
Andersson, et al [32]	Laparoscopy
Bringman, et al [33]	Laparoscopy
Colak, et al [34]	Laparoscopy
Lal, et al [35]	Laparoscopy
Eklund, et al [36]	Laparoscopy
Multicenter prospective randomized trials	
SCUR [39]	No difference
VA [40]	Laparoscopy

persisting pain 1 year after TAPP and TEP repair than open mesh repair. Therefore, evidence is solid that laparoscopic repair leads to less perioperative pain and is associated with similar or less risk of persisting pain than open mesh repair.

Return to work or activities

Complex confounding variables and tremendous subjectivity are incorporated in reporting the amount of time it takes a person to return to work or usual activities. However, recovery time is an important issue in terms of the degree of disruption to a patient's life and the cost to society calculated by days missed from productive work. With few exceptions, the literature has clearly proven that patients have a shorter convalescence and a faster return to work and activities after laparoscopic, compared with open mesh, inguinal hernia repair (Table 8). The impact of this difference on the lives of patients can be enormous. The overall economic effect is discussed in the Cost section.

Recurrence

Recurrence after inguinal hernia repair is one of the most important measurable outcomes. It is largely determined by technique and can only

Table 8

Comparison of time to return to work between laparoscopic (transabdominal preperitoneal and totally extraperitoneal) and open mesh repair

Investigator	Time to return to work (d)	
	Laparoscopic	Open
TAPP versus open mesh		
Payne, et al [18]	9	17
Heikkinen, et al [20]	14	19
Aitola, et al [21]	7	5
Heikkinen, et al [22]	14	21
Paganini, et al [23]	15	14
Wellwood, et al [24]	21	26
Picchio, et al [25]	46	43
TEP versus open mesh		
Champault, et al [29]	17	35
Heikkinen, et al [30]	12	17
Khoury, et al [31]	8	15
Andersson, et al [32]	8	11
Bringman, et al [33]	5	7
Colak, et al [34]	11	15
Lal, et al [35]	13	19
Eklund, et al [36]	7	12
Multicenter prospective randomized trials		
MRC [37]	10	14
SCUR [39]	15	18
VA [40]	4	5

accurately be reported with complete long-term follow-up. With the early laparoscopic mesh plug technique, Tetik and colleagues [4] reported a recurrence rate of 22% at 13-month follow-up. In the same study, the recurrence rate for TAPP and TEP repair was 0.7% and 0.4%, respectively. Table 9 shows that the recurrence rates after laparoscopic repair for most single-institution randomized trials is less than 5%. This result compares favorably with open repair, but the small number of patients in each individual study is insufficient to show statistical significance.

The SCUR trial [39] and the European Union meta-analysis [42] demonstrated no difference in recurrence rates between laparoscopic and open mesh repair. However, the other two multicenter randomized trials demonstrated significantly higher recurrence rates after laparoscopic repair [37,40]. At 1-year follow-up in the MRC trial [37], the recurrence rate after laparoscopic repair was 1.9%, compared with 0% in the open mesh group. The investigators did not provide details about surgeon experience or type of laparoscopic repair performed in the patients who had a recurrence. The recurrence rates at 2-year follow-up in the VA trial [40] were 10.1% and 4.9% after laparoscopic and open mesh repair, respectively. This rate is significantly higher than that quoted in other articles and information is not given linking the specific operation with the recurrence. However, when surgeon

Table 9
Comparison of recurrence rates between laparoscopic (transabdominal preperitoneal and totally extraperitoneal) and open mesh repair

	Recurrence rate	
Investigator	Laparoscopic	Open
TAPP versus open mesh		
Payne, et al [18]	0	0
Filipi, et al [19]	0	2 (7%)
Heikkinen, et al [20]	0	0
Aitola, et al [21]	13%	8%
Heikkinen, et al [22]	0	0
Paganini, et al [23]	2 (3.8%)	0
Wellwood, et al [24]	0	0
Douek, et al [26]	2 (2%)	3 (3%)
Anadol, et al [27]	0	0
TEP versus open mesh		
Champault, et al [29]	3 (6%)	1 (2%)
Heikkinen [30]	0	0
Khoury, et al [31]	3%	3%
Andersson, et al [32]	2 (3%)	0
Bringman, et al [33]	2 (2%)	0
Colak, et al [34]	2 (3%)	4 (6%)
Lal, et al [35]	0	0
Eklund, et al [36]	5 (1%)	0
Multicenter prospective randomized trials		
MRC [37]	7 (1.9%)	0
SCUR [39]	4	11
VA [40]	10.1%	4.9%

experience was taken into consideration, the recurrence rate for surgeons who had performed more than 250 laparoscopic repairs was not different than open repair (5.1% versus 4.1%). Although 250 repairs are many more than most experienced laparoscopic hernia surgeons consider necessary to become proficient, this may be testimony to differences in reported recurrence rates.

The mechanisms of recurrence have been studied by many investigators and are mostly related to technique [4,50–55]. As techniques have improved and surgeons have gained experience, recurrence rates have declined. One of the most common reasons for recurrence is incomplete dissection of the myopectineal orifice [54]. Incomplete dissection is more often associated with inadequate reduction of the hernia sac, missed hernias, missed lipomas or preperitoneal fat [53,56], or rolling of the mesh edges. Another common reason for hernia recurrence is inadequate overlap of the hernia defect from placement of a small mesh. The average mesh size in patients who had a recurrence was 6.0 cm × 9.2 cm in the trial by Fitzgibbons and colleagues [52]. It is now generally believed that the mesh size should be at least 10 cm × 14 cm [50,53] to cover all of the potential hernia sites, to provide at least 4 cm overlap with the hernia, and to avoid problems with mesh migration, shrinkage, and rolling.

Two techniques related to hernia recurrence after laparoscopic repair are debatable. Some surgeons cut a slit, or keyhole, in the mesh so it fits around the cord structures. Others have found that these mesh modifications place the patient at higher risk for recurrence [53,54]. The authors' preference is to slit the mesh for large indirect hernias and place the tails in the medial position. Most recurrences in these hernias occur laterally and this mesh configuration helps prevent abdominal contents from slipping under the mesh. The other debatable issue is the need for mesh fixation. Two randomized trials have demonstrated no difference in recurrence rates and postoperative pain after repairs using fixation versus no fixation [57,58]. However, other investigators support mesh fixation as a way of preventing hernia recurrence [52,53,55].

Cost

One of the major criticisms of laparoscopic hernia repair is increased cost compared with open repair, which has been consistently demonstrated by many studies (Table 10). It has also been shown that most of the increased cost is attributed to longer operative times and more expensive equipment [18,38].

Cost analysis comparing laparoscopic and open hernia repair is a complex task. Accurate evaluation of cost includes the integration of all operative, hidden, and indirect costs. Components of operative and hospital costs include operative time, type and length of anesthesia, equipment, and staffing.

Table 10
Comparison of cost between laparoscopic (transabdominal preperitoneal and totally extraperitoneal) and open mesh repair

| | Cost (US $) | |
Investigator	Laparoscopic	Open
TAPP versus open mesh		
Payne, et al [18]	3093	2494
Heikkinen, et al [20]	1395	875
Heikkinen, et al [22]	1299	851
Paganini, et al [23]	1249	306
Wellwood, et al [24]	747[a]	412[a]
Anadol, et al [27]	1100	629
TEP versus open mesh		
Heikkinen, et al [30]	1239	782
Andersson, et al [32]	2817	1726
Multicenter prospective randomized trials		
MRC [38]	1113[a]	789[a]
SCUR [39]	7063[b]	417[b]

[a] British pounds.
[b] Swedish krona.

Hidden costs are the administrative and overhead costs. The indirect costs are the most difficult to calculate because they include cost to society in terms of days missed from work. Other factors that affect cost are postoperative pain, recurrence rates, and surgeon experience.

Studies have attempted to incorporate many different factors into the evaluation of cost. Heikkinen and colleagues [20,22,30] published three articles that demonstrated a lower total cost for employed patients who have a laparoscopic repair when the shorter duration of time off from work was considered. Schneider and colleagues [59] suggested that the cost of laparoscopic repair could be dramatically reduced by the routine use of reusable equipment and the removal of unnecessary equipment such a balloon dissectors and expensive fixation devices. The MRC trial [38] found that the difference in cost between laparoscopic and open mesh repair decreased from 598 British pounds to 132 British pounds when disposable instruments were not used. In terms of operative time, they found that a 34-minute laparoscopic operation would make the cost of the two repairs equivalent. The same study balanced the increased cost with objective evidence of increased quality of life after laparoscopic hernia repair.

Data obtained from the VA Cooperative Study and published by Hynes and colleagues [60] demonstrated that the cost of the laparoscopic operation is higher than that of the open repair and that the costs for health care use through 2 postoperative years were similar. However, the laparoscopic repair of unilateral primary or recurrent hernias is more cost effective in terms of incremental cost per quality of adjusted life years gained, which reflects the importance of incorporating quality of life, morbidity, and mortality into patient and cost outcomes.

Transabdominal preperitoneal repair versus totally extraperitoneal repair

The learning curve for TAPP and TEP repair is long. The VA trial [40] found that surgeons who had performed more than 250 laparoscopic repairs had a 50% reduction in recurrence rate. However, most experienced laparoscopic hernia surgeons consider the number to be much lower. Some investigators have found that expertise is achieved after approximately 30 to 50 cases, when operative times, conversions to an open procedure, complications, and recurrences significantly decrease [46,47,61].

The TEP approach was developed in response to concerns about the need for intra-abdominal laparoscopic access required in the TAPP repair [62]. This method allows for access to the preperitoneal space and avoids the need for a peritoneal incision. However, this procedure is also felt to be more demanding technically, given the smaller working space provided compared with the one found in the TAPP repair. When Felix and colleagues [51] compared the two methods, they found that the TAPP repair had a higher incidence of intra-abdominal complications than the TEP repair. However, several TEP repairs needed conversion to a TAPP approach in the study. Additionally, the study showed no appreciable differences with regard to postoperative pain and return to normal activity.

In a review of the available literature comparing TAPP versus TEP repairs, Wake and colleagues [63] found no statistical difference in length of operation, length of stay, time to return to normal activity, or recurrence rates between the two techniques. The reviewed studies did report higher rates of intra-abdominal injuries and port site hernias in TAPP repairs. In another review, Leibl and colleagues [64] reported similar findings. However, they stated that the TAPP approach, in general, has a shorter learning curve than the TEP approach. They suggested that because of the shorter learning curve, the TAPP repair might be more easily adopted into further surgical education.

Further randomized controlled trials are needed comparing the TAPP and TEP repairs to determine whether one method is superior. Nevertheless, the authors do find the TAPP repair to be useful in certain clinical circumstances, such as when a patient has a large or incarcerated hernia or when a diagnostic laparoscopy is needed to see if a hernia is present in a patient whose history and physical examination are unclear. In addition, TAPP is the laparoscopic procedure of choice in patients with hernias who have had previous surgery in the preperitoneal space because this approach allows for wide exposure of the groin anatomy.

Summary

Laparoscopic hernia repair in 2007 still accounts for the minority of hernia repairs performed in the United States and around the world. The reasons for this are a demonstration in the literature of increased operative times, increased costs, and a longer learning curve. In addition are concerns about the need to use general anesthesia for laparoscopic operations and early reports of vascular and visceral injuries. As experience and knowledge have increased, these rare complications have become more important from a historical perspective.

The laparoscopic approach to hernia repair has clear advantages, including less acute and chronic postoperative pain, shorter convalescence, and earlier return to work. When performed by experienced surgeons, these results can be achieved with the same low rates of complications and recurrences as open mesh repair. Therefore, laparoscopic hernia repair has a beneficial role in recurrent, bilateral, and primary inguinal hernias. However, despite efforts to decrease cost and operating time, this approach will likely remain a less common operation than open mesh repair.

The laparoscopic revolution has fueled a vigorous debate over the safest and most effective inguinal hernia repair. This debate has broadened our understanding of inguinal anatomy and hernia repair. At the least, surgeons should be aware of the current indications and contraindications for laparoscopic inguinal hernia repair, because some hernias should have a laparoscopic repair. To increase versatility, surgeons should consider becoming skilled at both techniques, with the understanding that outcomes are optimal if one is committed to achieving expertise in laparoscopic repair.

References

[1] Ger R, Monroe K, Duvivier R, et al. Management of indirect inguinal hernias by laparoscopic closure of the neck of the sac. Am J Surg 1990;159:370–3.
[2] Schultz L, Cartuill J, Graber JN, et al. Transabdominal preperitoneal procedure. Semin Laparosc Surg 1994;1:98–105.
[3] Fitzgibbons RJ Jr, Salerno GM, Filipi CJ, et al. A laparoscopic intraperitoneal onlay mesh technique for the repair of an indirect inguinal hernia. Ann Surg 1994;219:144–56.
[4] Tetik C, Arregui ME, Dulucq JL, et al. Complications and recurrences associated with laparoscopic repair of groin hernias. A multi-institutional retrospective analysis. Surg Endosc 1994;8:1316–22 [discussion: 1322–3].
[5] Arregui ME, Davis CJ, Yucel O. Laparoscopic mesh repair of inguinal hernia using a preperitoneal approach: a preliminary report. Surg Laparosc Endosc 1992;2:53–8.
[6] McKernan JB, Laws HL. Laparoscopic repair of inguinal hernias using a totally extraperitoneal prosthetic approach. Surg Endosc 1993;7:26–8.
[7] Stoppa R, Petit J, Henry X. Unsutured Dacron prosthesis in groin hernias. Int Surg 1975;60:411–2.
[8] Lichtenstein IL, Shulman AG, Amid PK, et al. The tension-free hernioplasty. Am J Surg 1989;157:188–93.
[9] Shulman AG, Amid PK, Lichtenstein IL. The safety of mesh repair for primary inguinal hernias: results of 3,019 operations from five diverse surgical sources. Am Surg 1992;58:255–7.
[10] Amid PK, Shulman AG, Lichtenstein IL. Critical scrutiny of the open "tension-free" hernioplasty. Am J Surg 1993;165:369–71.
[11] Liem MS, van der Graaf Y, van Steensel C, et al. Comparison of conventional anterior surgery and laparoscopic surgery for inguinal hernia repair. N Engl J Med 1997;336:1541–7.
[12] EU Hernia Trialists Collaboration. Repair of groin hernia with synthetic mesh: meta-analysis of randomized controlled trials. Ann Surg 2002;235:323–32.
[13] Keidar A, Kanitkar A, Szold A. Laparoscopic repair of recurrent inguinal hernia. Surg Endosc 2002;16:1708–12.
[14] Mahon D, Decadt M, Rhodes M. Prospective randomized trial of laparoscopic (transabdominal preperitoneal) vs open (mesh) repair for bilateral and recurrent inguinal hernia. Surg Endosc 2003;17:1386–90.
[15] Feliu X, Jaurrieta E, Vinas X, et al. Recurrent inguinal hernia: a ten year review. J Laparoendosc Adv Surg Tech A 2004;14:362–7.
[16] Eklund A, Rudberg C, Leijonmarck CE, et al. Recurrent inguinal hernia: randomized multicenter trial comparing laparoscopic and Lichtenstein repair. Surg Endosc 2007;21:634–40.
[17] Sarli L, Iusco D, Sansebastiano G, et al. Simultaneous repair of bilateral inguinal hernias: a prospective randomized study of open, tension-free versus laparoscopic approach. Surg Laparosc Endosc Percutan Tech 2001;11:262–7.
[18] Payne JH, Grininger LM, Izawa M, et al. Laparoscopic or open inguinal herniorrhaphy? A randomized prospective trial. Arch Surg 1994;129:973–9.
[19] Filipi CJ, Gaston-Johansson F, McBride PJ, et al. An assessment of pain and return to normal activity: laparoscopic herniorrhaphy vs open tension-free Lichtenstein repair. Surg Endosc 1996;10:983–6.
[20] Heikkinen T, Haukipuro K, Leppala J, et al. Total costs of laparoscopic and Lichtenstein inguinal hernia repairs: a randomized prospective study. Surg Laparosc Endosc 1997;7:1–5.

[21] Aitola P, Airo I, Matikainen M. Laparoscopic versus open preperitoneal inguinal hernia repair: a prospective randomized trial. Ann Chir Gynaecol 1998;87:22–5.

[22] Heikkinen T, Haukipuro K, Hulkko A. A cost and outcome comparison between laparoscopic and Lichtenstein hernia operations in a day-case unit. Surg Endosc 1998;12:1199–203.

[23] Paganini AM, Lezoche E, Carle F, et al. A randomized, controlled, clinical study of laparoscopic vs open tension-free inguinal hernia repair. Surg Endosc 1998;12:979–86.

[24] Wellwood J, Sculpher MJ, Stoker D, et al. Randomised controlled trial of laparoscopic versus open mesh repair for inguinal hernia: outcome and cost. BMJ 1998;317:103–10.

[25] Picchio M, Lombardi A, Zolovkins A, et al. Tension-free laparoscopic and open hernia repair: randomized controlled trial of early results. World J Surg 1999;23:1004–9.

[26] Douek M, Smith G, Oshowo A, et al. Prospective randomized controlled trial of laparoscopic versus open inguinal hernia mesh repair: five year follow-up. BMJ 2003;326: 1012–3.

[27] Anadol AZ, Ersoy E, Taneri F, et al. Outcome and cost comparison of laparoscopic transabdominal preperitoneal hernia repair versus open Lichtenstein technique. J Laparoendosc Adv Surg Tech A 2004;14:159–63.

[28] Wright DM, Kennedy A, Baxter JN, et al. Early outcome after open versus extraperitoneal endoscopic tension-free hernioplasty: a randomized clinical trial. Surgery 1996;119:552–7.

[29] Champault GG, Rizk N, Catheline JM, et al. Inguinal hernia repair. Totally preperitoneal laparoscopic approach versus Stoppa operation: randomized trial of 100 cases. Surg Laparosc Endosc 1997;7:445–50.

[30] Heikkinen T, Haukipuro K, Koivukangas P, et al. A prospective randomized outcome and cost comparison of totally extraperitoneal endoscopic hernioplasty versus Lichtenstein hernia operation among employed patients. Surg Laparosc Endosc 1998;8:338–44.

[31] Khoury N. A randomized prospective controlled trial of laparoscopic extraperitoneal hernia repair and mesh-plug hernioplasty: a study of 315 cases. J Laparoendosc Adv Surg Tech A 1998;8:367–72.

[32] Andersson B, Hallen M, Leveau P, et al. Laparoscopic extraperitoneal inguinal hernia repair versus open mesh repair: a prospective randomized controlled trial. Surgery 2003;133: 464–72.

[33] Bringman S, Ramel S, Heikkinen TJ, et al. Tension-free inguinal hernia repair: TEP versus mesh-plug versus Lichtenstein: a prospective randomized controlled trial. Ann Surg 2003; 237:142–7.

[34] Colak T, Akca T, Kanik A, et al. Randomized clinical trial comparing laparoscopic totally extraperitoneal approach with open mesh repair in inguinal hernia. Surg Laparosc Endosc Percutan Tech 2003;13:191–5.

[35] Lal P, Kajla RK, Saha CR, et al. Randomized controlled study of laparoscopic total extraperitoneal vs open Lichtenstein inguinal hernia repair. Surg Endosc 2003;17:850–6.

[36] Eklund A, Rudberg C, Smedberg S, et al. Short-term results of a randomized clinical trial comparing Lichtenstein open repair with totally extraperitoneal laparoscopic inguinal hernia repair. Br J Surg 2006;93:1060–8.

[37] The MRC Laparoscopic Groin Hernia Trial Group. Laparoscopic versus open repair of groin hernia: a randomized comparison. Lancet 1999;354:185–90.

[38] The MRC Laparoscopic Groin Hernia Trial Group. Cost-utility analysis of open versus laparoscopic groin hernia repair: results from a multicentre randomized clinical trial. Br J Surg 2001;88:653–61.

[39] Johansson B, Hallerback B, Glise H, et al. Laparoscopic mesh versus open preperitoneal mesh versus conventional technique for inguinal hernia repair. A randomized multicenter trial (SCUR Hernia Repair Study). Ann Surg 1999;230:225–31.

[40] Neumayer L, Giobbie-Hurder A, Jonasson O, et al. Open mesh versus laparoscopic mesh repair of inguinal hernia. New Engl J Med 2004;350:1819–27.

[41] Chung RS, Rowland DY. Meta-analysis of randomized controlled trials of laparoscopic vs conventional inguinal hernia repairs. Surg Endosc 1999;13:689–94.

[42] Grant AM. The EU Hernia Trialists Collaboration. Laparoscopic versus open groin hernia repair: meta-analysis of randomized trials based on individual patient data. Hernia 2002;6: 2–10.

[43] Memon MA, Cooper NJ, Memon B, et al. Meta-analysis of randomized clinical trials comparing open and laparoscopic inguinal hernia repair. Br J Surg 2003;90:1479–92.

[44] Stengel D, Bauwens K, Ekkernkamp A. Recurrence risks in randomized trials of laparoscopic versus open inguinal hernia repair: to pool or not to pool (this is not the questions). Langenbecks Arch Surg 2004;389:492–8.

[45] Hawn MT, Itani KMF, Giobbie-Hurder A, et al. Patient reported outcomes after inguinal herniorrhaphy. Surgery 2006;140:198–205.

[46] Liem MS, van Steensel CJ, Boelhouwer RU, et al. The learning curve for totally extraperitoneal laparoscopic inguinal hernia repair. Am J Surg 1996;171:281–5.

[47] Voitk AJ. The learning curve in laparoscopic inguinal hernia repair for the community surgeon. Can J Surg 1998;41:446–50.

[48] Kieturakis MJ, Nguyen DT, Vargas H, et al. Balloon dissection facilitated laparoscopic extraperitoneal hernioplasty. Am J Surg 1994;168:603–7.

[49] Bringman S, Haglind E, Heikkinen T, et al. Is a dissection balloon beneficial in totally extraperitoneal endoscopic hernioplasty (TEP)? Surg Endosc 2001;15:266–70.

[50] Kapiris SA, Brough WA, Royston MS, et al. Laparoscopic transabdominal preperitoneal (TAPP) hernia repair. Surg Endosc 2001;15:972–5.

[51] Felix EL, Michas CA, Gonzalez MH. Laparoscopic hernioplasty: TAPP vs TEP. Surg Endosc 1995;9:984–9.

[52] Fitzgibbons RJ, Camps J, Cornet DA, et al. Laparoscopic inguinal herniorrhaphy: results of a multicenter trial. Ann Surg 1995;221:3–13.

[53] Felix E, Scott S, Crafton B, et al. Causes of recurrence after laparoscopic hernioplasty. Surg Endosc 1998;12:226–31.

[54] Lowham AS, Filipi CJ, Fitzgibbons RJ, et al. Mechanisms of hernia recurrence after preperitoneal mesh repair. Ann Surg 1997;225:422–31.

[55] Phillips EH, Rosenthal R, Fallas M, et al. Reasons for early recurrence following laparoscopic hernioplasty. Surg Endosc 1995;9:140–5.

[56] Gersin KS, Heniford BT, Garcia-Ruiz A, et al. Missed lipoma of the spermatic cord. Surg Endosc 1999;13:585–7.

[57] Ferzli GS, Frezza EE, Pecoraro AM, et al. Prospective randomized study of stapled versus unstapled mesh in a laparoscopic preperitoneal inguinal hernia repair. J Am Coll Surg 1999; 188:461–5.

[58] Smith AI, Royston MS, Sedman PC. Stapled and nonstapled laparoscopic transabdominal preperitoneal (TAPP) inguinal hernia repair. Surg Endosc 1999;13:804–6.

[59] Schneider BE, Castillo JM, Villegas L, et al. Laparoscopic totally extraperitoneal versus Lichtenstein herniorrhaphy: cost comparison at teaching hospitals. Surg Laparosc Endosc Percutan Tech 2003;13:261–7.

[60] Hynes DM, Stroupe KT, Luo P, et al. Cost effectiveness of laparoscopic versus open mesh hernia operation: results of a Department of Veterans Affairs randomized clinical trial. J Am Coll Surg 2006;203:447–57.

[61] Edwards CC, Bailey RW. Laparoscopic hernia repair: the learning curve. Surg Laparosc Endosc Percutan Tech 2000;10:149–53.

[62] Soper NJ, Swanstrom LL, Eubanks WS. Mastery of endoscopic and laparoscopic surgery. Philadelphia: Lippincott Williams & Wilins; 2005. p. 49.

[63] Wake BL, McCormack K, Fraser C, et al. Transabdominal preperitoneal (TAPP) vs totally extraperitoneal (TEP) laparoscopic techniques for inguinal hernia repair. Cochrane Database Syst Rev 2005;1:CD004703.

[64] Leibl BJ, Jager C, Kraft B, et al. Laparoscopic hernia repair—TAPP or/and TEP? Langenbecks Arch Surg 2005;390:77–82.

SURGICAL
CLINICS OF
NORTH AMERICA

ELSEVIER
SAUNDERS

Surg Clin N Am 88 (2008) 179–201

Prosthetic Material in Inguinal Hernia Repair: How Do I Choose?

David B. Earle, MD, FACS*, Lisa A. Mark, MD

Department of Surgery, Baystate Medical Center, Tufts University School of Medicine, 759 Chestnut Street, Springfield, MA 01199, USA

If we could artificially produce tissues of the density and toughness of fascia and tendon, the secret of the radical cure of hernia would be discovered.
Theodore Billroth (1829–1894)

Since the first description of treatment for inguinal hernia, many techniques have come and gone. Today, each surgeon clings to his or her technique like a favorite, comfortable piece of clothing. Over the years, those comforting techniques have evolved, such that most surgeons now use a prosthetic [1]. Prosthetics are widely used for different types of inguinal hernias because prosthetic techniques are comparatively easy to master and are associated with superior outcomes [2]. Prosthetic use tends to follow a geographic distribution pattern, likely due to local training and prosthetic variability (Table 1) [3–20].

The goals of treatment of any disease are relief of symptoms and cure of the disease to prevent adverse sequelae. In the case of hernia, the goals are to relieve pain and cure the hernia to prevent acute incarceration. Given these goals, correction of the underlying cause should provide the best chance for a successful long-term outcome. However, the etiology of groin hernia is often multifactorial and includes genetic, metabolic, and environmental factors—factors impossible to determine for each patient. Further complicating matters, an individual patient may have underlying causes that change over time, such as causes related to traumatic events, body mass index, activity levels, medications, immune status, or infection. Because the surgeon can only see the consequences of the disease process (ie, the hernia defect), tailoring the procedure to the individual patient based on the presumed

Disclosure: Dr. Earle has served as a consultant for Atrium Medical and has received grant support from Covidien for a fellowship.

* Corresponding author.

E-mail address: david.earle@bhs.org (D.B. Earle).

Table 1
Geographic patterns of prosthetic use and/or laparoscopy for inguinal hernia repair

Publication year	Location	Survey participants or data source	Use of prosthetic	Use of laparoscopy	Notes
1991	United Kingdom	240 consultant surgeons	<2.1%	0%	Maloney darn with nylon suture most common
1995	The Netherlands	448 surgeons	2%; mesh	2%	In Shouldice repair, 58% used absorbable sutures for the posterior wall repair
1998	Wales	79 surgeons	N/A	Lichtenstein most common	Increased use of laparoscopic approach since 1992 study, but still "majority" of surgeons use open techniques
1999	Canada	706 surgeons	Mean 59%	15%	Prosthetic use varied by hernia type: 52% primary unilateral; 71% primary bilateral; 78% recurrent; 36% femoral
2000	East Brandenburg, Germany	14 hospitals	60%	30%	
2001	Surrey, United Kingdom	1 hospital, 440 patients	83%	0%	Techniques included Shouldice (11%) and Bassini/Maloney darn (6%); increased use of mesh compared with 1991 United Kingdom survey (<2.1%)
2001	Denmark	26,304 hernia repairs	79%	5%	
2001	United States	555,954 hernia repairs	67%	N/A	ICD-9 mesh code data from Verispan for both inpatient and outpatient inguinal hernia repairs
2003	Gloucester, United Kingdom	78 consultant surgeons	>95%	8%	Use of laparoscopic approach with recurrent hernias, particularly if first operation done with mesh; other technique used was "darning"
2003	Japan	83 hospitals	83%	1%	
2003	United States	estimated 800,000	93%	14%	Data from ISM America[a], National Hospital Discharge Survey, and National Survey of Ambulatory Surgery
2004	United States	383,790 hernia repairs	77%	N/A	ICD-9 mesh code data from Verispan for both inpatient and outpatient inguinal hernia repairs[b]

Year	Location	Setting			Comments
2004	Kuala Lumpur, Malaysia	1 hospital, 103 patients	46%	0%	Mesh used (92%) if senior surgeon involved, usually with more difficult cases
2004	Lombardy, Italy	105 surgical departments, 16,935 hernia repairs	97%	N/A	Combination of laparoscopic and open; preperitoneal only for bilateral and recurrent hernias
2005	The Netherlands	97 hospitals, 3284 patients	78%	N/A	Mesh use increased from The Netherlands hernia survey published in 1995
2005	Amsterdam region	All hospitals in region; 3649 patients	91% (2001)	10% (2001)	Trend for prosthetic use increased from 17% in 1994; each year had higher prosthetic use for recurrent hernias
2005	Norway	57 hospitals	86%	3%	Data based on long term f/u of 2001 survey.
2005	Spain	46 hospitals, 386 patients	73%	5%	
2006	Aberdeen, United Kingdom	784 surgeons	94%	4%	
2005	Pakistan	65 surgeons	58%	N/A	Private hospitals more likely to use mesh; 71.4% recommend laparoscopic approach

Abbreviation: N/A, data not available.

[a] ISM America tracks supply sales to United States hospitals.

[b] Not all hernia repairs in United States included in data. Data based on coding, and hernia repairs "unspecified" may have used a prosthetic. Trend more accurate than absolute numbers.

etiology portends a higher failure rate compared with using a technique based on the physical properties and anatomy of the abdominal wall, regardless of the exact etiology. Prosthetic herniorrhaphy that addresses the physical and anatomic issues is more likely to be successful than the application of any of a wide range of primary repairs based on intraoperative assumptions. Therefore, it is prudent to hone a single prosthetic technique that yields the best results for the vast majority of inguinal hernias, and to have the capability of using one or two alternate techniques to accommodate clinical variability. This philosophy strikes a balance between optimal performance of one operation and having viable alternatives that may be more suitable for a given clinical situation.

Surgeons in training, who see a variety of prosthetics in use, must recognize that the technique of prosthetic implantation is far more important than the type of prosthetic. Once in practice, the surgeon must decide which combination of technique and prosthetic is most likely to provide a successful hernia repair. To help the surgeon choose, it is helpful to look at the prosthetic landscape with a perspective based on (1) the prosthetic's raw material and design, (2) the technique of implantation, and (3) the clinical scenario. It is also helpful to know the history of prosthetic use for inguinal hernia repair and the biologic reactivity of prosthetics in general. The debate on routine versus selective use of a prosthetic and which particular technique is best is beyond the scope of this article.

History

Why use a prosthetic for inguinal hernia repair? The answer lies in the history of its development. Trusses and other external prosthetics have been used for the treatment of inguinal hernia for thousands of years [21]. Internal, surgically placed prosthetics were probably first described by Billroth, but were not applied clinically until silver wire was used to repair inguinal hernias [22]. These prosthetics were associated with poor outcomes [23,24] and set the stage for the development, promulgation, and modification of a variety of primary suture repairs to avoid the use of a conventional prosthetic. Although there are still strong proponents of primary "tissue" repairs, these repairs are most frequently performed with permanent sutures—sutures made from the same raw materials that go into many prosthetics [25]. Given this fact, it's not the implantation of synthetic material that seems to be cause for argument. Rather, it's the amount, design, and placement of these foreign bodies that appears to provoke the strongest opinions amongst surgeons [26]. Since Usher first introduced polypropylene prosthetics for inguinal hernia in the late 1950s [27], they have dominated the field of prosthetic hernia repair. What has driven prosthetic use are the difficulties of teaching a variety of suture repairs as they were originally intended to be performed, as well as the comparably poor long-term results of primary suture repair in terms of treatment failure—namely, persistent pain and/or hernia recurrence [28,29]. Even Bassini's excellent results in terms of recurrence lack any information about postoperative symptom relief [30,31].

The invention of antibiotics, the development of biocompatible polymers, and advances in techniques to manufacture these polymers in a suitable form have helped to overcome hurdles that once stood in the way of widespread use of prosthetics. As prosthetic use became more commonplace, different designs and raw materials have been developed. The emergence and disappearance of a given prosthetic in the literature is one indicator of interest and acceptance in the surgical community. Table 2 illustrates this rise and fall of various prosthetics over time. While this research did not take into account all articles related to a given prosthetic or all available prosthetics, it accurately reflects the prevalence of prosthetic use and trends of development that we see clinically.

Biologic response

After any prosthetic is implanted, an extraordinarily complex series of events takes place (Fig. 1). Immediately after implantation, the prosthetic adsorbs proteins that create a coagulum around it. This coagulum consists of albumin, fibrinogen, plasminogen, complement factors, and immunoglobulins [32,33]. Platelets adhere to this protein coagulum and release a host of chemoattractants that invite other platelets, polymorphonucleocytes (PMNs), fibroblasts, smooth muscle cells, and macrophages to the area in a variety of sequences. Depending on a host of genetic and environmental factors, these chemoattractants may enhance or block a variety of receptors from initiating their specific sequence of events. Activated PMNs drawn to the area release proteases to attempt to destroy the foreign body in addition to organisms and surrounding tissue. PMN's also further attract fibroblasts, smooth muscle cells, and macrophages. The presence of a prosthetic within a wound allows the sequestration of necrotic debris, slime-producing bacteria, and a generalized prolongation of the inflammatory response of platelets and PMNs. Macrophages then increasingly populate the area to consume foreign bodies as well as dead organisms and tissue. These cells ultimately coalesce into foreign body giant cells that stay in the area for an indefinite period of time, their role being unclear. The fibroblasts and smooth muscle cells subsequently secrete monomeric fibers that polymerize into the helical structure of collagen deposited in the extracellular space. There is a general net production of collagen for about 21 days, after which there is a net loss and a changing proportion of type III (immature) to type I (mature) collagen. The collagen helices also undergo crosslinking to increase strength. The overall strength of this new collagen gradually increases for about 6 months, resulting in a relatively less elastic tissue that has only 70% to 80% of the strength of the native connective tissue [34,35]. It is for this reason that the permanent strength of a prosthetic is important for the best long-term success of hernia repair.

Table 2
Overview of the number of published articles by polymer type

Article year: first–last	Period	Search terms in addition to "hernia mesh"	No. of articles	Notes
1950–1974	23 years	Tantalum	48	Most recent article about ventral hernia repair in a horse
1950–1998	43 years	Stainless Steel Wire	25	Last article for migration of wire mesh into bowel lumen 30 years after implantation with a long time period from previous article
1951–1996	45 years	Nylon	20	Significant longevity; very few articles
1958–2007	49 years	Polypropylene Marlex Prolene	287	Longest experience and most articles of any hernia prosthetic
1962–2006	44 years	Polyester Dacron Mersilene	67	Significant longevity; distant second for number of articles
1987–2006	19 years	Polytetraflouroethylene PTFE Gore	63	Significant number of articles in a short period of time; most articles for ventral hernia repair
1989–2007	18 years	Polyglycolic acid Dexon Vicryl Polyglactin Absorbable	30	Most publications for ventral hernia or difficult-to-close abdomen
2002–2007	5 years	Partially absorbable Vypro Lightweight	25	No long-term data; significant number of articles in short period of time

PubMed database, August 2007. Date range: 1/1/1900 through 7/31/07. Total articles: 3378. Article selected if the terms appeared in the title or abstract.

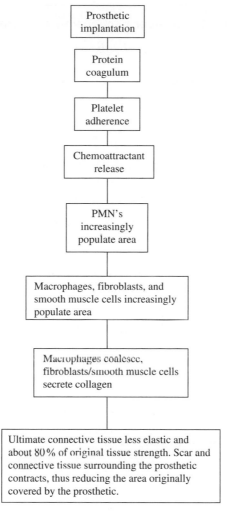

Fig. 1. Overview of the biologic response to a synthetic prosthetic. The presence of a prosthetic in a wound generally prolongs the inflammatory response, and can sequester necrotic debris and slime-producing bacteria. PMNs, polymorphonucleocytes.

Categories of prosthetics

To assist the surgeon in choosing prosthetic, a framework based on relevant variables may be useful. This framework should take into account (1) the raw material used to make the prosthetic, (2) the prosthetic's design, (3) the technique of implantation, and (4) the clinical scenario (Box 1). The surgeon must weigh the relative risks and benefits of each prosthetic for each given clinical scenario.

Box 1. Variables to consider in choosing a prosthetic

Raw material and design (and subsequent bioreactivity)
Synthetic nonabsorbable
Coated nonabsorbable
Partially absorbable
Biologic

Design (architecture)
Density (g/m^2)
Porosity
Strength

Technique
Anterior approach and prosthetic placement
Anterior approach with combined anterior–posterior prosthetic
    placement
Anterior approach with posterior prosthetic placement
Posterior approach: laparoscopic or open

Clinical scenario and patient factors
Symptoms: severity and duration of pain, limitation of activity
Concomitant diseases: immunologic, infectious
Past history: recurrence, prior prosthetic, infection
Urgency: hernia reducible, acute and chronic incarceration,
    bowel obstruction
Anatomy: defect size and location, hernia sac size, previous
    operation
Future risk: need for prostatectomy

Raw material

General considerations
   By taking into account the raw materials that go into a prosthetic, the surgeon can better evaluate the risks of the prosthetic, as well as its proposed benefits, which are usually based on claims related to specific aspects of the prosthetic's bioreactivity and handling characteristics. Also, processes involved in manufacturing of polymeric prosthetics vary [36] and may potentially alter clinical performance. That is, all woven, monofilament polypropylene prosthetics are not the same. This means that factors other than the raw material are also at play in determining how well an implanted prosthetic functions, and the surgeon should take these into consideration when choosing the prosthetic. These factors include the thickness of the fibers, the architecture of the fibers, the overall density and strength of the material, the implantation technique [37,38], and the biologic and physical

response to the prosthetic (Box 2). Because there are so many variables and experimental models, the literature generally makes it difficult if not impossible to make an equivalent comparison of available prosthetics.

Synthetic nonabsorbable prosthetics

Synthetic polymers are the most commonly used prosthetics. Hence, more data is available regarding their biologic response and clinical outcomes than for other comparable prosthetics. Each polymer induces a biologic response that varies slightly because of both the polymer composition and structure [39].

By far the most widely used raw material is polypropylene (PP). Propylene is an ethylene with an attached methyl group, and was developed and polymerized in 1954 by the Italian scientist, Giolo Natta. The position of the methyl groups during polymerization affects overall strength, being maximal when they are all on the same side of the polymeric chain [40]. This polymer is hydrophobic, electrostatically neutral, and resistant to significant biologic degradation. Prosthetics made from polypropylene induce

---

Box 2. Factors associated with prosthetic performance

Raw material and design
    Polymer/tissue
    Strength
    Elasticity
    Architecture
        Pore size
        Fiber size
        Density
        "Weave"
    Bioreactivity
Implantation technique:
    Position in relation to structures of the abdominal wall
        Muscle layers
        Ligaments
    Folding of the prosthetic
    Fixation method
Clinical situation and host factors
    Physical activity
    Obesity
    Immunologic response to foreign bodies
    Propensity for infection
    Need for reoperation
    Other diseases

biologic reactivity, which varies depending on the weight, filament size, pore size, and architecture of the prosthetic, as well as on the individual host response [39]. Common brand names include Marlex (Davol, Cranston, Rhode Island), Prolene (Ethicon, Somerville, New Jersey), SurgiPro (Covidien, Norwalk, Connecticut), and Prolite (Atrium Medical, Hudson, New Hampshire). These hernia prosthetics are manufactured in a variety of forms, each with either mono- or multifilament strands along with unique overall density and pore sizes. To reduce the inflammatory response, yet maintain the benefits of a prosthetic repair, there has been a trend toward lighter weight, more porous polypropylene prosthetics, which are designed to enhance the formation of a scar "net" rather than a scar "plate" [41,42]. This trend has a sound foundation and can be applied to inguinal hernia repair. However, the optimal density and porosity remain unknown.

The biologic response to PP begins with protein adherence that ultimately envelops the polypropylene in scar tissue. In the clinical arena, there is concern that scar tissue and adhesions at the prosthetic–tissue interface cause chronic pain and discomfort [43,44]. Additionally, direct contact of the polypropylene with the abdominal viscera can lead to the complications of bowel obstruction or fistula formation [45,46]. Studies have shown increased adhesion formation with polypropylene versus adhesion formation involving composite prosthetics with a physical or chemical adhesion barrier. However, the adhesion formation may be independent of the mesh composition, and more related to the structure of the prosthetic [47]. The intensity of the host response has been shown to be related to the density and coating of the prosthetic as well [48].

Polyester, the common textile term for polyethylene terephthalate (PET), is a combination of ethylene glycol and terephthalic acid, and was patented by the English chemists J.R. Whinfield and J.T. Dickson in 1941 at the Calico Printers Association Ltd. in Lancashire, the United Kingdom [49]. Mersilene (Ethicon) and Parietex (Covidien) are both manufactured from this polymer. PET is hydrophilic and thus has the propensity to swell. The inflammatory response attracts predominately macrophages, but also PMNs, and is heavily influenced by the adsorbed protein coagulum [32,33]. This response is generally similar to that for other implants in both the acute and chronic inflammatory responses, scar tissue formation, and prosthetic contracture after implantation [50–52]. PET, which is the same polymer used for plastic beverage bottles, also can degrade over time, particularly in an infected environment [53], but it is doubtful that this has clinical significance for inguinal hernia repair. Like polypropylene, PET is manufactured in a variety of forms as a medical textile for use in hernia repair.

Polytetraflouroethylene (PTFE) was discovered at a DuPont laboratory serendipitously by Roy Plunkett in 1938. While researching tetraflouroethylene gas as a refrigerant, he discovered that the gas spontaneously polymerized into a slippery, white, powdery wax. After some time on the shelf, it was eventually used as a coating for cables. While still working at DuPont, William Gore subsequently saw the potential for medical applications, and ultimately started his own company, W.L. Gore and Associates, in 1958. That company developed and manufactured expanded PTFE under the brand name Gore-Tex (W.L. Gore and Associates, Flagstaff, Arizona) for hernia repair products, among other things. There are other manufacturers of PTFE hernia prosthetics, each with a different manufacturing process, and hence a slightly different architecture. Few PTFE prosthetics have been designed specifically for inguinal hernia repair, and although there is little use of PTFE in this setting, there are reports of good clinical outcomes [54]. Because PTFE is relatively compatible with viscera, its use in transabdominal preperitoneal (TAPP) laparoscopic hernia repair allows the surgeon to leave the peritoneum open once the prosthetic is in place. It is also useful for inguinal hernias that coexist with incisional hernias in the lower abdomen when approached form the peritoneal cavity.

Other polymers, such as carbon fiber [55] and polyvinylidenflouride [56], have been studied extensively both clinically and in the laboratory, but they have not significantly penetrated the clinical market for use in hernia repair.

Coated nonabsorbable prosthetics

To attenuate the host response to the prosthetic, yet still provide adequate strength for repair, some prosthetics use an absorbable or nonabsorbable coating over polypropylene or polyester [57]. These products have been primarily designed for ventral hernia repair in cases where the prosthetic is exposed to the viscera. However, they potentially have a role in inguinal hernia repair for reducing chronic pain and recurrence due to prosthetic shrinkage [58]. These types of prosthetics are also of interest to laparoscopic surgeons using the TAPP approach, as these types of prosthetics may eliminate the need to close the peritoneum. The basic premise of these prosthetics is that the coating should decrease the adherence of the protein coagulum, thus partially inhibiting the initiation of the inflammatory cascade (see Fig. 1) and decreasing the overall intensity of the response.

C-Qur mesh (Atrium Medical) is a midweight polypropylene mesh (50 or 85 g/m^2) coated with an absorbable omega-3 fatty acid preparation derived from fish oil. The coating is about 70% absorbed in 120 days and has had all protein removed to avoid an immune response. The same mesh without the coating has been analyzed in the laboratory and found to be acceptable in terms of inflammatory response compared with more heavyweight polypropylene prosthetics [59].

Glucamesh (Brennen Medical, St. Paul, Minnesota), only available in Europe, is a midweight polypropylene mesh (50 g/m^2) coated with the absorbable complex carbohydrate, oat beta glucan. A prospective study of 115 patients undergoing Lichtenstein or laparoscopic (totally extraperitoneal or TAPP) hernia repair with this prosthetic evaluated postoperative pain compared with pain following repair involving a heavyweight polypropylene prosthetic [44]. With a mean 24-month follow-up, 90% of patients returned a pain-related questionnaire. There was significantly less severe pain at 2-year follow-up with the lighter weight, coated polypropylene, regardless of technique. Despite the statistical analysis, it is unclear the degree to which each variable (prosthetic or technique) contributed. Recurrence rates were assessed by questionnaire, a relatively inaccurate method of detecting a recurrent hernia [60,61].

TiMESH (GFE Medizintechnik, Nürnberg, Germany) is a polypropylene mesh coated with titanium. Like any prosthetic, this product is manufactured in a variety of forms, and pushes the limits of density with one model as low as 16 g/m^2. While there are some conflicting data, there are no obvious differences in connective tissue and inflammatory markers with this compared with bare polypropylene [62]. Clinically, there are minor symptom improvements with this compared with heavyweight and partially absorbable prosthetics placed laparoscopically (TAPP) [63].

Partially absorbable prosthetics

To reduce the density of polymer (and subsequent inflammatory response), yet maintain the intraoperative handling characteristics and long-term wound strength, prosthetics have been developed that mix nonabsorbable polymers (eg, polypropylene) with absorbable polymers. There are conflicting results of the reduced inflammatory response. Comparing partially absorbable polypropylene–polyglactin (Vypro II) with pure polypropylene, Schumpelick and colleagues [41] showed statistically significant differences in a variety of inflammatory markers at 3, 21, and 90 days. Most of the values revealed less inflammation from polypropylene–polyglactin, but some favored polypropylene. Fibroblast morphometry and tensile strength, thought to be important in hernia repair, favored polypropylene [64]. In contrast, Bellon and colleagues [65] used a rabbit model to compare partially absorbable polypropylene meshes (Vypro and Ultrapro) with bare polypropylene (Surgipro). There were no statistically significant differences in postimplantation type-I/type-III collagen ratio, macrophage counts, shrinkage, and fixation. Despite the statistically significant advantages seen in the laboratory, it was still unknown if these prosthetics would have a clinically significant advantage. O'Dwyer and colleagues [66] randomized 321 patients undergoing an open Lichtenstein repair to a pure, "heavyweight" 85-g/m^2 polypropylene Atrium Medical prosthetic with a pore size of 1000 μm or the 32-g/m^2 (after absorption) Ethicon Vypro II partially absorbable polypropylene–polyglactin prosthetic with a pore size of 4000 μm. This study found no difference in the severity of pain preoperatively and at 1 and 3 months postoperatively. At 12 months postoperatively, severe pain was present in 3% to 4% of each group, and the statistically significant difference in mild pain was not clinically significant in that the pain did not affect physical function or limit roles. The lightweight, partially absorbable mesh group did, however, have a significant increase in recurrence rate (5.6% versus 0.4%). This underscores the fact that we do not know the optimal balance between weight and porosity of mesh as it relates to prosthetic fixation and long-term outcomes.

Biologic prosthetics

The emerging biologic prosthetics have primarily been designed for use in contaminated fields, limiting their role in inguinal hernia repair because the vast majority of these operations are clean. They may play an important role for acutely incarcerated groin hernias associated with tissue necrosis and/or infection. The basic concept behind these types of prosthetics is that they provide a matrix for native cells to populate and generate connective tissue that will replace the tissue in the hernia defect. The cost of these prosthetics is generally much higher than that of polypropylene or PET prosthetics. Given that newly formed connective tissue is only 70% to 80% as strong as native connective tissue, and that hernia patients may have an inherent defect in their native connective tissue, biologic (or absorbable synthetic) prosthetics would theoretically have a higher risk of recurrence than would permanent prosthetics. Nonetheless, some have advocated their use in elective inguinal hernia repair. One investigator [67] used a laparoscopic totally extraperitoneal approach to place Surgisis (Cook Medical, Bloomington, Indiana), a porcine intestinal submucosal graft. With 92% 5-year follow-up, this study claimed a recurrence rate similar to those from studies using synthetic prosthetics. However, the study used the relatively poor method of telephone interview as the method of detection [60,61]. No patients in this study had long-term or chronic pain, although in a previous study by the same investigator, the rate of postoperative discomfort in patients with Surgisis compared with patients with a polypropylene prosthetic was no different [68]. With a theoretic increased risk of long-term recurrence, relatively high cost, and no clear benefit, the use of these products for elective inguinal hernia repair should be considered investigational.

Design: density, porosity, and strength

To gauge the value of currently available and emerging prosthetics, it is helpful for a surgeon to know the design requirements of the ideal prosthetic. The ideal prosthetic should (1) possess good handling characteristics in the operating room, (2) invoke a favorable host response, (3) be strong enough to prevent recurrence, (4) place no restrictions on postimplantation function, (5) perform well in the presence of infection, (6) resist shrinkage or degradation over time, (7) make no restrictions on future access, (8) block transmission of infectious disease, (9) be inexpensive, and (10) be easy to manufacture [69]. All commercially available synthetic prosthetics today have long-term foreign-body reactions [59]. The differences in biologic response from the host do not seem to make major discernable clinical differences [66,70–72]. Data suggest that the density of the prosthetic—whether the prosthetic is "lightweight" or "heavyweight"—has an impact, but the optimal density is unknown [43]. Given the existing products and body of evidence, the overall density should probably be somewhere between 28 g/m^2 and 90 g/m^2 to minimize recurrence and adverse effects of the host foreign-body response [66]. Methods to decrease the density of the prosthetic include reduction in fiber diameter (ie, strength) and number of fibers (ie, increase in pore size). Laboratory studies suggest that the prosthetic should have at least 16 N/cm strength to avoid disruption and maintain proper fixation to the tissues [59]. Studies have also shown that a polypropylene mesh with a pore size greater than 600 to 800 μm should result in more of a scar "net" rather than a scar "plate" [41]. The "net," compared to the "plate," is less prone to contracture and stiffness of the abdominal wall. Not all small-pore prosthetics are stiff. Consider what is seen clinically with microporous PTFE, and the maintenance of pliability even with encapsulation. It may then be that the architecture (woven versus solid) of the prosthetic is a more significant contributor to performance than the polymer itself. The upper limits of pore size for adequate fixation to prevent recurrence have not been adequately investigated. Very large pore size (4000 μm) combined with a partially absorbable component doesn't appear to have any clinical benefits in terms of pain, and may not be sufficient to prevent higher recurrence rates when used with a Lichtenstein technique [66]. For making comparisons, it would be helpful to uniformly classify density (weight) and pore size in a standard fashion. Box 3 is a proposal of such a standard based on currently available data.

By technique

Techniques can be categorized in a range moving from anterior to posterior. There are prosthetics designed specifically for each approach, for

---

Box 3. Categories of prosthetic size and density

Heavyweight: >90 g/m^2
Mediumweight: 50–90 g/m^2
Lightweight: 35–50 g/m^2
Ultra-lightweight: <35 g/m^2

Very large pore: >2000 μm
Large pore: 1000–2000 μm
Medium pore: 600–1000 μm
Small pore: 100–600 μm
Microporous (solid): <100 μm

Although listed here as absolute values, the limits of each range are approximate values. The optimum combination of density and pore size is still unknown. Pore sizes less than 600 μm consistently cause scar bridging. Density greater than 90 g/m^2 consistently has the most severe host response.

example, flat prosthetics that can be tailored at the time of operation to meet the requirements of a given approach.

For strictly anterior repairs, the widely used Lichtenstein technique can use any flat sheet of mesh that is approximately 5 × 10 cm [73]. Additionally, the prosthetic should have properties that maximize chances of long-term hernia repair as well as minimize the negative aspects of the foreign-body response that may cause chronic pain or excessive scarring.

For techniques using a partial posterior repair combined with an anterior repair, there are a variety of "plug and patch" prosthetics. The "plug and patch" technique popularized by Rutkow and Robbins [74] uses a prosthetic "plug" placed in the defect and a flat mesh placed over the inguinal floor in a way similar to that used with the Lichtenstein technique. The concept of this repair is that the plug is an immediate, but relatively temporary repair, and the flat mesh serves to prevent long-term recurrence. As this technique became more widespread, concern developed regarding the fate of the conical polypropylene plug, as reports emerged regarding plug migration, hernia recurrence, and penetration into other organs [75]. The original Perfix plug (CM Bard, Murray Hill, New Jersey) is made of relatively heavyweight polypropylene, and thus is prone to contract and possibly migrate as scar tissue decreases its size [76,77]. In response to this concern, new "plug" prosthetics have been developed. The ProLoop Ultra plug (Atrium Medical) uses a lightweight, porous polypropylene with filaments designed to anchor to surrounding tissue and minimize contracture. The Gore Bioabsorbable plug (W.L. Gore and Associates) uses the copolymer polyglycolic acid–trimethylene carbonate, which was first introduced as the absorbable suture Maxon (American Cyanamid, Wayne, New Jersey) in 1982. Because of the bioabsorbable nature of this plug, it is supposed to incorporate with native connective tissue while avoiding problems with long-term contracture or plug migration. Both plugs are designed for placement in the defect under a flat polypropylene mesh (Fig. 2).

Another prosthetic designed for a more extensive, but still partial, posterior repair combined with an anterior repair is the Prolene Hernia System (Ethicon). It is manufactured from heavyweight polypropylene and has a flat, round, preperitoneal component physically attached to an oval, anterior flat prosthetic by a column. A partially absorbable, ultra-lightweight product with the same design, dubbed the Ultrapro Hernia System (Ethicon), is also available.

For completely posterior repairs, there are prosthetics specifically designed according to whether the approach is via open or laparoscopic techniques. For open techniques, any flat sheet of mesh large enough to cover the entire myopectineal orifice should suffice. For the classic giant prosthetic reinforcement of the visceral sac (GPRVS) performed through a lower midline or Pfannenstiel incision, any flat mesh that is of appropriate size and conformability can be used. The first surgeons who performed GPRVS with this technique preferred polyethylene terephthalate because

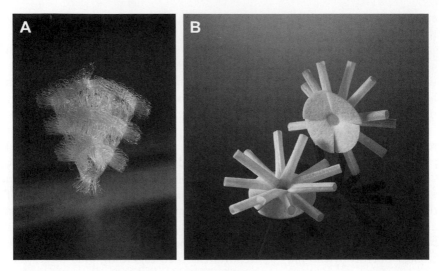

Fig. 2. New "plugs" for partially posterior combined with anterior repair for inguinal hernia. (*A*) Lightweight polypropylene. (*B*) Absorbable polyglycolic acid–trimethylene carbonate.

of its favorable handling characteristics [78,79]. For bilateral hernias, the width of the prosthetic should be 2 cm shorter than the distance between the anterior superior iliac spines, equal in length to the distance from the symphysis pubis to the umbilicus, and fashioned in the shape of a chevron [80]. Another posterior repair via an anterior incision was developed by Kugel. The basic premise of his procedure is the same as that for the GPRVS, but uses a much smaller incision and prosthetic [81]. The smaller size of both the prosthetic and incision make this a relatively difficult operation to master. Additionally, the commercially available Bard Kugel Hernia Patch (CM Bard) is made of two layers of heavyweight polypropylene with an additional polypropylene recoil ring designed to assist deployment. One study of 386 hernia repairs with 87% of the patients followed up for a median of 42 months revealed an overall recurrence rate of 7.7% [82]. Recurrence was more likely in cases involving repair of recurrent hernias, large direct hernias, and surgeons with less experience. A laparoscopic approach to posterior repair more closely mimics the GPRVS approach in that it uses a conformable prosthetic, typically larger than that for the Kugel repair, but still smaller than that for the GPRVS. Any flat prosthetic of adequate size (10 × 15 cm) should suffice. Prosthetics are available with a slit to accommodate the spermatic cord. There is no consensus regarding optimal location of the slit, and some come with an additional, smaller prosthetic intended to be placed over the slit. 3D Max (CM Bard) is a heavyweight polypropylene mesh that is slightly curved to conform to the shape of the myopectineal orifice. This does not require fixation, according to the manufacturer, and there are reports of series with good results [83].

Recently approved by the Food and Drug Administration, Rebound HRD (MMDI, Minneapolis, Minnesota) is a polypropylene prosthetic with a conformable nitinol frame intended to minimize the need for fixation and help maintain the original shape and size of the prosthetic.

By clinical scenario

To lower the chances of choosing the wrong prosthetic, it is useful to categorize prosthetics according to the clinical situation and patient factors. Additionally, the patient and the surgeon should agree preoperatively on what the desired outcome of the hernia repair should be. Achieving these goals may then guide a prosthetic choice.

Symptoms

If a patient is asymptomatic, the primary goal is cure of the hernia to prevent complications of acute incarceration or hernia enlargement. The surgeon should therefore use his or her best technique to accomplish this. The choice of prosthetic should be from among those best suited for this technique. If the patient presents with significant pain, a prosthetic that will theoretically reduce the inflammatory response may be best.

Medical history

The presence of significant cardiopulmonary disease may guide the approach as well, and hence the prosthetic choice. Other factors to consider are whether or not the patient has an ongoing infectious process elsewhere, a history of wound infection after operation, and whether or not the hernia is recurrent. Recurrent hernias often require a different approach than that for the first repair, thus guiding the prosthetic choice. A prior history of lower abdominal surgery or preperitoneal hernia repair may also change the approach, and thus the prosthetic choice.

Urgency

Emergency settings clearly differ from elective settings. In an emergency setting, the clinical course guides the urgency of surgical repair. When bowel strangulation is present, a prosthetic that performs relatively well in a contaminated field should be chosen. For a bowel obstruction, a posterior approach may be preferred to allow examination of the intestine for viability, at which time any prosthetic suitable for a posterior repair can be used.

Hernia size

Large inguinal-scrotal hernias may also dictate the approach. In addition to the size of the sac and reducibility of its contents, the defect size also plays a role in determining the approach. While defect size for inguinal hernias does not have the same variability as that for ventral hernias, larger defects require a prosthetic large enough to prevent recurrence.

Future risk

Some oppose a preperitoneal approach for inguinal hernia in men because such an approach increases the technical difficulty of subsequent radical prostatectomy in the presence of a prosthetic placed for hernia repair [84]. Others, however, have shown that, while the technical difficulty of subsequent prostatectomy is increased, it can be performed safely with a retropubic approach laparoscopically, or via a perineal approach [85,86]. There are many reports of safely performing inguinal hernia repair and radical prostatectomy at the same operative setting [87–89]. If performing an inguinal hernia repair concomitantly with a radical prostatectomy, once again the approach dictates the choice of prosthetic.

Summary

With numerous prosthetic options and a changing landscape of prosthetic development, a systematic approach to choosing a prosthetic is more sensible than trying to memorize all the details of each prosthetic. The surgeon should hone a single technique for the vast majority of inguinal hernia repairs to maximize proficiency. This limits the number of prosthetics to those suitable for that technique. Narrowing the choice further should be based on the likelihood that a given prosthetic will achieve the preoperative goals of the hernia repair for both the surgeon and the patient [90]. These goals should be symptom relief and/or hernia cure. For alternative clinical scenarios, a different approach may be necessary, and hence a different prosthetic. Reducing the negative consequences of the inflammatory response to the prosthetic, yet maintaining the strength to prevent recurrence, is the subject of much research and debate. The optimal way to accomplish this goal is unknown, and current strategies include reducing the prosthetic density, mixing the permanent prosthetic with an absorbable component, and coating the prosthetic. Cost is another issue that invariably factors in to the clinical availability of a prosthetic at a given institution, and should also be considered. A cost analysis is more than financial, and the amount of potential clinical benefit should be commensurate with any increase in cost. Long-term benefits of any new prosthetic are theoretical, and the surgeon should decide the likelihood of realizing these long-term benefits based on the existing experimental and clinical data.

How do I choose?

First, align the goals of operation (symptom relief and/or hernia cure) with those of the patient. Next, give consideration to the expected acute inflammatory response and long-term performance of the prosthetic. Then plan the technique according to your practice standard and clinical scenario. Once the technique is decided upon, a prosthetic that best suits the technique should be selected.

If the surgeon chooses to use a prosthetic that alters his or her routine, the reasons for this change should be sound and discussed with the patient. If the prosthetic is new to the market or type of hernia, the surgeon must assess whether the new prosthetic will achieve the goals of the particular case and weigh the uncertainty of long-term outcomes for the new prosthetic against more certain outcomes of existing products. If the prosthetic is used for investigational purposes, an approval from the institutional review board should be sought. Using a newly FDA-approved prosthetic for presumed clinical benefit does not require institutional review board approval, but must be discussed with the patient. If this is too much to undertake, then reconsider the choice of prosthetic.

References

[1] Rutkow IM. Demographics and socioeconomic aspects of hernia repair in the United States in 2003. Surg Clin North Am 2003;83(5):1045–51.
[2] EU Hernia Trialists Collaboration. Repair of groin hernia with synthetic mesh: a meta-analysis of randomized controlled trials. Ann Surg 2002;235(3):322–32.
[3] Morgan M, Reynolds A, Swan AV, et al. Are current techniques of inguinal hernia repair optimal? A survey in the United Kingdom. Ann R Coll Surg Engl 1991;73(6):341–5.
[4] Abatek U, Spence RK, Pello M, et al. A survey of preferred approach to inguinal hernia repair: laparoscopic or inguinal incision? Am Surg 1994;60(4):255–8.
[5] Simons MP, Hoitsma HF, Mullan FJ, et al. Primary inguinal hernia repair in The Netherlands. Eur J Surg 1995;161(5):345–8.
[6] Ciampolini J, Boyce DE, Shandall AA. Adult hernia surgery in Wales revisited: impact of the guidelines of The Royal College of Surgeons of England. Ann R Coll Surg Engl 1998;80(5): 335–8.
[7] DesCoteaux JG, Sutherland F. Inguinal hernia repair: a survey of Canadian practice patterns. Can J Surg 1999;42(2):127–32.
[8] Ziesche M, Manger T. Determining the status of laparoscopic surgery in East Brandenburg. Results of a survey. Zentralbl Chir 2000;125(12):997–1002.
[9] Metzger J, Lutz N, Laidlaw I. Guidelines for inguinal hernia repair in everyday practice. Ann R Coll Surg Engl 2001;83(3):209–14.
[10] Bay-Nielsen M, Kehlet H, Strand L, et al. Danish Hernia Database Collaboration. Quality assessment of 26,304 herniorrhaphies in Denmark: a prospective nationwide study. Lancet 2001;358(9288):1124–8.
[11] Data from Verispan. Available at: www.verispan.com.
[12] Richards SK, Earnshaw JJ. Management of primary and recurrent inguinal hernia by surgeons for the South West of England. Ann R Coll Surg Engl 2003;85(6):402–4.
[13] Onitsuka A, Katagiri Y, Kiyama S, et al. Current practices in adult groin hernias: a survey of Japanese general surgeons. Surg Today 2003;33(2):155–7.
[14] Chan KY, Rohaizak M, Sukumar N, et al. Inguinal hernia repair by surgical trainees at a Malayasian teaching hospital. Asian J Surg 2004;27(4):306–12.
[15] Ferrante F, Rusconi A, Galimerti A, et al. Lombardia Hernia Study Group. Hernia repair in the Lombardy region in 2000: preliminary results. Hernia 2004;8(3):247–51.
[16] Mjaland O, Johnson E, Myrvold H. Hernia surgery in Norway. Tidsskr Nor Laegeforcn 2001;121(21):2481–3.
[17] de Lange DH, Aufenacker TJ, Roest M, et al. Inguinal hernia surgery in The Netherlands: a baseline study before the introduction of the Dutch Guidelines. Hernia 2005;9(2):172–7.
[18] Rodriguez-Cuellar E, Villeta R, Ruiz P, et al. National project for the management of clinical processes. Surgical treatment of inguinal hernia. Cir Esp 2005;77(4):194–202.

[19] Ravindran R, Bruce J, Debnath D, et al. A United Kingdom survey of surgical technique and handling practice of inguinal canal structures during hernia surgery. Surgery 2006;139(4): 523–6.

[20] Shamim SM, Shamim MS, Jaffary SA, et al. Trends in the management of inguinal hernia in Karachi, Pakistan: a survey of practice patterns. Singapore Med J 2006;47(6):512–7.

[21] Lau WY. History of treatment of groin hernia. World J Surg 2002;26:748–59.

[22] Skandalakis JE, Colborn GL, Skandalakis LJ, et al. Historic aspects of groin hernia repair. In: Fitzsgibbons RJ, Greenburg AG, editors. Nyhus and condon's hernia. 5th edition. Philadelphia: Williams and Wilkins; 2002. p. 39.

[23] McClusky DA, Mirilas P, Zoras O, et al. Groin hernia: anatomical and surgical history. Arch Surg 2006;141(10):1035–42.

[24] Kux M, Fuchsjäger N, Schemper M. Shouldice is superior to Bassini inguinal herniorrhaphy. Am J Surg 1994;168(1):15–8.

[25] Farooq O, Batool Z, Bashir-ur-Rehman. Prolene darn: safe and effective method for primary inguinal hernia repair. J Coll Phys Surg Pak 2005;15(6):358–61.

[26] Thorbjarnarson B, Goulian D. Complications from use of surgical mesh in repair of hernias. N Y State J Med 1967;67(9):1189–92.

[27] Usher FC. Further observations on the use of Marlex mesh: a new technique for the repair of ingiuonal hernias. Am Surg 1959;25:792–5.

[28] Butters M, Redecke J, Kooninger J. Long term results of a randomized clinical trial of Shouldice, Lichtenstein, and transabdominal preperitoneal hernia repairs. Br J Surg 2007; 94:562–5.

[29] Liem MS, van Duyn EB, van der Graaf Y, et al. Recurrences after conventional anterior and laparoscopic inguinal hernia repair. Ann Surg 2003;237(1):136–41.

[30] Bassini E. Nuovo metodo operativo per la cura dell'hernia inguinale. Padova. R. Stabilimento Prosperini 1989.

[31] Nicolo E. Presented at the Annual Meeting of the American Hernia Society. Hollywood (FL): March 2007.

[32] Tang L, Ugarova TP, Plow EF, et al. Molecular determinates of acute inflammatory response to biomaterials. J Clin Invest 1996;97(5):1329–34.

[33] Busutill SJ, Ploplis VA, Castellino FJ, et al. A central role for plasminogen in the inflammatory response to biomaterials. J Thromb Hemost 2004;2(10):1798–805.

[34] Woloson SK, Greisler HP. Biochemistry, immunology, and tissue response to prosthetic material. In: Bendavid, et al, editors. Abdominal wall hernias, principles and management. New York: Springer-Verlag; 2001. p. 201–7.

[35] Diegelmann RF. Collagen metabolism. Wounds 2000;13(5):177–82.

[36] McDermott MK, Isayeva IS, Thomas TM, et al. Characterization of the structure and properties of authentic and counterfeit polypropylene surgical meshes. Hernia 2006;10:1313–4.

[37] Amid PK, Shulman AG, Lichtenstein IL, et al. Experimental evaluation of a new composite mesh with the selective properties of incorporation to the abdominal wall without adhering to the intestines. J Biomed Mater Res 1994;28:373–5.

[38] Stengel D, Bauwens K, Ekkernkamp A. Recurrence risks in randomized trials of laparoscopic versus open inguinal hernia repair: to pool or not to pool (this is not the question). Langenbecks Arch Surg 2004;389(6):492–8.

[39] Langenbeck MR, Schmidt J, Zirngibi H. Comparison of biomaterials in the early postoperative period: polypropylene meshes in laparoscopic inguinal hernia repair. Surg Endosc 2003;17:1105–9.

[40] Kossovy N, Freiman CJ, Howarth D. Biomaterials pathology. In: Bendavid, et al, editors. Abdominal wall hernias, principles and management. New York: Springer-Verlag; 2001. p. 225.

[41] Schumpelick V, Klinge U, Rosch R, et al. Light weight meshes in incisional hernia repair. J Min Access Surg 2006;3:117–23.

[42] Novitsky YW, Harrell AG, Hope WW, et al. Meshes in hernia repair. Surg Technol Int 2007; 16:123–7.

[43] Cobb WS, Kercher KW, Heniford BT. The argument for lightweight polypropylene mesh in hernia repair. Surg Innov 2005;12(1):63–9.

[44] Champault G, Barrat C. Inguinal hernia repair with beta glucan-coated mesh: results at two-year follow up. Hernia 2004;9:125–30.

[45] Losanoff JE, Richman BW, Jones JW. Entero-colocutaneous fistula: a late consequence of polypropylene mesh abdominal wall repair: case report and review of the literature. Hernia 2002;6:144–7.

[46] Chuback JA, Sigh RS, Sill D, et al. Small bowel obstruction resulting from mesh plug migration after open inguinal hernia repair. Surgery 2000;127:475–6.

[47] Bellon JM, Rodriguez M, Garcia-Honduvilla N, et al. Peritoneal effects of prosthetic meshes use to repair abdominal wall defects: monitoring adhesions by sequential laparoscopy. J Laparoend Tech 2007;17(2):160–6.

[48] Langer C, Schwartz P, Krause P, et al. In-vitro study of the cellular response of human fibroblasts cultured on alloplastic hernia meshes. Influence of mesh material and structure. Chirurg 2005;76(9):876–85.

[49] Hounshell DA, Smith JK. Science and corporate strategy: DuPont r and d, 1902–1980. 1st edition. Cambridge: Cambridge University Press; 2006. p. 411.

[50] Bussitil SJ, Drumm C, Plow EF. In vivo comparision of the inflammatory response induced by different vascular biomaterials. Vascular 2005;13(4):230–5.

[51] Van Bilsen PH, Popa ER, Brouwer LA, et al. Ongoing foreign body reaction to subcutaneous implanted (heparin) modified Dacron in rats. J Biomed Mater Res 2004;68(3):423–7.

[52] Zieren J, Neuss H, Muller J. Introduction of polyethylene terephthalate mesh (KoSa hochfest) for abdominal hernia repair: an animal experimental study. BioMed Mater Eng 2004;14(2):127–32.

[53] Gumargalieva KZ, Mosieev YuV, Daurova TT, et al. Effects of infections on the degradation of polyethylene terephthalate implants. Biomaterials 1982;3(3):177–80.

[54] Athanasakis E, Saridaki Z, Kafetzakis A, et al. Surgical repair of inguinal hernia: tension free technique with prosthetic material (Gore-Tex Mycro Mesh Expanded Polytetrafluoroethylene). Am Surg 2000;66(8):728–31.

[55] Minns RJ, Claque MB, Ward R, et al. The repair of inguinal hernias using carbon fibre patches—a five year follow-up. Clin Mater 1993;14(2):139–44.

[56] Junge K, Kinge U, Rosch R, et al. Improved colalgen type I/III ration at the interface of gentamicin-supplemented polyvinylidenfluoride mesh materials. Langenbecks Arch Surg 2007; 392(4):465–71.

[57] Klinge U, Klosterhalfen B, Muller M, et al. Influence of ployglactin-coating on functional and morphologic parameters of ploypropylene-mesh modifications for abdominal wall repair. Biomaterials 1999;20:613.

[58] Scheidbach H, Tamme C, Tanapfel A, et al. In vivo studies comparing the biocompatibility of various polypropylene meshes and their handling properties during endoscopic total extraperitoneal (TEP) patchplasty. An experimetnal study in pigs. Surg Endosc 2004; 18(2):211–20.

[59] Kosterhalfern B, Klinge U, Hermanns B, et al. [Pathology of traditional surgical nets for hernia repair after long-term implantation in humans]. Chiurg 2000;71:43–51 [in German].

[60] Vos PM, Simons MP, Luitse JS, et al. Follow-up after inguinal hernia repair: questionnaire compared with physical examination: a prospective study of 299 patients. Eur J Surg 1998; 14:533–6.

[61] Haappaniemi S, Nilsson E. Recurrences and pain three years after groin hernia repair. Validation of postal questionnaire and selective physical examination as a method of follow-up 2002;168:22–8.

[62] Junge K, Rosch R, Klinge U, et al. Titanium coating of a polypropylene mesh for hernia repair: effect on biocompatibility. Hernia 2005;9:115–9.

[63] Horstmann R, Hellwig M, Classen C, et al. Impact of polypropylene amount on functional outcome and quality of life after inguinal hernia repair by the TAPP procedure using pure, mixed, and titanium-coated meshes. World J Surg 2006;30(9):1742–9.

[64] Junge K, Klinge U, Rosch R, et al. Functional and morphologic properties of a modified mesh for inguinal hernia repair offer advantages over nonabsorbable meshes. Am J Surg 2002;26:1472–80.

[65] Bellon JM, Rodriguez M, Garcia-Honduvilla N, et al. Partially absorbable meshes for hernia repair offer advantages over nonabsorbable meshes. Am J Surg 2007;194:68–74.

[66] O'Dwyer PJ, Kingsnorth AN, Molloy RG, et al. Randomized clinical trial assessing impact of a lightweight or heavyweight mesh on chronic pain after inguinal hernia repair. Br J Surg 2005;92:166–70.

[67] Edelman DS, Hodde JP. Bioactive prosthetic materials for treatment of hernias. Surg Technol Int 2006;15:104–8.

[68] Edelman DS. Laparoscopic herniorrhaphy with porcine small intestine submucosa: a preliminary study. JSLS 2002;6:203–5.

[69] Earle DB, Romanelli J. Prosthetic materials for hernia: What's new. How to make sense of the multitude of mesh options for inguinal and ventral hernia repairs. Contemp Surg 2007; 63(2):63–9.

[70] Bracco P, Brunella V, Trossarelli L, et al. Comparison of polypropylene and polyethylene terephthalate (Dacron) meshes for abdominal wall hernia repair: a chemical and morphological study. Hernia 2005;9(1):51–5.

[71] Klinge U, Conze J, Limberg W, et al. Pathophysiology of the abdominal wall. Chirurg 1996; 67:229.

[72] Cobb WS, Burns JM, Peindl RD, et al. Textile analysis of heavy weight, mid-weight, and light weight polypropylene mesh in a porcine ventral hernia model. J Surg Res 2006;136:1–7.

[73] Lichtenstein IL, Shulman AG, Amid P, et al. The tension-free herniaplasty. Am J Surg 1989; 157(2):188–93.

[74] Rutkow IM, Robbins AW. The Marlex mesh Perfix plug groin heriaplasty. Eur J Surg 1998; 164(7):549–52.

[75] Murphy JW, Misra DC, Silverglide B. Sigmoid colonic fistula secondary to Perfixplug, left inguinal hernia repair. Hernia 2006;19(5):436–8.

[76] Moorman ML, Price PD. Migratig mesh plug: cmplication of a well-established hernia repair technique. Am Surg 2004;70(4):298–9.

[77] Mayagoitia JC, Prieto-Diaz Chavez E, Suarez D, et al. Predictive factors and comparison of complications and recurrences in three tension-free herniorrhaphy techniques. Hernia 2006; 10(2):147–51.

[78] Rives J, Stoppa R, Fortesa L, et al. Les pieces en Dacron et leur place dans la chirurgie des hernies de l'aine. Ann Chir 1968;22:59.

[79] Wantz GE. Giant reinforcement of the visceral sac. Surg Gynecol Obstet 1989;169:408.

[80] Wantz GE. Atlas of hernia surgery. New York: Raven Press; 1991. p. 120.

[81] Kugel RD. The Kugel repair for groin hernias. Surg Clin North Am 2003;83(5):1119–39.

[82] Schroeder DM, Lloyd LR, Boccaccio JE, et al. Inguinal hernia recurrence following preperitoneal Kugel patch repair. Am Surg 2004;70(2):132–6.

[83] Bell RCW, Price JG. Laparoscopic inguinal hernia repair using an anatomically contoured three-dimensional mesh. Surg Endosc 2003;17:1784–8.

[84] Katz EE, Patel RV, Sokoloff MH, et al. Bilateral laparoscopic inguinal hernia repair can complicate subsequent radical retropubic prostatectomy. J Urol 2002;167:637–8.

[85] Stolzenburg JU, Anderson C, Rabenalt R, et al. Endoscopic extraperitoneal radical prostatectomy in patients with prostate cancer and previous laparoscopic ingunal mesh placement for hernia repair. World J Urol 2005;23(4):295–9.

[86] Borchers H, Brehmer B, van Poppel H, et al. Radical prostatectomy in patients with previous groin hernia repair using synthetic nonabsorbable mesh. Urol Int 2001;67(3):213–5.

[87] Lee BC, Rodin DM, Shah KK, et al. Laparoscopic inguinal hernia repair duting laparoscopic radical prostatectomy. BJU Int 2007;99(3):637–9.

[88] Manorhan M, Vyas S, Araki M, et al. Concurrent radical retropubic prostatectomy and Lichtenstein inguinal hernia repair through a single modified Pfannenstiel incision: a 3-year experience. BJU Int 2006;98(2):341–4.

[89] Drachenberg DE, Bell DG. Preperitoneal mesh plug herniorraphy during radical retropubic prostatectomy. Can J Urol 2002;9(4):1602–6.

[90] Franneby U, Gunnaraaon U, Wollert S, et al. Discordance between the patient's and surgeon's perception of complications following hernia surgery. Hernia 2005;9(2):145–9.

ELSEVIER
SAUNDERS

SURGICAL
CLINICS OF
NORTH AMERICA

Surg Clin N Am 88 (2008) 203–216

Postherniorrhaphy Groin Pain and How to Avoid It

George S. Ferzli, MD, FACS[a,b,c,*], Eric Edwards, MD[d],
Georges Al-Khoury, MD[e], RoseMarie Hardin, MD[b]

[a]Department of Surgery, Lutheran Medical Center, 150 East 55th Street,
Brooklyn, NY 11201, USA
[b]Department of Surgery, SUNY Health Sciences Center at Brooklyn,
450 Clarkson Avenue, Brooklyn, NY 11203, USA
[c]65 Cromwell Avenue, Staten Island, NY 10304, USA
[d]St. Mary Medical Center, 1205 Langhorne-Newtown Road, Langhorne, PA 19047, USA
[e]6225 Monitor Street, Apartment E, Pittsburgh, PA 15217, USA

Henry Kissinger once stated that, "soccer is a game that hides great complexity in the appearance of simplicity"; he could have very well been describing an inguinal hernia repair. Few other anatomic dissections in general surgery can prove as challenging as an inguinal hernia repair. Despite the procedure's seemingly straightforward steps, if strict adherence to anatomic planes of dissection is not followed as well as the use of precise knowledge of potential pitfalls, morbidity can easily result. One of the most common sources of postoperative morbidity in surgical patients is the occurrence of postherniorrhaphy chronic groin pain, defined as pain that persists after the normal healing process has occurred—typically 3 months after surgery. Chronic groin pain is most often a result of nerve injury sustained during improper dissection. Careful dissection of the five major nerves encountered during this procedure and their protection can help to reduce this complication substantially and its concomitant adverse effects on quality of life.

The complexity of nerve dissections in the inguinal region is increased by the varied patterns of distribution. It has been shown that there is direct communication between branches of the major innervations of the groin. In fact, only approximately 20% of patients were found to have the "normal" pattern of sensory distribution of the iliohypogastric and ilioinguinal nerves, as outlined by modern anatomic references. This is further

---

* Corresponding author. Department of Surgery, Lutheran Medical Center.
E-mail address: gferzli@aol.com (G.S. Ferzli).

0039-6109/08/$ - see front matter © 2008 Elsevier Inc. All rights reserved.
doi:10.1016/j.suc.2007.10.006

complicated by the fact that these patterns of innervation are only symmetrical in approximately 40% of patients [1].

The true incidence of postherniorrhaphy groin pain has not been fully elucidated, in part because most surgeons have been more concerned with recurrence rates than with this seemingly insignificant symptom. However, with the advent of tension-free mesh repairs, inguinal hernia recurrences are uncommon, unless underlying patient factors predispose to the development of hernias. Furthermore, not all patients suffering with chronic groin pain seek medical assistance, especially for mild symptoms. Few are referred back to the operating surgeon, and only a small percentage of patients seek help from a pain specialist [2]. In fact, one study demonstrated that after 24 to 36 months of follow-up, approximately 30% of patients undergoing inguinal herniorrhaphy reported pain or discomfort and nearly 6% reported high-intensity pain resulting in inability to perform activities of daily living. This was in comparison with a recurrence rate of only 4.5% [3]. The point of maximal tenderness is usually at the pubic tubercle, usually from incorporation of a stitch or staple into the peritosteum [2]. In recent years, emphasis has shifted toward evaluation of the patient's quality of life after surgical intervention and relief of symptoms, with presence of inguinal pain viewed as an endpoint in evaluating hernia surgery. This emphasis is of particular importance: if a patient is undergoing herniorrhaphy to reduce inguinal pain, it would be a disservice to cause undue pain secondary to improper groin dissection. It is also crucial to determine whether any other associated pathology exists and can contribute to the sensation of inguinal pain because this will lead to persistent pain after surgical intervention.

This article aims to provide a thorough review of pertinent anatomic landmarks for the proper identification of the nerves that, if injured, result in chronic groin pain and to provide a treatment algorithm for patients suffering with this morbidity.

Anatomic considerations

To prevent technical errors resulting from improper nerve dissection, a thorough understanding of the innervation to the groin and the anatomic location of the nerves is essential for their preservation and protection from injury. This will help to not only better understand the etiology of the problem, but also to provide a means of preventing this complication. Interestingly, according to the present author's residents, only the ilioinguinal nerve is routinely sought in groin dissections and protected from injury. This may be the fundamental problem in the technical approach to inguinal herniorrhaphy that predisposes to chronic groin pain. In fact, there are five main nerves that must be identified and preserved during an inguinal herniorrhapy: the ilioinguinal, the iliohypogastric, the genitofemoral, the lateral femoral cutaneous, and the femoral nerves. Table 1 presents a complete review of the origin and course of these vital structures.

Table 1
Inguinal region nerve descriptions

Nerve	Origin	Course	Function
Ilioinguinal	T12-L1 nerve roots	It emerges from the border of the psoas major, passes the quadratus lumborum and iliacus, perforates the transverses abdominis, and then accompanies the spermatic cord	Supplies sensory innervation to the proximal and medial thigh. In females it innervates the mons pubis and labium majus; in males it innervates the root of the penis and upper scrotum.
Iliohypogastric	T12-L1 nerve roots	Same as ilioinguinal	Same as ilioinguinal
Genitofemoral	L1-L2 nerve roots	It emerges from the medial border of the psoas muscle and subsequently divides into a genital and femoral branch. The genital branch pierces the transversalis fascia, where it travels with the spermatic cord to the scrotum; the femoral branch travels with the external iliac artery and passes beneath the inguinal ligament and extends to the anterior surface of the thigh.	The genital branch supplies sensation to the mons pubis and labium majus. In males it supplies sensation to the scrotum and motor fibers to the cremasteric muscle. The femoral branch supplies innervation to the anteriorlateral thigh.
Lateral femoral cutaneous	L2-L3 nerve roots	It emerges from the lateral border of the osoas muscles, goes toward the anterior superior iliac spine, and passes under the inguinal ligament	Provides sensory innervation to the anteriorlateral thigh. Injury most commonly results in severe burning sensation along its course.
Femoral	L2-L3 nerve roots	Emerges at the inferior border of the psoas muscle and passes beneath the inguinal ligament to innervate the thigh	Provides sensory branches to the anterior thigh. Predominant function is motor innervation to the quadriceps resulting in muscle atrophy if injured.

When the groin is explored via the anterior approach, one may encounter the ilioinguinal nerve, the genital branch of the genitofemoral nerve, and the iliohypogastric nerve (Fig. 1). The ilioinguinal nerve can usually be identified lateral to the internal ring. The genital branch of the genitofemoral can be identified in the lateral crus of the internal ring. Another possible anatomic location of this nerve is between the spermatic cord and inguinal ligament. The iliohypogastric nerve can be identified by separating the aponeurosis of the external oblique from the internal oblique muscle. The iliohypogastric nerve is the regional nerve that is at highest risk during tension-free repair because it can be trapped by the overlapping mesh in the scar tissue that forms between the mesh and the muscle plane along which the nerve runs [4].

When the groin is explored with minimally invasive techniques, the nerves that are prone to injury include the lateral femoral cutaneous, the femoral branch of the genitofemoral nerve, and the femoral nerve (Fig. 2). During a laparoscopic repair, one must identify the "triangle of pain," appropriately named because of the many nerves that course through it and the potential for injury if careful dissection is not performed. This

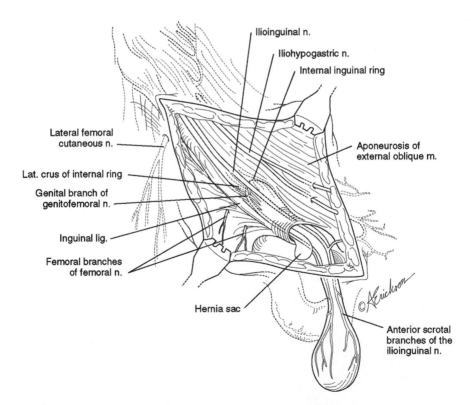

Fig. 1. Nerves encountered during the anterior inguinal herniorrhaphy approach. (*Courtesy of* A. Erickson, Brooklyn, NY.)

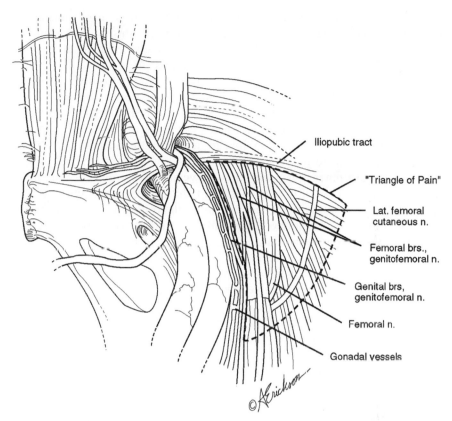

Iliopubic tract

"Triangle of Pain"

Lat. femoral
cutaneous n.

Femoral brs.,
genitofemoral n.

Genital brs,
genitofemoral n.

Femoral n.

Gonadal vessels

Fig. 2. Nerves prone to injury during laparoscopic inguinal herniorrhaphy. (*Courtesy of* A. Erickson, Brooklyn, NY.)

triangle is a theoretical space bounded by the gonadal vessels medially, the reflected peritoneum laterally, and the iliopubic tract superiorly.

Risk factors for chronic pain following inguinal herniorrhaphy

One study sought to understand the phenomenon of postoperative inguinodynia with a population-based study involving more than 9000 patients undergoing inguinal hernia repair. Patients were given a questionnaire designed to identify postoperative inguinal pain and determine severity and impact on quality of life—specifically in impeding functional daily activities and ability to work and exercise. In multivariate logistic analyses, severe preoperative groin pain and presence of postoperative complications such as infection or hematoma were found to independently predict postoperative inguinal pain in a statistically significant manner ($P = 0.001$ and $P = .003$, respectively) [3]. Preoperative pain may indicate complicated disease pathology prior to surgical intervention resulting in stretching, entrapment, or inflammation of inguinal nerves. It may also indicate the presence of psychologic predisposition and lowered pain thresholds among these patients, increasing potential for postoperative pain [3]. There may be an underlying cycle of chronic pain that is difficult to break.

Direct injury to nerves that results in either partial or complete transaction can lead to neuroma formation and the subsequent development of chronic pain. Some have implicated the role of mesh as well. It has been demonstrated experimentally that when peripheral nerve tissue comes in contact with polypropylene mesh, myelin degeneration, edema, and fibrosis result and can lead to neuralgia and peripheral neuropathy [5,6]. Multiple studies have examined this issue and the weight of the evidence seems to favor a lack of association with mesh and the occurrence of chronic pain [7–9]. In fact, one study sought to determine the outcomes of hernia repair with the use of biocompatible, "light" meshes and the potential for reduction of postoperative pain. These light meshes have been constructed with an aim to improve tissue integration into the mesh, thereby reducing the foreign body reaction thought to be partly responsible for postherniorrhaphy groin pain. In a prospective, randomized clinical trial, light meshes were associated with similar rates of chronic groin pain compared with traditional meshes, 3% and 4%, respectively [10]. These data are largely preliminary, and research into alternatives to polypropylene will surely continue.

Operative technique has been implicated in the etiology of groin pain following inguinal herniorrhaphy. There are numerous published reports of nerve entrapment by tacks placed during laparoscopic repair [11–13].

Laparoscopic herniorrhaphy without the use of a tacker has been described and eliminates the risk of misplaced tacks [1,14,15]. It has been accepted, however, that laparoscopic hernia repairs result in less chronic pain syndromes in comparison with open repairs, predominately owing to failed identification of the ilioinguinal nerve in the latter approach. Furthermore, laparoscopic repair requires limited dissection and avoids undue stress and trauma to the ilioinguinal and iliohypogastric nerves [10].

Avoiding chronic pain following inguinal herniorrhaphy

The cornerstone of avoiding postoperative pain following inguinal hernia surgery is precise knowledge of groin anatomy and careful dissection and preservation of inguinal nerves. Some have even gone to the extreme of advocating "watchful waiting" for asymptomatic hernias to avoid postoperative pain, but this must be carefully weighed against the potential for incarceration or strangulation. Judicious clinical judgment would advocate early intervention with careful dissection to avoid preventable nerve injury, thereby minimizing this potentially debilitating morbidity.

Care must be taken to avoid placement of sutures at the medial insertion of the inguinal ligament to avoid excessive tightness of the inguinal ligament at the pubic tubercle. Most somatic pain following inguinal herniorrhaphy results from damage to the pubic tubercle during stapling or suturing of the mesh prosthesis with incorporation of the periosteum of the pubic tubercle [16]. A description of six specific maneuvers to reduce the risk of nerve injury during open herniorrhaphy has been described [17]: avoiding indiscriminate division of the subcutaneous tissue, avoiding removal of the cremasteric muscle fibers, avoiding extensive dissection of the ilioinguinal nerve, identifying and preserving all neural structures, avoiding making the inguinal ring too tight, and avoiding placement of sutures in the lower edge of the internal oblique muscle. Nerve trauma can be caused by several mechanisms, including partial or complete transaction, stretching, contusion, crushing, cautery damage, or suture compression [16].

Of interest, a study performed by Lichtenstein that investigated the prevention of postherniorrhaphy neuralgia proposed that transection of the ilioinguinal and genitofemoral nerves may prove to be a useful solution [18]. Several groups have attempted to avoid chronic postoperative pain by the use of selective neurectomy during elective repair of groin hernias. A small number of patients undergoing resection of the iliohypogastric and ilioinguinal nerves during open, tension-free mesh repair have been studied [19]. It was demonstrated that none of these patients developed chronic groin pain; however, 6.2% reported numbness at the 1-year follow-up A retrospective review found that ilioinguinal neurectomy during open, tension-free mesh repair resulted in significantly less pain after 1 year compared with routine nerve preservation, 3% and 25%, respectively [20]. A double-blinded, randomized controlled trial to investigate the effects of prophylactic ilioinguinal neurectomy following tension-free mesh repair of inguinal hernia was conducted with 100 male patients randomized into two groups: prophylactic ilioinguinal neurectomy or ilioinguinal nerve preservation. The findings demonstrated that the incidence of chronic groin pain at 6 months was significantly lowered compared with the nerve preservation group (8% versus 28.6%, $P = .0008$). No significant difference was found in the incidence of neurosensory complaints, including groin numbness and sensory loss [21]. The authors advocated that prophylactic neurectomy should be incorporated into the essential steps of a Lichtenstein hernia repair. However, this remains controversial because other studies have failed to demonstrate a statistically significant difference in incidence of postoperative pain between nerve division versus preservation. A recent study was conducted to determine whether prophylactic neurectomy might prevent persistent pain after inguinal herniorrhaphy. Unilateral iliohypogastric neurectomy was performed on 100 men requiring bilateral inguinal hernia repair, with each patient also serving as a control. Pain was evaluated on postoperative days 1 and 7 and at years 1 and 2 with established pain scale tools to compare pain on the neurectomized and non-neurectomized sides and to assess altered sensation, including both hypoesthesia and paraesthesia on both sides. The study found that although patients complained of less pain on the neurectomized side after postoperative day 7, no statistical significance was reached. Interestingly, no significant difference was found in the incidence of sensory abnormalities between the two sides [4]. The authors concluded that studies involving larger patient samples are warranted to definitively demonstrate, with statistical significance, whether prophylactic neurectomy can help to alleviate persistent pain after inguinal herniorrhaphy. In fact, the only difference between these two groups was a decrease in touch sensation and numbness in the group that underwent routine division of the ilioinguinal nerve. One major criticism of prophylactic neurectomy is the resulting neurosensory disturbances that cause loss of sensation and groin numbness. However, it has been postulated that the sensory loss that may result following prophylactic neurectomy might be compensated for by cross-innervation provided by cutaneous nerves from the contralateral side and, therefore, the morbidity following neurectomy would be negligible [21].

The most crucial preventative step to reduce the incidence of postoperative groin pain is careful dissection and preservation of the ilioinguinal, iliohypogastric, and genitofemoral nerves [22]. It has been demonstrated that when all three nerves are identified and preserved, no cases of chronic pain were identified at 6-month follow-up. This was in stark contrast to the 40% of patients who reported moderate to severe pain when all three nerves were divided.

Evaluating and treating chronic pain following inguinal herniorrhaphy

Although chronic groin pain following inguinal herniorrhaphy may be mild and nondebilitating, a subset of patients will suffer with severe groin pain that significantly inhibits their ability to perform activities of daily living. A brief trial of conservative management is appropriate in all cases of groin pain; however, when symptoms are persistent, surgical intervention is warranted and this presents a difficult and challenging dilemma to surgeons. It is hoped that this article provides a useful algorithm to evaluate these patients and to effectively treat inguinodynia. It is important to remember, however, that each treatment plan must be individualized to every patient on the basis of the surgeon's judgment and that management of these patients will never fall into a standard regimental protocol.

When evaluating a patient with postoperative groin pain, it should be remembered that, although the most likely source of morbidity is the repair itself, the differential for symptoms is broad and must be considered carefully (Table 2). Causes of chronic pain related to herniorrhaphy can be divided into neuropathic and non-neuropathic etiologies. The most common non-neuropathic etiologies include, most commonly, hernia recurrence, excessive scar formation, and pressure from the bulk of the mesh.

The neuropathic etiologies of chronic pain include nerve entrapment by sutures or staples (Fig. 3) and neuroma formation with partial or complete

Table 2
Differential diagnosis of chronic groin pain

Dermatology	Gynecology	Orthopedic	Surgery
• Lymphadenitis	• C-section	Hip disorders	• Compensation
• Psoriasis/burn	• Cervical cancer	• Acetabular labral	(workman's)
• Sebaceous cyst/	• Endometriosis	tears	• Hernia
hioradenitis	• Tubal/ovarian	• Avascular necrosis	• Recurrent hernia
• Thrombophlebitis/	disorders	• Chondritis dissecans	• Posthernia
cellulites		• Legge-Calve Perthes	Open
		disease	• Neuropathic
		• Osteoarthritis	• Non-neuropathic
		• Pelvic stress fractures	Laparoscopic
		• Slipped femoral	• Neuropathic
		capsule epiphysis	• Non-neuropathic
		• Snapping hip	
		syndrome	
		• Synovitis	
Infectious disease	Neurology	Rheumatology	Urology
• Herpes zoster	• Lumbosacral	• Connective tissue	• Cystitis
• HIV/tuberculosis	disorders	disease	• Epididymitis
• Lyme disease	• Neurofibromatosis	• Iliopsoas bursitis	• Nephrolithiasis
• Psoas abscess		• Osteitis pubis	• Prostatitis
		• Systemic lupus	• Torsion of testes
		eritematous	• Urethral
			extravasation
			• Urinary tract
			infection
			• Vas granuloma/
			fibrosis
Gastroenterology	Neurosurgery	Sports medicine	Vascular
• Appendicitis/	• Disc disease	• "Sports hernia"	• Abscess hematoma
adhesions	• Spinal injuries,	(adductor strains)	• Postvein stripping
• Diverticulitis	inflammation,	• Gilmore's groin	• Pseudoaneurysm
• Inflammatory	tumors		• Vascular graft
retroperitoneal	• Spondylosisthesis		
phlegmon	• Spondylolysis		
(pancreatitis)			
• Meckel diverticulitis			
• Granulomatous			
colitis			

transection of the involved nerve [6,23]. Neuropathic pain related to the genitofemoral nerve may result in testicular pain in men and labial pain in women. In these patients, a thorough urologic evaluation aimed at identification of underlying testicular or epididymal pathology in men and careful gynecologic examination in women is also necessary [24].

Hernia recurrence may be a source of chronic pain and should be ruled out early in the evaluation. CT scan may be helpful for establishing a diagnosis in cases of recurrence that are not readily apparent on physical examination [25]. Ultrasound is another potential diagnostic modality to help

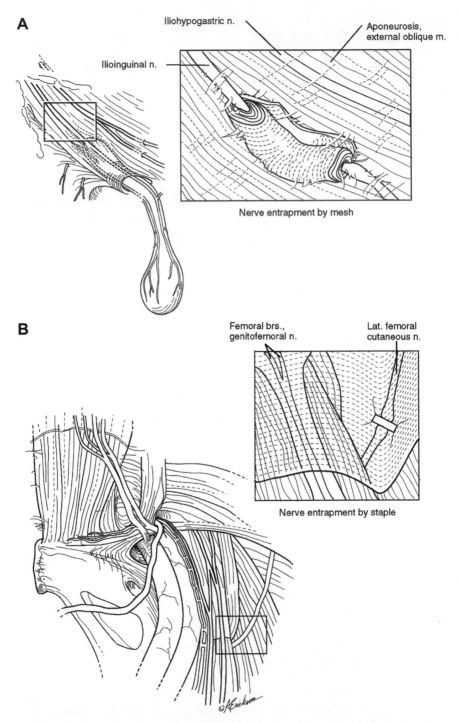

Fig. 3. Neuropathic etiologies of postherniorrhaphy groin pain. (*Courtesy of* A. Erickson, Brooklyn, NY.)

determine occult recurrences as a potential cause of postoperative pain [26]. MRI has also been used to detect recurrence, delineate mesh position, and demonstrate non–hernia-related causes of pain [27,28]. One may or may not be able to elicit a history of pain presenting in a classic distribution of a particular nerve. One can specifically elicit ilioinguinal nerve entrapment by having the patient hyperextend and twist the trunk of the body—twisting toward the affected side does not reproduce symptoms, whereas twisting away from it does [29].

The best modality for treatment of chronic groin pain is yet to be elucidated and is an area that continues to perplex even the most competent of surgeons. Treatment modalities include oral analgesics, regional nerve blocks, re-operation with mesh excision, and surgical neurectomy. Continued experience with this long-term complication of inguinal herniorrhaphy will undoubtedly result in other proposed solutions. Some have described performing selective nerve blocks for both diagnostic and therapeutic purposes [30,31]. For example, if physical examination suggests involvement of the ilioinguinal nerve, a nerve block may help to confirm relief of symptoms followed by definitive surgical neurectomy. Acupuncture, tricyclic antidepressants, and gabapentin have been useful in the treatment of chronic pain syndromes, but their utility in management of chronic groin pain is unclear. Pulsed radiofrequency techniques have also been described and have become an accepted modality for neurodestructive treatment of severe pain syndromes. This technique applies a high-frequency and high-temperature electrical current to the affected tissue, resulting in neurodestruction and prevention of the transmission of pain signals [32]. However, this treatment is not without its own potentially debilitating complications—in particular, the formation of a neuroma and a neuritis reaction that can increase the sympathetic discharge and exacerbate pain. Therefore, this modality remains highly controversial. Unfortunately, a large percentage of patients with chronic groin pain fail to experience symptomatic improvement with nonoperative management strategies. The question arises as to who needs an operation and what is the preferred procedure that will relieve the symptoms without causing worsening of pain. If the pain persists for 6 months to 1 year, operative intervention should be discussed with the patient. The surgical approach of identification and resection of neuromas involving the ilioinguinal, iliohypogastric, and lateral femoral cutaneous nerves results in 80% success rates in pain relief as well as the ability to resume activities and return to work [24].

For patients with chronic pain resulting from laparoscopic repair with mesh and probable improper placement of securing tacks, it may by necessary to re-operate laparoscopically and remove the offending tacks. This may prove to be challenging because re-operating in the preperitoneal space may be difficult, but certainly feasible. Success has been reported with this technique [23,33,34].

The best surgical option to date may in fact be open-groin exploration with neurectomy and possible mesh removal. A thorough description of operative technique in re-operation for testicular pain has been described and involves careful exposure of the operative field with an incision over the inguinal canal. In these cases, injury to the genitofemoral nerve was suspected. Given its anatomic variations, steps to careful identification of the nerve were developed following careful examination and dissection of cadavers. The technique that has been postulated includes following the nerve distally along the canal to exclude other communications and then following it proximally to the preperitoneum, where it is resected [24]. The authors stress the importance of high resection of the nerve, allowing it to retract behind the peritoneum and preventing the nerve end from rescarring (which would result in continued groin pain following re-exploration) [24]. On a reported series of 54 patients who underwent groin exploration with triple neurectomy that included the ilioinguinal, iliohypogastric, and genitofemoral nerves, 68% were relieved of pain [35]. This was confirmed in another study, which demonstrated that triple neurectomy resulted in a 72% complete pain relief and 25% partial relief [29]. In the largest series to date, 225 patients underwent triple neurectomy resulting in an 80% complete resolution of pain [35]. Despite these high rates of success, surgical intervention for chronic groin pain remains a source of distress for both patient and surgeon.

Summary

The number of patients afflicted with chronic groin pain following inguinal herniorrhaphy is grossly underestimated and unacceptably high. Despite attempts to predict who may or may not develop this complication, it is not entirely understood who is at risk and why. For this reason, the present authors emphasize the importance of a preoperative discussion of the possibility of this complication with the patient. To date, evidence suggests that the best prevention for this morbidity is avoiding inguinal nerve injury. All measures should be taken to ensure meticulous technique and careful dissection, with particular attention to avoiding incorporation of the inguinal nerves into stitches or staples. This will not only decrease the potential for recurrence, but will likely also result in decreased incidence of postoperative inguinal neuralgia.

It must be recognized that groin pain may be multifactorial, and it is quite possible that no specific etiology is identifiable. Given that a significant number of patients may improve with nonoperative management, the authors advocate observation with supportive care. However, if after 1 year the patient continues to suffer from this potentially debilitating symptom, operative intervention is the only solution, with triple neurectomy offering the most acceptable results.

References

[1] Rab M, Ebmer J, Dellon AL. Anatomic variability of the ilioinguinal and genitofemoral nerve: implications for the treatment of groin pain. Plast Reconstr Surg 2001;108(6):1618–23.

[2] O'Dwyer PJ, Norrie J, Alani A, et al. Observation or operation for patients with an asymptomatic inguinal hernia: a randomized clinical trial. Ann Surg 2006;244(2):167–73.

[3] Franneby U, Sandbloom G, Nordin P, et al. Risk factors for long-term pain after hernia surgery. Ann Surg 2006;244(2):212–9.

[4] Pappalardo G, Frattaroli FM, Mongardini M, et al. Neurectomy to prevent persistent pain after inguinal herniorrhaphy: a prospective study using objective criteria to assess pain. World J Surg 2007;31:1081–6.

[5] Heise CP, Starling JR. Mesh inguinodynia: a new clinical syndrome after inguinal herniorrhaphy? J Am Coll Surg 1998;187(5):514–8.

[6] Demirer S, Kepenekci I, Evirgen O, et al. The effect of polypropylene mesh on ilioinguinal nerve in open mesh repair of groin hernia. J Surg Res 2006;131(2):175–81.

[7] Poobalan AS, Bruce J, King PM, et al. Chronic pain and quality of life following open inguinal hernia repair. Br J Surg 2001;88(8):1122–6.

[8] Courtney CA, Duffy K, Serpell MG. Outcomes of patients with severe chronic pain following repair of groin hernia. Br J Surg 2002;89(10):1310–4.

[9] Koninger J, Redecke J, Butters M. Chronic pain after hernia repair: a randomized trial comparing Shouldice, Lichtenstein and TAPP. Langenbecks Arch Surg 2004;389(5):361–5.

[10] Weyhe D, Belyaev O, Muller C, et al. Improving outcomes in hernia repair by the use of light meshes–a comparision of different implant constructions based on a critical appraisal of the literature. World J Surg 2007;31(1):234–44.

[11] Grant AM, Scott NW, O'Dwyer PJ. Five-year follow-up of a randomized trial to assess pain and numbness after laparascopic or open repair of groin hernia. Br J Surg 2004;91(12):1570–4.

[12] Cobb WS, Kercher KW, Heniford BT. The argument for lightweight polypropylene mesh in hernia repair. Surg Innov 2005,12(1).63–9.

[13] Douek M, Smith G, Oshowo A, et al. Prospective randomized controlled trial of laparascopic versus open inguinal hernia mesh repair: five year follow up. Br Med J 2003; 326(7397):1012–3.

[14] Ferzli GS, Frezza EE, Pecoraro Am Jr, et al. Prospective randomized study of stapled versus unstapled mesh in laparascopic preperitoneal inguinal hernia repair. J Am Coll Surg 1999; 188(5):461–5.

[15] Choy C, Shapiro K, Patel S, et al. Investigating a possible cause of mesh migration during totally extraperitoneal (TEP) repair. Surg Endosc 2004;18(3):523–5.

[16] Poobalan A, Bruce J, Cairns W, et al. A review of chronic groin pain after inguinal herniorrhaphy. Clin J Pain 2003;19:48–54.

[17] Amid PK. Causes, prevention, and surgical treatment of postherniorrhaphy neuropathic inguinodynia: triple neurectomy with proximal end implantation. Hernia 2004;8(4):343–9.

[18] Lichtenstein IL, Shulman AG, Amid PK, et al. Cause and prevention of postherniorrhaphy neuralgia: a protocol for treatment. Am J Surg 1988;155:786–90.

[19] Tsakayannis DE, Kiriakopoulos AC, Linos DA. Elective neurectomy during open, "tension free" inguinal hernia repair. Hernia 2004;8(1):67–9.

[20] Dittrick GW, Ridl K, Kuhn JA, et al. Routine ilioinguinal nerve excision in inguinal hernia repairs. Am J Surg 2004;188(6):736–40.

[21] Mui WL, Ng CS, Fung TM. Prophylactic ilioinguinal neurectomy in open inguinal hernia repair: a double-blind randomized controlled trial. Ann Surg 2006;244(1):27–33.

[22] Alfieri S, Rotondi F, Di Giorgio A, et al. Influence of preservation versus division of ilioinguinal, iliohypogastric, and genital nerves during open mesh herniorrhaphy: prospective multicentric study of chronic pain. Ann Surg 2006;243(4):553–8.

[23] Lantis JC, Schwaitzberg SD. Tack entrapment of the ilioinguinal nerve during laparoscopic hernia repair. J Laparoendosc Adv Surg Tech A 1999;9(3):285–9.

[24] Ducic I, Dellon AL. Testicular pain after inguinal hernia repair: an approach to resection of the genital branch of the genitofemoral nerve. J Am Coll Surg 2004;198:181–4.

[25] Aguirre DA, Santosa AC, Casola G. Abdominal wall hernias: imaging features, complications, and diagnostic pitfalls at multi-detector row CT. Radiographics 2005;25(6):1501–20.

[26] Lilly MC, Arregui ME. Ultrasound of the inguinal floor for evaluation of hernias. Surg Endosc 2002;16(4):659–62.

[27] Leander P, Ekberg O, Sjoberg S, et al. MR imaging following herniorrhaphy in patients with unclear groin pain. Eur Radiol 2000;10(11):1691–6.

[28] van den Berg JC, Go PM, de Valois J, et al. Preoperative and postoperative assessment of laparoscopic inguinal hernia repair by dynamic MRI. Invest Radiol 2000;35(11):695–8.

[29] Madura JA, Madura JA II, Copper CM, et al. Inguinal neurectomy for inguinal nerve entrapment: an experience with 100 patients. Am J Surg 2005;189(3):283–7.

[30] Deysine M, Deysine GR, Reed WP. Groin pain in the absence of hernia: a new syndrome. Hernia 2002;6(2):64–7.

[31] Bower S, Moore BB, Weiss SM. Neuralgia after inguinal hernia repair. Am Surg 1996;62(8): 664–7.

[32] Rozen D, Ahn J. Pulsed radiofrequency for the treatment of ilioinguinal neuralgia after inguinal herniorrhaphy. Mt Sinai J Med 2006;73(4):716–8.

[33] Wong J, Anvari M. Treatment of inguinodynia after laparoscopic herniorrhaphy: a combined laparoscopic and fluoroscopic approach to the removal of helical tackers. Surg Laparosc Endosc Percutan Tech 2001;11(2):148–51.

[34] Seid AS, Amos E. Entrapment neuropathy in laparoscopic herniorrhaphy. Surg Endosc 1994;8(9):1050–3.

[35] Lee CH, Dellon AL. Surgical management of groin pain of neural origin. J Am Coll Surg 2000;191(2):137–42.

ELSEVIER
SAUNDERS

Surg Clin N Am 88 (2008) 217–222

SURGICAL
CLINICS OF
NORTH AMERICA

Index

Note: Page numbers of article titles are in **boldface** type.

0039-6109/08/$ - see front matter © 2008 Elsevier Inc. All rights reserved.
doi:10.1016/S0039-6109(08)00014-5

surgical.theclinics.com

Moving?

Make sure your subscription moves with you!

To notify us of your new address, find your **Clinics Account Number** (located on your mailing label above your name), and contact customer service at:

 E-mail: elspcs@elsevier.com

 800-654-2452 (subscribers in the U.S. & Canada)
407-345-4000 (subscribers outside of the U.S. & Canada)

 Fax number: 407-363-9661

 Elsevier Periodicals Customer Service
6277 Sea Harbor Drive
Orlando, FL 32887-4800

*To ensure uninterrupted delivery of your subscription, please notify us at least 4 weeks in advance of move.